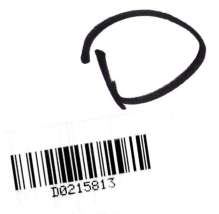

ENCYCLOPEDIA OF ATTENTION DEFICIT HYPERACTIVITY DISORDERS

ENCYCLOPEDIA OF ATTENTION DEFICIT HYPERACTIVITY DISORDERS

Evelyn Kelly

GREENWOOD PRESS
An Imprint of ABC-CLIO, LLC

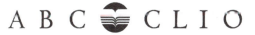

A B C ⬤ C L I O

Santa Barbara, California • Denver, Colorado • Oxford, England

Library of Congress Cataloging-in-Publication Data
Kelly, Evelyn B.
    Encyclopedia of attention deficit hyperactivity disorders / Evelyn Kelly.
        p. ; cm.
    Includes bibliographical references and index.
    ISBN 978-0-313-34249-3 (hard copy : alk. paper) —
ISBN 978-0-313-34250-9 (ebook)
1. Attention-deficit hyperactivity disorder—Encyclopedias. I. Title.
    [DNLM: 1. Attention Deficit Disorder with Hyperactivity—
Encyclopedias—English. WS 13 K29e 2009]
    RJ506.H9K447 2009
    616.85'89003—dc2   2009020451

13 12 11 10 9   1 2 3 4 5

This book is also available on the World Wide Web as an eBook.
Visit www.abc-clio.com for details.

ABC-CLIO, LLC
130 Cremona Drive, P.O. Box 1911
Santa Barbara, California 93116-1911

This book is printed on acid-free paper ∞

Manufactured in the United States of America

CONTENTS

LIST OF ENTRIES

INTRODUCTION

Frazzled and befuddled, the mother of 5-year-old John brought him to the specialist's office. His teacher said he was the terror of the kindergarten, and his parents were concerned about his nonstop destructive behavior at home. In the doctor's office he jumped from chair to chair, climbed under a table, and flailed his arms like an animated rag doll. He picked up the tape and stapler from the receptionist's desk and then began to flip the light switch off and on, to everyone's annoyance. He ambled over to a group of children and butted into a game they were playing. They complained about his bossiness and moved away from him. The doctor immediately suspected John had attention-deficit hyperactivity disorder (ADHD). Is it really ADHD or is it something else?

The words "attention-deficit hyperactivity disorder" or ADHD are on the lips of many teachers, parents, and physicians. Generally, the child displays a persistent pattern of inattention and/or hyperactivity and impulsivity, which developed in the early years. When other symptoms such as forgetfulness, poor impulse control, and distractibility begin to interfere with the child's performance in the classroom or at home, parents become concerned. Unfortunately, the condition may persist into adulthood.

In 1998 the American Medical Association stated that ADHD is one of the best researched disorders in medicine. It is also one of the most controversial. Yet, with all the interest and research, no one knows what causes ADHD or how to cure it.

According to the January 2002 "International Consensus Statement on ADHD," ADHD affects 3–5 percent of the population, and boys are diagnosed two to three times more than girls. ADHD is considered to be a developmental disorder largely neurological in origin. The term "developmental" means that certain traits, such as impulse control are slower to develop in these children than in the general population. That degree of lag appears to relate to the degree of severity of the disease. The compound terms "neurobehavioral" or "neurodevelopmental" disorders are frequently used to describe the disorder. The Greek root *neuro* means "nerve." ADHD is not thought to be a disorder relating to the brain and nervous system. However, the origin, causes, and treatments are subjects of debate and controversy.

ADHD is not just a fad that has been created in the latter half of the 20th century. It is documented in history. In 493 B.C. Hippocrates, the great physician on the Greek island of Cos, described a condition in patients who had quick sensory experience and their souls moved quickly on to the next impression. Believing that an imbalance of the four humors—water, fire, earth, and air—cause all diseases, Hippocrates attributed this condition to an overbalance of fire over water. He recommended a diet of barley rather than wheat bread and fish rather than meat; he also recommended adding water drinks and natural and diverse physical activities. Even Shakespeare referred to a serious malady of attention in King Henry VIII.

In 1845 a German, Dr. Heinrich Hoffman, wrote an illustrated book of children's poetry that described a boy named Fidgety Phillip, who obviously had all the symptoms of ADHD and who met a tragic end when he pulled all the food on the table over on top of him. Dr. Hoffman attributed the problem to bad behavior and certainly never considered it could be inherited from parents.

ADHD was first observed clinically in 1902. Sir George F. Still described a group of impulsive children who had behavioral problems. He added the idea that the problems of these children could be traced to a genetic disorder and not poor parenting. Still called the condition a "morbid defect of moral control." Others studied the condition and found the condition to be one that had identifiable symptoms.

Twentieth century scientists began to look for the causes of ADHD. In 1918, a terrible influenza epidemic left many survivors with neurological dysfunctions; some survivors exhibited behaviors that corresponded to ADHD. Dr. Bradley made a chance discovery in 1937; he found that a group of children with behavioral problems in Providence, Rhode Island, improved after receiving stimulant medication. In 1957 the stimulant methylphenidate (Ritalin) became available and in various forms and is still one of the most prescribed medications.

Studying the results of the survivors of the great flu epidemic, some researchers began to propose that injury caused the behavior conditions and not genetics. In 1960 Stella Chess proposed this idea as "hyperactive child syndrome." A rift developed in the scientific community. In Europe scientists supported the idea that the disorder, which is called hyperkinesis, is associated with retardation, brain damage, and conduct disorders. This term comes from two Greek words: *hyper* meaning "above and beyond" and *kine* meaning "movement." This perspective of the relationship between hyperactivity and retardation was not changed until 1994. However, in the United States, observations that the condition occurred without any observed pathological injury led researchers to change the terminology from minimal brain damage to minimal brain dysfunction (MBD).

Here are some of the names that have been given to the condition now identified as ADHD throughout the 20th century:

- 1940s: Brain dysfunction
- 1950s: Hyperkinetic syndrome

- 1960s: Minimal brain dysfunction
- 1968: Hyperactive child
- 1980s: Attention-deficit disorder with or without hyperactivity; introduced in the DSM-III
- 1994: Attention-deficit hyperactive disorder in DSM-IV
- 2002: The International Consensus Statement on ADHD was signed by 80 of the world's leading experts to counteract media misrepresentation.
- 2005: More than 100 European experts added their signatures to the document asserting the validity of ADHD as a mental disorder.

Although it does affect 3–5 percent of school-age children, no simple test exists for ADHD. According to the American Psychiatric Association (2004), the condition is more common in boys with a ratio of two to one. Girls may hide the condition by sitting back and refusing to participate and consequently go undiagnosed. An estimated 60 percent of children diagnosed with ADHD retain the disorder as adults.

In a classroom not paying attention, losing things, making careless mistakes, and forgetting to turn in homework are normal to some degree, and taken individually may not indicate anything problematic. However, the child with ADHD may have a constellation of symptoms that interfere with school, home, and friends. Many of these children will carry the disorder into adulthood, when it will also cause tremendous problems. Sometimes the diagnosis of ADHD in adults is done when their kids are discovered in school to have the disorder.

This *Encyclopedia of Attention-Deficit Hyperactivity Disorder* was written to assist interested high school and college students, parents, teachers, and other nonspecialist users of school, university, and public libraries in learning about topics relating to ADHD. The writer acknowledges that the book will not be read cover to cover, so some ideas may be repeated as necessary to throw light on the topic. At times the reader may be directed to refer to other entries for additional information.

The information here is straightforward and objective; the writer is not arguing theories or interpreting them and does not take sides in the discussions. Provided here are unbiased summaries of major ideas and positions, focusing on the claims, arguments, and evidence offered by the proponents of certain theories and techniques. Medical information is presented with reference to researchers in the field and Web sites are provided that report their findings.

Although this volume is practical in most aspects, it is solidly based on the research of specialists in many areas who have substantiated the following conclusions:

- ADHD is associated with numerous developmental, cognitive, academic, and health risks and impairments.
- In cognitive and academic domains, ADHD is specifically associated with moderate or greater deficiencies in domains of adaptive function and academic achievement skills and a considerably higher risk for learning disabilities.

- Research findings suggest deficiencies in planning ability in conjunction with ADHD.
- ADHD is strongly related to difficulties with emotion regulation, particularly the management of frustration. Children with ADHD show higher levels of aggression, anger, and sadness, while possibly showing lower levels of empathy.
- Concerns have begun to arise that ADHD may be associated with reduced life expectancy.

ADHD is a serious condition that causes disruption in the life of a child and the family.

This encyclopedia seeks to present a comprehensive look at many options that people may have. This encyclopedia presents many ideas about ADHD and the people involved in the debates. The book does not give medical advice. For information on treatments for an individual, consult a physician or other qualified health professional.

ADHD is one of the most studied neuropsychological disorders. A literature research at the end of 2003 found more than 200 published studies that compared groups with and without ADHD on neuropsychological measures. These studies show that a rapid accumulation of knowledge is a tool to refine understanding of the issues relating to ADHD. However, these studies underscore the complexities and clearly demonstrate that much remains to be learned.

Some of the selections in this volume are overviews of a particular topic, such as nutrition or drug therapy, but topics within a long entry may include short sections with additional information. For example, the entry titled "Teaching Children with ADHD" contains "Tips for Teachers," but some of the principles also can be used by parents.

There is a Further Reading list at the end of each entry a Bibliography, a list of conditions that may be confused with ADHD, a directory of organizations that includes Web sites, and an index.

Disclaimer

The author and publisher of this encyclopedia do not endorse, recommend, or make representations with respect to the research, services, medication, treatments, or products mentioned in this volume. The information is provided to give readers the scope of the medical, psychological, social, and legal implications of the disorder. The information provided here is with the understanding that the author and publisher are not engaged in rendering medical or legal advice or recommendation. The information is not to replace consultations with qualified health care or legal professionals to meet any individual need. References to any treatment or therapy option, to any program, or to service provided are not endorsement but to provide awareness of the existence of such therapy, program, or service. Parents and professionals are encouraged to fully investigate treatment options and provide those most appropriate for a specific individual.

ABBREVIATIONS

ACA	American Chiropractic Association
ADD	Attention Deficit disorder
ADHD	Attention-deficit hyperactivity disorder
AMA	American Medical Association
CD	Conduct disorder
CDC	Centers for Disease Control and Prevention
D.C.	Doctor of Chiropractic
D.N.	Doctor of Naturopathy
D.O.	Doctor of Osteopathy
FDA	United States Food and Drug Administration
MAOI	Monoamine oxidase inhibitor (used to treat depression)
MBD	Minimal brain dysfunction
M.D.	Doctor of Medicine
NIH	National Institutes of Health
NIMH	National Institute of Mental Health
ODD	Oppositional defiant disorder
SUD	Sudden unexplained death
SAD	Seasonal affective disorder
SAD	Substance abuse disorder
TCM	Traditional Chinese medicine

A

Accidents

Because of the inattentive, impulsive, and hyperactive traits, children with attention-deficit hyperactivity disorder (ADHD) are considerably more likely to experience injuries due to accidents than other children. Hartsough and Lambert (1985) found that up to 57 percent of children with ADHD were described as accident prone, and 15 percent had at least four or more serious accidental injuries, such as broken bones, lacerations, head injuries, severe bruises, lost teeth, or accidental poisonings. Children with ADHD may be admitted to intensive care units or have an injury result in disabilities more frequently than other children.

Several studies indicate that children with ADHD have an elevated risk of physical injuries or more frequent injuries and more severe injuries than other children. About 15.6 percent of hyperactive children have had at least four accidental injuries, whereas only 4.8 percent of children in the general population sustain such injuries. At the same time, 68.4 percent of children with ADHD have experienced physical trauma sufficient to warrant sutures, hospitalization, or extensive and painful injuries; only 39.5 percent of the general population of children have these injuries. Bone fractures are common. In addition, children with ADHD have an approximately threefold greater likelihood of accidental poisoning.

Some studies have related the degree of aggressiveness to the likelihood of accidental injury in preschoolers. Because some children with ADHD are more likely to be oppositional, the proneness may be due to this trait rather than just a level of impulsivity. A 2004 study of 10,000 children in Britain found that ADHD was more likely to be related to fractures, whereas oppositional defiant disorder (ODD) was more closely related to burns and poisonings. Thus both ADHD and ODD appear to be related to accidental injuries, but of different forms.

Parents report that their children with ADHD are inattentive and will engage in risky activities, are more heedless or thoughtless of the consequences, and thus place themselves in situations or engage in activities that are more likely to result in harm. For example, children with ADHD who are riding a bicycle may weave in and out of cars and may not look both ways before venturing into the street. They may be engage in risky behavior such as darting into the street, daring cars, or seeing how close they can come without colliding. They appear to be completely unaware of the danger or receive some thrill by challenging the edge of danger.

Teenagers with ADHD who drive automobiles are more dangerous because they have thousands of pounds of steel that they are taking chances with. They often enjoy the thrill of speeding and may have more speeding tickets and traffic violations than other students their age. These teenagers are twice as likely to have their driver's licenses suspended than drivers without ADHD.

Russell Barkley (2006) lists several other reasons that deserve consideration:

- Motor coordination. Children with ADHD may demonstrate more clumsiness, awkwardness, rapid and ill-timed motor movements, and slower reaction times.
- Comorbid ODD and conduct disorder (CD). Children with ODD and CD have more accidents than other children. Although sometimes the disorders are correlated with ADHD, it is these disorders that probably account for more accidents than hyperactivity itself.
- Poor parental supervision and monitoring of activities. Several studies have found that children who have more accidents have less supervision, especially out of doors than other children do.

Barkley believes that these factors must be considered in evaluating and preventing accidents among these children.

In a 2002 report Barkley also warns about summer events and activities when many children do not take stimulant medication because they are not in school. He suggests that children with ADHD continue to take medication in nonacademic setting and points to fewer behavioral problems at home, fewer disagreements with friends and siblings, and less irritability.

An event relating to accidents and ADHD is driving. Actually, driving is a major activity in the life of teens and adults, facilitating the ability for employment, family and work responsibilities, education, social engagement, shopping, and entertainment. All these activities are hampered if one cannot drive, especially in the United States. Driving is the one domain that can open up many possibilities in areas of living. However, it is also is an instrument that can lead to great harm to oneself and to other because there is a one- to two-ton projectile that can move at speeds of 80 miles per hour.

Barkley et al. (2003) conducted a series of studies of driving problems associated with ADHD that included surveys of nondisabled adolescents and adolescents with ADHD. The researchers found the following about teens and young adults and driving:

- They were more likely to have driven before the legal age without a license.
- According to the parents, they were not good drivers.
- They were more likely to have their licenses suspended or revoked.
- They were more likely to have been issued citations for driving infractions especially for speeding.
- They were four times more likely to have an accident while driving a vehicle.

Although some of the difficulties appeared related to ADHD, they were also connected with the degree of oppositional and conduct problems.

The Centers for Disease Control and Prevention (CDC) offers several suggestions for injury prevention that can be applied to people with ADHD:

- Ensure bicycle helmet use. Remind children as often as necessary to watch for cars and to avoid unsafe activities.
- Supervise children when they are involved in high-risk activities or are in a risky setting, such as climbing or when in or around a swimming pool.
- Keep potentially harmful household products, tools, equipment, and objects out of the reach of young children.
- Parents may want to enroll their teens in driving safety courses before they get their driver's license.
- Teens with ADHD may need to limit the amount of music listened to in the car while driving and drive without passengers or keep the number of passengers to a chosen few.
- Plan trips well ahead of time and know the best routes for short trips.
- Avoid the use of cellular phones, alcohol, and drugs.

Further Readings: Barkley, Russell. 2002. ADHD and accident proneness. *ADHD Report* May:2–5; Barkley, R. A. et al. 2003. Driving-related risks and outcomes of attention deficit hyperactivity disorder in adolescents and young adults: A 3–5 year follow-up survey. *Pediatrics* 92:212–18; Barkley, R. A. 2006. *Attention-deficit hyperactivity disorder: A handbook for diagnosis and treatment.* 3rd ed. New York: Guilford Press; Hartsough, C. S., and N. M. Lambert. 1985. Medical factors in hyperactive and normal children: Prenatal, developmental, and health history findings. *American Journal of Orthopsychiatry* 55:190–210; "Public Health Issues in ADHD." http://www.cdc.gov/ncbddd/adhd/facts.html. Accessed 6/17/2009; Rowe, R. et al. 2004. Childhood psychiatric disorder and unintentional injury: Findings from a national cohort study. *Journal of Pediatric Psychology* 29:119–30.

Acupuncture

Children with ADHD may sometimes have unpleasant side effects when taking medications. Some physicians and families have found complementary treatments such as acupuncture an adjunct therapy for these disorders. This therapy may be a helpful tool to calm the disruptive symptoms of ADHD and address some of the unpleasant side effects of the medications used to treat the disorder.

Acupuncture, one of the strategies of traditional Chinese medicine (TCM), was developed at least 3,000 years ago and can be traced back to the Stone Age. The word "acupuncture" comes from the roots *acus* meaning "needle" and puncture meaning "pierce the skin." Then acupuncture literally means to puncture with needles. By placing hair-fine needles into the skin at strategic points in the body known at "acupuncture points," the acupuncturist seeks to promote healing, alleviate pain, calm spasms and tics, bolster the immune system, and encourage good health in a multitude of ways.

Acupuncture works in this way, according to its practitioners. The flow of energy in the body known as qi or ch'i (pronounced *chee*) flows in 14 specific channels called meridians. Twelve major meridians are associated with the twelve major systems of the body including the lungs, large intestine, stomach, spleen, heart, small intestine, kidney, pericardium (the tissues surrounding the heart), gall bladder, liver, and the san jiao, recognized as an acuan only in TCM and thought to be the seat of heat in the body. Through these meridians flow qi, the source that promotes life and well-being and affects the quality of the physical, mental, spiritual, and emotional health. If the flow of energy is blocked or impeded, the acuans and tissues along in that line of flow will be disturbed. There are two main energies: Yin, which is designated as female, and Yang, designated as male. The two energies must be in balance for health.

Treatment consists of inserting fine, stainless steel, sterile, disposable needles into specific points along the meridians. The practice is based on the belief that certain areas of the skin affect the functioning of the body's internal acuans. The acupuncturist places needles into the acupuncture points, which correspond with the meridians and the presumed source of pain. This allows qi to flow freely again, restoring the balance and alleviating symptoms.

In order to affect the qi and return body systems to order, the acupuncturist applies specific herbs, which are heated and smolder above the acupuncture points. This procedure called moxibustion sends warmth down into specific points. Cupping is the placement of small glass cups on the skin of the back. Smoke fills the inside of the cups and draws the skin up into the cup as the air inside cools. A suction gun connects to the outside of the cup, which pulls the air out. This suctioning of the skin draws out toxins from the body and promotes healing and balance. Sometimes a small amount of electrical current is applied to the end of the need and sends a current down into the point to provide added stimulus.

Some of the examination procedures may appear strange to patients who are accustomed to Western medicine. For example, when the practitioner takes the person's pulse, he or she does three readings, alternating the finger used to read the pulse. The patient's tongue is examined carefully, as deficiencies in the shape, color, and texture of the tongue indicate that qi is not in order. After the complete examination, the patient is told to lie down on the massage table, and the practitioner places needles into the body; the number varies with the patient, who usually feels no pain. Once the needles are in place, the patient lies quietly in a dim room, listening to soft music for 10 to 30 minutes.

Because acupuncture works with the energy force in the body and regulates the flow of energy, it addresses a host of behavioral and social disorders related to ADHD. However, Oriental medicine looks at ADHD much differently than Western medicine, which views ADHD as a neurodevelopmental disorder. According to Chinese medicine, ADHD is either due to insufficient nourishment of the spirit or spirit agitation by some type of heat or as an orifice (body opening) disorder in which static blood or phlegm obstructs a body opening. In Chinese medicine hyperactivity is a symptom of heat in the body that is caused by food such as cow's milk, oranges, sugar, and artificial flavors and colorings. Heat may linger after a condition with a fever or after an immunization; tension in the family may generate heat. In addition, a shock during or after birth or the mother's diet during pregnancy may cause heat. Heat causes restlessness, agitation, violence, and insomnia. The poor diet or allergic reactions to food that generate heat affect the heart. Because the heart is presumed to be the house of the mind and spirit, heat in the heart affects the spleen, leading to the production of mucus or phlegm. The combination of heat and phlegm results in severe disturbances in the mind and behavior. Treatment with acupuncture targets the heat to calm the child.

A subspecialty of acupuncture is auricular medicine, which uses the human ear as a means of diagnosing and treating dysfunctional systems in the body. The procedure stimulates certain points on the ear with a mild, electrical pulse. According to the practitioner, the symptoms disappear after 1 to 4 months of weekly treatment sessions.

Acupuncture points for ADHD depend on whether the child has a weak or strong constitution, whether stress or lack of energy is present, and whether the child is hot or cold. Often hyperactive children have pale faces with red cheeks and tongues; these children usually respond well to treatment, according to acupuncturists. If there is no mucus, about five to ten sessions will be required; if there is mucus, more treatments will be necessary. The speed of improvement varies according to the patient and the complaint.

States control the practice and licensing of practitioners of acupuncture. Since the 1980s numerous clinics using acupuncture and herbal remedies have developed. The American Academy of Medical Acupuncture (AAMA) has over 2000 licensed Doctors of Medicine (M.D.s) and Doctors of Osteopathy (D.O.s) who integrate Western medicine with alternative treatment modalities may practice medical acupuncture.

Further Readings: "American Academy of Medical Acupuncture (AAMA)." http://www.medicalacupuncture.org; Cauldwell, K. 2008. "Acupuncture for Attention Deficit Disorder and ADHD." http://www.associatedcontent.com/pop_print.shtml?content_type=article&content_type_id. Accessed 4/26/2008; Cooper, Paul, and Katherine Bilton. 1999. *ADHD: Research, practice and opinion.* London: Whurr Publishers; Duke, M. 1973. *Acupuncture, the Chinese art of healing.* London: Constable; "Medical Acupuncture Treats ADHD without Drugs." August 16, 2000. http://www.medicalacupuncture.org/acu_info/pressrelease/adhd.html. Accessed 4/26/2008; Seller, Wanda. 1992. *Directory of essential oils.* London: C. W. Daniel Co; Scott, Julian, and Teresa Barlow. 1999. *Acupuncture in the treatment of children.* Vista, CA: Eastland Press; "Treating ADHD &ADD with Acupuncture." 2007. http://www.healthy.net/scr/news/asp?id=9235&action=print. Accessed 4/26/2008; Wormwood, V. A. 1991. *The fragrant pharmacy: A complete guide to aromatherapy and essential oils.* London: Bantam.

Adderall

Stimulant compounds are often prescribed for people with ADHD, and if used properly under the close supervision of a physician, the drugs can be beneficial. Adderall and AdderallXR, amphetamine compounds, are the registered trademarks of Shire, Inc., a pharmaceutical company located in Florence, Kentucky. Adderall is a central nervous stimulant that is used to treat ADHD in children 6 years of age and older and in adults.

The mode of therapeutic action of the stimulants is not exactly known. The neurotransmitters norepinephrine and dopamine are thought to be involved in the development of the symptoms of ADHD. These stimulant drugs are thought to block the reuptake of the neurotransmitters. The drugs are part of a class called noncatecholamine sympathomimetic amines, which affect the release of norepinephrine and dopamine into the presynaptic neuron and increase the release of these monoamines into extraneuronal space (or space outside the neurons), where the transmitters are not effective.

The drug is administered as Adderall tablets, which are mixed amphetamine salts with immediate release available in 5-, 7.4-, 10-, 10.5-, 12.5-, 15-, 20-, and 30-mg doses. The drug is also available in Adderall XR capsules, which are mixed amphetamine salts with extended release available in 5-, 10-, 15-, 20-, 25-, and 30-mg doses. The salts include dextroamphetamine saccharate, amphetamine aspartate monohydrate, dextroamphetamine sulfate USP, and amphetamine sulfate USP, in different amounts according to the dosage strength.

Adderall should be taken by mouth in the morning with or without food exactly as the health care professional prescribes. The capsules may be taken whole, or the contents may be sprinkled on a spoonful of applesauce. It is recommended to take the drug immediately without chewing. It is not recommended to take the drug later in the afternoon because of the potential for insomnia. Immediate release Adderall reaches maximum potential in about 4 hours and in Adderall XR in about 7 hours.

Adderall has been tested in clinical trials. A double-blind, randomized, placebo-controlled, parallel-group study was conducted in 584 children aged 6–12 who met DSM-IV criteria for ADHD (either the combined type or the hyperactive-impulsive type). (Clinical Trials and Medical Approval.) A double-blind randomized trial means that neither the scientist nor those administering the drug knows who is getting the drug or a placebo and the participants have been chosen at random with no bias of who would be in what class. A placebo is a pill that is made to look just like the study pill but does not have any of the active ingredients. A parallel study means that it was conducted at the same time. Patients were randomized to receive doses of 10, 20, or 30 mg or placebo in the morning for 3 weeks. Significant improvements in patient behavior, based on teacher rating of attention and hyperactivity, were observed for all Adderall XR compared to patients who received placebo. Those in the study group showed behavioral improvements in both morning and afternoon assessments compared to patients on placebo. A similar study was conducted on 255 adults, who met the Diagnostic and Statistical Manual (DSM-IV-TR) criteria for ADHD. Significant improvements, measured with the ADHD-RS, an 18-item scale that measures the core symptoms of ADHD, were compared to those who received placebo for 4 weeks. There was no adequate evidence that doses greater than 20 mg/day conferred additional benefit.

What are the risks? There are several groups that should not take Adderall: people with a heart defect or other heart problems and those with overactive thyroids, glaucoma, or a history of drugs abuse. Also, someone who has taken a drug called a monoamine oxidase inhibitor (MAOI) to treat depression or one who has stopped taking the MAOI in the last 14 days should not take Adderall. MAOI drugs include Nardil (phenelzine sulfate), Parnate (tranylcypromine sulfate), Marpan (isocarboxid), and other brands. Taking Adderall close in time to an MAOI can result in serious, sometimes fatal reactions, including high body temperature, coma, and seizures.

There are several risks for taking Adderall. Health Canada suspended marketing of Adderall in February 2005 because of reports of sudden unexplained death (SUD) in children taking the drugs. SUD has been associated with amphetamine abuse and has been reported in children with underlying cardiac abnormalities who were taking recommended doses of amphetamines. In addition, a small number of cases of SUD have been reported in children without structural cardiac abnormalities. However, the U.S. Food and Drug Administration (FDA) did not conclude that recommended doses of Adderall can cause SUD, but continued to monitor the data. In August 2005 Health Canada announced that they were returning the drug to the market but would revise the Canadian Product Monograph to include warning about the misuse of Adderall and that it should not be generally used in patients with structural cardiac abnormalities.

The term "black box warning" is used for a warning of serious potential and is written on a sheet of information that is placed in the package insert for physicians. The information is inserted in a box surrounded by black lines and is written in capital letters. The following is the black box warning for Adderall and Adderall XR:

> Amphetamines have a high potential for abuse. Administration of amphetamines for prolonged periods of time may lead to drug dependence. Particular attention should be paid to the possibility of subjects obtaining amphetamines for nontherapeutic use for distribution to others, and the drugs should be prescribed or dispensed sparingly. Misuse of amphetamine may cause sudden death and serious cardiovascular adverse events.

In February 2006, the FDA warned of several serious cardiac and cardiovascular risks including sudden unexplained death associated with the use of amphetamine or dextroamphetamine in children, adolescents, and adults. In addition to sudden death and abuse potential, additional risks include the following:

- Worsening mental illness or psychosis. Adderall may make symptoms of existing mental illness worse.
- Possible decreased growth and weight loss. Adderall may decrease growth and cause weight loss. Children who take it for a long time should have their growth and body weight measured regularly.
- Increased tics. Adderall may worsen tics and Tourette's disorder.
- Pregnancy. A woman who is pregnant should not take Adderall. The baby may be premature or have a low birth weight Also, the baby may show withdrawal symptoms, such as agitation and drowsiness.

- Breast feeding. A mother should not take Adderall while breast feeding because the drug can pass into the breast milk.

Other side effects include loss of appetite, difficulty sleeping, dry mouth, headaches, and mood changes. The physician should be told immediately if the person taking the medication has any of these symptoms or medical conditions.

What are the interactions with other drugs or foods? Adderall may interact with other medicines, which may cause serious side effects. The physician should be told about all medicines, vitamins, and herbal supplements that one is taking, especially the following:

- Medicines used to treat depression known as tricyclic antidepressants and MAOIs
- Antacids, including over-the-counter medicines
- Medicines used to treat urinary problems
- Diuretics
- Pain killers such as Darvon and Darvocet that contain propoxyphene.

Individual patients differ in their response to amphetamines. Toxic symptoms may occur at low doses. Overdosage should be treated as with any poison. Consult a Certified Poison Control Center. Specialists at the center may use stomach lavage or washing out the contents of the stomach, administer activated charcoal, and administer a cathartic and sedative.

Further Readings: "Adderall." http://www.adderallxr.com. Accessed 5/18/2009; "Adderall Package Insert." U.S. Food and Drug Administration; "Attention-Deficit/Hyperactive Disorder." National Alliance on Mental Illness. http://www.nami.org/Content/ContentGroups/Policy/Issues_Spotlights/Children/FDA_Warning_On_ADHD_Medications_Talking_Points.htm. Accessed 6/17/2009; "Patient Information Sheet: Adderall and Adderall XR Extended-Release Capsules." http://www.realmentalhealth.com/medications/adderall_patient.asp. Accessed 6/17/2009.

Additives. *See* Food Additives.

Adolescence

Most people find the teen years very challenging. The issue of peer pressure, the threat of failure in both school and socially, and low self-esteem make the years difficult for most individuals. For those with ADHD, the years appear very difficult. Although a person with ADHD may successfully navigate the early school years, the teenage years can provide a challenge for parents, teachers, and students. The desire to be independent and to try new and forbidden things such as alcohol, drugs, and sex can lead to unforeseen consequences. Rules that once were followed are often now flaunted, and parents may find themselves disagreeing on how to handle the teenager's behavior. This is a good time for a complete evaluation of the individual's health.

Now it is important for rules to be communicated in a straightforward and easy-to-understand manner. Communication between the adolescent and parents can help the person know the reasons for each rule. When it is set, it should be explained and then reinforced consistently. If rules are broken, respond in a calm and matter of fact manner. Use punishment sparingly. Even with teenagers, time out can be effective. The impulsivity and temper that accompany ADHD can often benefit from a short time alone.

As a teenager spends more time away from home, parents may see the demand for communication of the rules increase. Listening to his or her opinions, negotiating, and compromising can often prove helpful. Parenting the Child with ADHD.

Teenagers and Cars

Both male and female teenagers relish the idea of the independence that driving affords. Most states allow beginner's permits at about the age of 15 with full licensing at 16. According to Barkley's study (2001), 16-year-old drivers have more accidents per driving mile than any other age. For example, in the year 2000, 18 percent of those who died in speed-related crashes were youth aged 15 to 19. Barkley cites the facts that youth with ADHD, in their first 2 to 5 years of driving have nearly four times as many automobile accidents, are more likely to cause bodily injury in accidents, and have three times as many accidents as those without ADHD. Looking at these statistics, most states have begun to use a graduated drivers licensing (GDL) system that eases young drivers onto the roads by a slow progression of exposure to more difficult driving experiences. The program developed by the National Highway Traffic Safety Administration and the American Association of Motor Vehicle Administrators consists of three stages: learner's permit, intermediate license (provisional), and full licensures. Drivers must demonstrate responsible driving behavior at each stage before advancing to the next level. It is important for the teenager with ADHD to realize the dangers that can be involved with impulsivity and recklessness in a motor vehicle. *See also* Accidents.

Further Readings: Barkley, R. A. 2001. *Taking charge of ADHD*. New York: Guilford Press; Hallowell, Edward M., and John J. Ratey. 1994. *Driven to distraction: Recognizing and coping with attention deficit disorder from childhood through adulthood*. New York: Touchstone Press.

Adult ADHD

The idea of adult ADHD is fairly new and somewhat controversial. Papers dealing with an adult equivalent of childhood hyperactivity/minimal brain dysfunction were found in the late 1960s and 1970s, but they did not get widespread acceptance of the adult equivalents in the fields of psychiatry and clinical psychology. In 1994 Edward Hallowell and John Ratey wrote *Driven to Distraction*, which became a best seller and brought adult ADHD to the public's attention. Scientists, such as S. Goldstein (1997), K. Nadeau (1995), and Paul Wender (1995) conducted serious and rigorous scientific research on adults with ADHD. During the 1990s more and more scientists began to consider the disorder as a real condition worthy of diagnosis and treatment.

Adults with ADHD in the Workplace

Adults with ADD or ADHD may find both positive and negatives in the workplace and adapt to those strengths and weaknesses. Kathleen Nadeau, Ph.D., suggests some of the following hints:

- If you are in a job that requires intense concentration, request or find a quiet spot where disturbances and movement are not obvious.
- Many offices offer flex time where one can arrive later or earlier and be at work at times when people are not around.
- Take the opportunity to request assignments that interest you. For example, if you are creative, high energy, and intelligent, avoid jobs that are dull or detail oriented.
- Set goals and prioritize your work and inform your supervisor for suggestions on being more productive.
- Do not hesitate to ask for instructions to be repeated if you do not know what is meant. You may want to write the instructions down.
- Move around when possible. Instead of calling someone on the telephone, walk down the hall. Walk and exercise on breaks.
- Work on more than one project at a time. When you get bored with one, switch to the other.

Remember that if you were the one who was hyperactive in school, that attribute can translate into high energy and drive. If you were the one who talked too much in class, you may be very successful at networking, promoting, and sales.

Source: Adapted from ADDvance. "ADD (ADHD) in the workplace." 2004. http://www.addvance.com/help/adults/workplace.html. Accessed 5/18/2009. *See also* Nadeau, Kathleen. 1997. *ADD in the workplace: Choices, changes, and challenges.* Florence, KY: Brunner/Mazel.

Several other popular books, as well as the media, also called attention to ADHD in adults. Internet chat rooms, Web pages, and bulletin boards were dedicated to this topic, and support groups such as ADDA and CHADD began to include adults with ADHD in their discussions. Adults with the disorder began to ask questions that challenged the old idea of the 1960s that they would outgrow the condition. The adult form of ADHD was found to share many of the attribute of childhood ADHD and was found to respond to similar medications and treatments. The acceptance of ADHD in adults continues at the present time and is likely to increase in the decades ahead.

Many adults realize they have ADHD when they seek diagnosis for a son or daughter. Up to 65 percent of children diagnosed with ADHD will continue to manifest symptoms of the disorder in adulthood. Barkley (1990) found that antisocial behavior can be seen in 20–45 percent of adults with ADHD; 25 percent of these adults develop an antisocial personality. Twelve percent may develop substance abuse disorders. Interpersonal problems were reported by 75 percent of adults with ADHD, and sexual adjustment problems in about 20 percent. Serfontein in a 1994 study suggested that up to 10 percent of the jail population are adult sufferers of ADHD.

Adults are diagnosed under the same criteria as young people, including the fact that the symptoms began prior to age 7. Adults with ADHD may face challenges in self-control, self-motivation, executive functions, and inattention. They usually exhibit fewer of the impulsive and hyperactive tendencies that children have. However, they exhibit secondary symptoms such as disorganization, lack of follow-through, thrill-seeking, and impatience. These attributes may cause numerous problems in the work world.

Joseph Biederman, professor of psychiatry, Harvard Medical School, in a 2004 AMA briefing, observed that adults with ADHD had significant problems in the quality of their lives. According to Biederman, eight million adult Americans are estimated to struggle with inattention, impulsivity, and hyperactivity. He referred to his study of a large-scale survey that estimates yearly loss of household earning potential due to ADHD in the United States to be $77 billion. In the study he matched patients by educational levels. ADHD patients with high school education earn significantly less than their non-ADHD counterparts. On the average those with ADHD had household incomes $10,000 lower for high school graduates and $4,334 lower for college graduates. About 50 percent of those with ADHD reported they have lost or changed jobs because of the disorder.

Biederman also found that compared with people without ADHD, those with ADHD had the following problems:

- Higher divorce rates
- More substance abuse
- Lower level of satisfaction with all aspects of their lives
- Less positive self-image or optimistic point-of-view

He was struck by the fact that only about one-third of the adults who had been diagnosed in the past were now being treated for their disorder.

Adults that suspect they have ADHD may ask themselves some of the following questions:

- Did you have developmental delays in walking, talking, or sitting up?
- In the early grades, did your teachers complain that you were noisy or disruptive?
- Were you accused of daydreaming a lot at school?
- Did your teachers claim you were not living up to your potential?
- Did you often fail to complete homework?
- Did you have poor study habits?
- Did you experiment with drugs and alcohol?
- Do you frequently feel upset about lost opportunities of the past?

Diagnosing ADHD in an adult is very difficult because there are so many variables. It is important to contact a trained health professional who keeps up with the field. An organization like Children and Adults with Attention Deficit Disorder (CHADD) can provide information. The psychologist and physician can determine the appropriate treatment, which may involve medication, vocational and family counseling, or behavioral modification.

ADHD in adults is just beginning to be researched and reported. Dr. Russell Barkley, ADHD authority, in his book *ADHD in Adults: What Science Says,* has determined that adult ADHD is not well known and embarked on an educational tour in 2008 to proclaim how the seriousness of not knowing about the disease can lead to major problems in adults compared to their non-ADHD peers. According to Dr. Barkley, adults with ADHD are

- three times more likely to be currently unemployed;
- two times more likely to have problems keeping friends;
- four times more likely to have contracted a sexually transmitted disease.

Barkley's book is based on two studies:

1. A University of Massachusetts study conducted from 2003 to 2004 examined lifestyle outcomes among three cohorts of adults patients: 146 clinic-referred adults with ADHD, 97 adults seen in the same clinic who were not diagnosed with ADHD, and a general sample of 109 adults without ADHD. The study found that adults with ADHD were three times more likely to sell drugs illegally (21 percent compared to 6 percent) and that 67 percent of adults with ADHD compared to the control group (15 percent) had trouble managing their money.
2. The Milwaukee study has been ongoing since 1977, with the most recent following up from 1999 to 2003. This longitudinal study followed individuals over a period of years. The study looked at secondary life outcomes of 158 children who had been diagnosed with ADHD and who as adults either continue to experience the symptoms or who no longer have the disorder at age 27. They compared the results to a community control group of 81 children without ADHD. They found that adults with ADHD were about three times as likely to initiate physical fights (30 percent compared to 9 percent), destroy other's property (31 percent compared to 8 percent), and break and enter (20 percent compared to 7 percent).

Both studies documented behavior through a combination of data gathering techniques, such as self-reporting, patient interviews, and observation. ADHD has an impact on the lives of many people. However, Dr. Barkley encourages people with adult ADHD to seek help from their physicians to manage these destructive behaviors.

Although the existence and burden of ADHD have previously been questioned, ample data now support the validity of ADHD as diagnosis. Many successful people proclaim their struggle with ADHD as children and adults. James Carville, a political consultant whose skills as an organizer of campaigns and television commentator are well known, told of his difficulties with the condition but how it has given him positive creativity and ability to think out of the box. He revealed his ADHD in and interview on CNN in 2004 and is featured in the book *Positively ADD: Real Stories to Inspire Your Dreams.* David Neeleman, founder of JetBlue Airways, discussed his ADHD in "Career Advice from Powerful ADHD Executives: Flying High" in

Successful People with ADHD: James Carville, Political Consultant (1944–)

Just one glimpse at James Carville, television personality, author, and famous political consultant, and one knows that he cannot sit still. He is known for his strategies in the successful campaigns of Bill Clinton and Israeli Prime Minister Ehud Barak. But as a child, it was a different story. He was known as the "Ragin'Cajun" because of his fiery personality and Louisiana roots. He was impulsive, impatient, and eager to talk to others. According to his account told in *Positively ADD*, he was always in trouble at school, and the nuns made him sit at the front of the class. If he misbehaved, they swatted him with a piece of wood.

After a stint in the marines, he decided to get serious about school and eventually went to law school and began to practice law, which he disliked. When he started volunteering for campaigns, he really found his niche. Here he brought all his interests and abilities together and found something that he was really good at. He then began to view having ADD as a positive thing. He figures that falling down flat on one's face and then getting up again is part of life; eventually you will get things right.

Source: Corman, C. A., and E. Hallowell. 2006. *Positively ADD: Real stories to inspire your dreams.* New York: Walker and Company.

the December/January 2005 issue of *ADDitude* magazine. Several athletes have ADHD; Scott Eyre, pitcher for the Chicago Cubs, acknowledged his ADHD as an adult.

Medications for the treatment of adult ADHD are being developed. On April 24, 2008, Shire, a global biopharmaceutical company, announced that the FDA had approved Vyvanse or lisdexamfetamine dimethysylate for the treatment of ADHD. Vyvanse was introduced in July 2007 for treatment in children, aged 6 to 12. Currently, it is the only once-only prodrug stimulant approved to treat adults with ADHD. The Phase III trial that led the FDA to approve the drug for adults was a double-blind, placebo-controlled, 4-week study with 414 adults aged 18 to 55 years. Within this study adults' ADHD symptoms improved within 1 week of treatment with once-daily Vyvanse. Clinical Trials and Medical Approval.

In May 2008 a presentation at the 161st Annual Meeting of the American Psychiatric Association reported new insights into treatment of adult ADHD with OROS methylphenidate extended-release tablets. The findings included efficacy and safety analyses from a randomized, double-blind, placebo-controlled, dose-titration trial completed in 2007 and final results from a long-term open-label safety trial. In the placebo-controlled trial 226 patients with ADHD ages 18 to 65 were randomized to receive placebo or OROS for 7 weeks. The patients showed significant results, with improvements in symptom management compared to the placebo group.

Patient education is the heart of therapeutic success in adults. When people with ADHD realize that perceived shortcomings have a neurological basis, they can begin to accept that training can assist in changing those shortcomings. Personal coaching can provide strategies and encouragement and help individuals set and achieve goals. Physicians are just now beginning to recognize the challenge of adult ADHD in America. Proper screening and education will continue to be the imperative for the mental health of our society. However, the outlook is good because treatment for adult ADHD comes at a relatively low annual cost and does not require inpatient treatment, but has the potential to improve the human condition.

Further Readings: Barkley, R. A. 1990. *ADHD adolescents: Family conflicts and their management.* Grant from National Institute of Mental Health, MH41583; Barkley, Russell, Kevin R. Murphy, and Mariellen Fischer. 2007. *ADHD in adults: What the science says.* New York: Guilford Press; Biederman"?, J. 2004. "Breaking News: The Social an Economic Impact of ADHD." Discussion presented at the Attention Deficit Hyperactive Disorder (ADHD) AMA Briefing: September 9; New York, NY; Corman, C. A., and E. Hallowell. 2006. *Positively ADD: Real stories to inspire your dreams.* New York: Walker and Company; Gilman, Lois?. "Career advice from powerful ADHD executives." (December/January 2005). *ADDitude.* http://www.additudemag.com/adhd/article/754.html. Accessed May 18, 2009; Goldstein, S. 1997. *Managing attention and learning disorders in late adolescence and adulthood.* New York: Wiley; Murphy, Kevin R. 1995. *Out of the fog treatment option and coping strategies for adult attention deficit disorder.* New York: Hyperion; Nadeau, K. 1995. *A comprehensive guide to adults with attention deficit hyperactivity disorder.* New York: Brunner/Mazel; Serfontein, Gordon. 1994. *ADD in adults.* New York: Simon & Schuster; Wender, Paul. 1995. *Attention deficit hyperactive disorder in adults.* New York: Oxford University Press.

Allergies

Dr. Benjamin F. Feingold linked allergies and ADHD in the 1970s. Since that time, the debate has continued. Alternative practitioners consider allergies as a cause of ADHD. With the advent of more studies in nutrition, more doctors of medicine are accepting the two as possible comorbid conditions. Therefore, conflicting information about allergies may exist.

Researchers in traditional medicine do not consider allergies as a cause of ADD because they do not have the studies that show it. However, the Center for Science in the Public Interest (CSPI) counters that the studies show no correlation because they were poorly designed and executed and often were paid for by the food industry. For example, when researchers tested whether children reacted to artificial food dyes made from petroleum, they tested only one dye at a time although children may eat foods with the dyes at the same time. The amount tested was probably only a fraction of the dyes that children actually eat because no one calculated the actual food intake of children.

About 15 to 20 percent of the population has some type of allergy. If a car receives fuel that it is not compatible with, it will not run properly. This analogy describes what happened when people food they are allergic to and that may affect their behavior.

When the individual encounters an allergen, the item that evokes the allergic reaction, the body releases a chemical known as histamine, which works to increase the removal of blood serum from around the brain tissue. The adequate flow to the tiny capillaries of the tiny capillaries in the brain is affected and the brain becomes unbalanced. Thus, there may be a loss of memory, attention, and cognitive function.

Here are some signs that indicate allergies (Thumell-Read 2005):

1. Dark circles or bags under the eyes called allergy shiners
2. Dark flaky lips; lips are often involved in allergic reactions
3. Sweaty feet may indicate the allergic reactions; the liver is coping with an overload of toxins
4. One or both ears may be red or burn; the reaction often starts about 1 hour 45 minutes after exposure.
5. Children with allergies may appear pale and anemic.
6. A child may be a fussy eater; the child may be allergic to the food he will not eat.
7. Babies with food allergies may be very good tempered or very ill-tempered the first thing in the morning.
8. There may be a family history of allergies with near relatives suffering from hay fever or eczema.
9. Allergic children and adults often like peculiar smell; they may sniff felt pens or like the smell of gas. They are nearly always allergic to the smell.

Symptoms of ADHD may worsen with a seasonal allergy. Doctors at Long Island Hospital studied 20 children with ADHD between the ages of 5 and 18. They found that 40 percent of the children were diagnosed with asthma or atopical dermatitis; 23 percent with allergic rhinitis, and 9 percent had a positive allergy test. The researchers concluded that a high percentage of children with ADHD may also harbor behavior problems because of sleep problems caused by allergy symptoms—especially nasal obstruction. The study urged that all children diagnosed with ADHD be tested and treated for seasonal and environmental allergies.

Using a diary or journal to log the foods eaten by the person over a 30-day period will often provide insight into the items that may be creating complex ADHD symptoms. Diets such as the Feingold diet recommend that one perform trial and error with foods to discover allergies and how they are related to behavior. *See also* Feingold Diet; Nutrition.

Further Readings: Bouchez, Collette. "Seasonal Allergies Affect ADHD." http://preventdisease.com/news/articles/Seasonal_Allergies_Affect_ADHD.shtml. Accessed 8/7/2008; "Can Allergies Cause Behavior Problems?" http://borntoexplore.org/allergies.htm. Accessed 8/7/2008; Center for Science in the Public Interest. "Diet, ADHD & Behavior." http://www.cspinet.org. Accessed 7/13/2008; "Food Intolerance and Allergies in the ADHD Child." http://www.associatedcontent.com/article/155824/food_intolerance_allergies_in_the_adhd.html?cat=25. Accessed 6/17/2009; Thumell-Read, Jane. "9 Allergy Signs in Children." November 2005. http://ezinearticles.com/?9-Allergy-Signs-In-Children&id=97360. Accessed 5/18/2009.

Alpha-2A-agonist. *See* Guanfacine; INTUNIV.

Alternative Medicine

Many individuals are attracted to alternative medicine for treatment for ADHD because of adverse reactions from stimulants or other drugs. Others may be attracted because of the philosophies and health beliefs of these treatments. The term "alternative medicine" refers to healing practices that generally do not fall with the realm of conventional medicine. In the history of medicine in the Western world of Europe and the United States, a system of medicine developed that uses scientific of evidence-based trials to show the effectiveness of a treatment or medication. This system of evidence-based medicine or trial-based medicine has been dubbed "Western medicine." Alternative medicine then encompasses any healing practice that does not fall within the realm of conventional medicine.

Several alternative medical treatments tout help for children with ADHD. These examples include naturopathy, Ayurveda, meditation, yoga, biofeedback, chiropractic, herbal medicine, traditional Chinese medicine (TCM), hypnosis, bodywork and massage, homeopathy, and diet-based therapies. Alternative medical practices are diverse philosophies and methodologies. Some practices are based on prescientific traditional medicine, folk knowledge, spiritual practices, and even newly conceived methods of healing. Alternative medicine is often grouped with complementary medicine, which generally refers to alternative techniques used in conjunction with mainstream medicine. The umbrella term complementary and alternative medicine (CAM) describes the combination of the two.

Some scientists reject the use of the term "alternative medicine" on the grounds that the techniques or treatments have not been adequately tested to determine what works and what does not work. Although proponents of alternative medicine cite a large number of studies, critics point out that the statistics were not the result of controlled, double-blind, peer-reviewed experiments. The advocates may deny that there is a need for such testing. The advocates claim that stories and anecdotes of the treatment's effectiveness are sufficient.

The National Center for Complementary and Alternative Medicine (NCCAM) defines CAM as a group of diverse medical and health care systems, practices, and products that are not currently part of conventional medicine. NCCAM divides the therapies into five major groups:

- Whole medical systems that cut across many groups, such as traditional Chinese medicine and Ayurveda
- Mind-body medicine that focuses on holistic health and explores the interconnection between mind, body, and spirit
- Biologically based practices that use substances found in natures such as herbs, vitamins, and other natural substances
- Manipulative and body-based practices that are based on movement of body parts, such as chiropractic and osteopathic manipulation
- Energy medicine are of two kinds: energy fields that purportedly surround and penetrate the bodies and bioeletromagnetic-based therapies uses the magnetic energy fields that supposedly surround and penetrate the body

Because of the uncertain nature of alternative therapies and the dependence on anecdotes and lack of scientific research, alternative medicine remains a source of serious debate. Forms of alternative medicine that are biologically active may interfere with conventional treatments or produce serious side effects. Debates about alternative and mainstream medicine spill over into freedom of expression and even freedom of religion discussions. Government regulators continue to attempt to find a regulatory balance.

The success of treating ADHD with alternative or complementary medicine varies. Typically parents use a trial-and-error approach to evaluate effectiveness. The most commonly used alternative treatments for ADHD are neurofeedback, homeopathy, herbal medicines, iron supplements, and dietary modifications and supplements. *See also* Complementary Medicine.

Further Readings: Bratman, Steven. 1997. *The alternative medicine sourcebook.* Los Angeles, CA: Lowell House; "Complementary and Alternative Medicine." http://www.nccam.nih.gov/. Accessed 6/17/2009; "Medline Abstracts"?: Complementary and Alternative Therapies for ADHD." http://www.medscape.com/viewarticle/438960_print; "White House Commission on Complementary and Alternative Medicine Policy." Final report: March 2002. Washington, D.C. http://www.whccamp.hhs.gov/. Accessed 5/18/2009.

Americans with Disabilities Act

Title II of the Americans with Disabilities Act (ADA), which became effective January 26, 1992, prohibits discrimination in services, programs, and activities provided by state and local governments. Schools must make programs available and accessible to all disabled individuals who are otherwise qualified to participate in the program.

Two federal laws require public schools to provide additional educational services to children who need them, at no cost to the parents. To qualify under ADA and the Individuals with Disabilities Education Act (IDEA), a child must meet the criteria for thirteen specific disability categories, which include learning disabilities and developmental delays. ADHD is not one of these categories. However, some children with ADHD may also have these disabilities and will qualify under IDEA or he or she may qualify under IDEA's "other health impairments." Just having ADHD or a learning disability does not guarantee eligibility for special services. To qualify, the disorder must substantially affect the ability to function in school.

Children who qualify under IDEA are entitled to special services, including individual instruction by educational specialists. Parents, teachers, and other school staff work together to develop an Individualized Education Program (IEP), a plan for best delivering these services. The plan describes the individuals learning problems, details the services, sets annual goals, and defines how progress will be measured. Parents have a right to ask for changes in the plan.

ADA applies to a district regardless of federal funding. IDEA, Section 504, and ADA all cover students with disabilities and place legal obligations on schools. Laws concerning special education have led educators to do what they have not done on their own. *See also* Individuals with Disabilities Education Act (IDEA); Discrimination in Employment; Section 504.

Further Reading: Kelly, Evelyn B. 2006. *Legal basics: A handbook for educators.* 2nd ed. Bloomington, IN: Phi Delta Kappa International; "Know Your Child's Educational Rights." *ADDitude* August/September 2006. http://www.additudemag.com/adhd/article/1623.html Accessed 5/19/2009.

Amphetamine

Amphetamine, dextroamphetamine, and mixed amphetamine salts are prescription medications that have been shown effective in the treatment of ADHD in children, adolescents, and adults. These compounds increase effective use of the transmitters of dopamine and norepinephrine in parts of the brain that regulate attention and behavior in order to control symptoms associated with ADHD and improve functioning. Scientific literature shows that stimulant medications including amphetamine and dextroamphetamine are the most effect treatment options for ADHD. The American Academy of Pediatrics and the American Academy of Child and Adolescent Psychiatry consider these medicines to be the best treatment options.

Amphetamines are used in the treatment of people who have been diagnosed with ADHD through rigorous evaluations. The symptoms are associated with severe inattention, hyperactivity, and impulsivity that interfere with the person's every day living activities, such as school, home, and work. Adults with ADHD may be prone to procrastination, become easily frustrated, and take on many tasks while accomplishing none. A person with inattentive symptoms only can respond equally well to amphetamine or dextroamphetamine, as well as someone who has both inattentive and hyperactive symptoms.

Amphetamines are available in the following compounds:

- Amphetamine sulfate (racemic amphetamine sulfate) for immediate release
- Dextrostat (dextroamphetamine), immediate release 5- or 10-mg tablets
- Dexedrine (dextroamphetamine), immediate release 5-mg tablets
- Dexedrine spansules (dextroamphetamine), 5-, 19-, and 15-mg sustained release capsules
- Adderall (mixed amphetamine salts), 5-, 7.5-, 19-, 12.5-, 15-, 20-, and 30-mg immediate release tablets
- Adderall XR (mixed amphetamine salts), 5-, 10-, 15-, 20-, 25-, and 30-mg extended release capsules
- Concerta (OROS methylphenidate), 18-, 27-, 36-, and 54-mg sustained release capsules
- Vyvanse (lisdexamfetamine dimesylate), 30-, 50, and 70-mg patch

Amphetamine medications start working within 1 to 3 hours of ingesting the medications. The effect generally lasts about 4 to 5 hours for the immediate release forms and 8-12 hours for the sustained release forms.

What are the Concerns about Amphetamines?

These drugs should be avoided in individuals who have the following conditions:

- Psychotic symptoms caused by schizophrenia, schizoaffective disorder, bipolar disorder, or any other brain disorder, because they are likely to worsen the condition

- People with cardiovascular disorders such as abnormal heart defects, uncontrolled high blood pressure, or any disorder of the blood vessels or the heart
- Overactive thyroid
- Glaucoma
- Uncontrolled seizures
- History of drug abuse
- Women who are pregnant or planning to become pregnant

Sudden unexplained death (SUD) has been associated with amphetamine abuse, and SUD has been reported in children and adults with and without underlying cardiac abnormalities taking the recommended doses of amphetamines, including Adderall and AdderallXR.

Amphetamine and dextroamphetamine are known to produce euphoria or feeling high, increased energy, and wakefulness, which carry a potential for abuse if more of the drug is used than prescribed. Therefore, the potential for abuse has made it a highly regulated drug in the United States. Pharmacies carefully regulate the storage and dispensing of these medications, and in some states, physicians must write prescriptions on tamper-proof pads. Several studies have shown that taking stimulants for ADHD may prevent an individual from developing a substance abuse problem. The high risk for developing substance abuse lies in not treating the ADHD. However, if a person does have an active substance abuse disorder and is not motivated to get off the drugs, the health care provider should not prescribe amphetamines but should look for another medication without abuse potential.

Amphetamines should not be used within 14 days of taking drugs called monoamine oxidase inhibitors (MAOIs) to treat depression. Taking these two drugs together can cause serious and sometimes fatal reactions, which include high fevers, high blood pressure, seizures, and possibly coma.

If a woman is pregnant or planning on becoming pregnant, amphetamines are not a good choice. Studies in mice have shown that these drugs can cause fetal malformation and death when administered at high doses. One report showed severe congenital deformity in a baby born to a woman who took dextroamphetamine along with other medications during the first trimester of pregnancy. Infants have an increased risk of premature delivery and low birth weight and may show symptoms of withdrawal such as agitation and lack of energy. Several case reports indicate that the use during pregnancy may influence the development of children up to at least 10 years. Amphetamines are excreted in breast milk and should be avoided by mothers who are breast-feeding.

Amphetamines must be taken orally, in the morning, with or without food, and exactly as the healthcare provider prescribes. Different forms are available for easier swallowing, fewer side effects, and for taking the medication fewer times during the day. The following forms are available:

- Tablets. Swallow whole because chewing gives an unpleasant taste and can irritate the mouth and throat. Take one to three times daily as instructed by the doctor.

- Sprinkle capsules. Dexedrine spansules may be swallowed whole or opened and sprinkled onto food such as applesauce or pudding. These capsules should not be chewed and taken once daily as the doctor has prescribed.
- Long-acting capsules. AdderallXR and Dexedrine spansule can be taken once daily. Do not cut, crush, or chew these capsules.

The absorption of amphetamine medications can be reduced if strong organic acids are present in the stomach at the time of taking the drug. The following foods should be avoided for 1 hour before and after taking the medication: citrus fruit, citrus juices, soda/carbonated beverages, lemonade, Gatorade, and vitamins and food supplements containing vitamin C.

If a dose of amphetamine is missed, it may be taken as soon as remembered as long as it is not too close to the time for the next dose. If it is close to the time, wait until that time. Do not double the dose or take more than has been prescribed. If an overdose does occur, immediate attention is necessary because high fever, abnormal heart rhythms, high blood pressure, seizure, coma, and death can occur.

The following address the side effects of amphetamines:

- Upset stomach is one of the most common side effects. Taking it on a full stomach or lowering the dose can manage the effect.
- Loss of weight and appetite can be improved by serving the person favorite foods when the stimulant effects are low. This time is in the morning before medication or at night when the medication effects are lower. Use nutritional supplements.
- Give the medication as early in the day as possible to avoid afternoon or evening dosing. Some physicians may prescribe sedative medications at night. Melatonin may effectively manage insomnia related to the ADHD medicine.
- If abnormal movements or muscle twitches develop, the medication does should be lowered. These movements may include excessive eye blinking, nose scrunching, or shoulder shrugging.
- Reducing the dosage or changing medications usually manages mild anxiety or restlessness.
- Severe anxiety, panic attacks, mania, hallucinations, paranoia, and delusions are all possible with this medication. If these occur, discontinue use and contact the health care provider immediately.
- Certain medications, such as those used to treat depression, antacids, or urinary medications, can interact with amphetamines with serious reactions.

Amphetamines can be useful medications for some people with ADHD. Following the guidance of the health care provider is imperative to avoid side effects and abuse.

Further Readings: Food and Drug Administration. http://www.fda.gov; "National Alliance on Mental Illness (NAMI)." http://www.nami.org. Accessed 5/18/2009.

Anxiety

Anxiety, a normal reaction to stress, helps people deal with tense situations at school and at work. It helps them stay focused to study harder for an exam, keep focused on an important speech, or perform tasks in a timely manner. However, if anxiety becomes excessive or takes the form of an irrational dread of everyday situations, it becomes a debilitating disorder.

Childhood ADHD is commonly comorbid with anxiety disorders at an estimated rate of 20 to 40 percent. There are three types of anxiety disorders:

1. Generalized anxiety disorder (GAD), thought to be the most prevalent disorder
2. Social phobia or fear of relating to others
3. Separation anxiety disorder, which occurs when a child is separated from a loved one

Of these disorders, GAD is considered to be the most prevalent, followed by social phobia and separation anxiety disorder. Some children may have more than one anxiety disorder.

Studies have shown that children with anxiety and ADHD are less likely to display the off-task and hyperactive behavior and have longer reaction times than those children with pure ADHD. Because of this difference, some researchers have suggested that this is a separate subtype of ADHD and is pathologically different from the other subtypes. Also for this reason, it may be easy to overlook ADHD in children with anxiety. These children may often be preoccupied with fears that impair their ability to focus on the task at hand. For anxious children who do not have ADHD, when the anxiety improves, so will the inattention; children with ADHD will continue to struggle with inattention even in the absence of anxiety.

Some have suggested that the anxiety associated with ADHD is a product of the inability to function in daily life, rather than the typical phobic and anxious behavior. This idea highlights the fact that early recognition and intervention of ADHD can lead to the improvement of anxiety. Because of the close connection between ADHD and anxiety, children need to be closely monitored for symptoms.

According to Kunwar et al. (2007), if a child has comorbid ADHD/anxiety, initial treatment should be with a stimulant or atomoxetine. In cases where ADHD symptoms improve but anxiety persists, psychotherapy targeting the anxiety symptoms should be added. If anxiety is severe, specific treatments for anxiety symptoms with a medication, psychotherapy, or both should be started first and ADHD treated next.

Anxiety and panic attack are sudden surges of overwhelming fear that come without warning and for no obvious reason. According to the National Institute of Mental Health, the prevalence of anxiety attacks disorder is approximately 2.4 million Americans. Annual incidence of panic disorder is 1.7 percent or 4.6 million people in the United States. Panic attacks are the most prevalent emotional disorder and are more common than bipolar disorder, obsessive compulsive disorder, schizophrenia, ADHD, phobias, alcohol abuse, and depression. The condition is also the one that has the lowest rates for seeking help and finding it. The symptoms include the following:

- Raging heartbeat
- Difficulty breathing

- Feeling of terror that is almost paralyzing
- Nervousness and shaking
- Dizziness, lightheadedness, and nausea
- Trembling and sweating
- Choking
- Hot flashes or sudden chills
- Fear that one is going crazy or about to die

Adult ADHD is common among patients that seek help in anxiety disorder clinics. A study of consecutive patients seen in an anxiety-disorder clinic found that 33 percent met criteria for adult ADHD, which is much higher than the 4.4 percent prevalence of adults with ADHD in the U.S. population. Michael Van Amerigen and colleagues from McMaster University Medical Center in Canada looked at 97 people referred to their clinic. Although these patients had not come for treatment of ADHD, they completed an assessment called the Mini International Neuropsychiatric Interview (MINI) for ADHD. The researchers found that 32 of the 97 or 33 percent of adults met the MINI criteria. Most reported that they knew they had some symptoms, but no one had formally diagnosed the condition.

Further Readings: "Anxiety and Panic Attacks." 2008. http://www.anxiety/panic. com. Accessed 5/19/2008; Busco, Marlene. 2008. Adult ADHD is common among patients in anxiety-disorders clinic. http://www.medscape.com/viewarticles/571537. Accessed 5/19/2008; Faraone, Stephen. 2007. "ADHD in Children with Comorbid Conditions: Diagnosis, Misdiagnosis, and Keeping Tabs on Both." *Medscape Psychiatry and Mental Health.* http://www.medscape.com/viewarticle/555748. Accessed 5/19/2008; Kunwar, A. et al. 2007. Treating common psychiatric disorders associated with attention-deficit/hyperactive disorder. *Expert Opinion Pharmacotherapy* 8:555–62; Van Amerigen, M. et al. 2008. "Adult ADHD is common among patients that seek help in anxiety disorder clinics." Discussion presented at the 28th Annual Meeting of the Anxiety Disorders Association of America; March 6–9; Savannah, Georgia. http://www.medscape.com/view article/571537_print, Accessed 5/19/2009.

Aromatherapy

Some practitioners recommend aromatherapy for ADHD. Aromatherapy, an ancient treatment, dates back more than 3,000 years to the Egyptians and Greeks. Aromatherapy exerts its effects through the sense of smell or olfaction. The olfactory nerves lie in the upper part of the nose and are connected directly to the brain. This sense of smell is the most immediate of a human's senses. When smells vaporize, minute particles dissolve in the moist secretions inside the nasal passages and pass to the olfactory cells at the back of the nose. The molecules have different shapes and when they meet receptors that match, a signal is transmitted to the limbic area of the brain where it is perceived as smell. The nose can register about 10,000 types of smell sensations.

The link of smell to the limbic system is the hypothalamus at the base of the brain. The right side of the brain is believed to be associated with intuitive thought and behavior; the left side of the brain is thought be relate to logical and intellectual processes. If the two hemispheres are in harmony, aromatherapists believe the person experiences calm and well-being. Pleasant aromatic experiences promote this well-being.

Practitioners use about 300 aromatic oils, each with its own range of properties that target antiviral, anti-inflammatory, antitoxic, uplifting, and calming efforts. These essential oils are extracted from certain plants, herbs, grasses, and flowers. Some oils are expensive because the extraction process is extremely laborious. For example, it takes 60,000 rose blossoms to produce 1 ounce of rose oil. The most common use of oils is in therapeutic massage, which has the dual benefit of relaxing muscles and stimulating pleasant aromas.

Aromatherapists recommend that a parent massage the child. For the ADHD child, massage has the benefit of positive physical contact between parent and child. Recommended for babies and small children are Roman chamomile and lavender. Other useful oils for babies are mandarin, tangerine, and geranium. For children who may have angry aggressive tendencies, lavender is often effective, and ylang ylang is useful for poor self-esteem. Several other oils may be useful in ADHD, depending on the child's personality and behavior.

The U.S. Food and Drug Administration (FDA) is an agency of the federal government charged with guarding and determining safety of consumer products and drugs. Fragrance products are sometimes marketed with claims or implications that their use will improve personal well-being in a variety of ways. These products of aromatherapy fit into this description if they are intended in the diagnosis, mitigation, treatment, or prevention of disease and intended to affect the structure or any function of the body. Both cosmetics and drugs are under the FDA's jurisdiction, but the legal requirements may differ. A claim that a perfume's aroma makes a person feel more attractive in general does not require approval before a product is sold. However, if someone tries to market a scent suggesting effectiveness as an aid in treating a disease or condition or affect the body's structure or function, such a claim may cause the product to be regulated as a drug. The agency makes judgments on a case-by-case basis. The Federal Claims Commission regulates claims made in advertising but not on product labeling.

Further Readings: Davis, P., and Waldon Saffron. 1988. *Aromatherapy from A-Z.* Essex, England: Daniel Publishers; U.S. Food and Drug Administration. "Aromatherapy." http://vm.cfsan.fda.gov/. Accessed 5/20/2008; Wormwood, V. A. 1991. *The fragrant pharmacy: a complete guide to aromatherapy and essential oils.* London: Bantam.

Assessment Tools

The purpose of assessment tools is to help the physician address three things that relate to a diagnosis of ADHD:

1. Is the diagnosis of ADHD justified?
2. If the diagnosis is not justified, then are there other explanations for the symptoms?
3. If the diagnosis of ADHD is not justified, are there other conditions such as depression or anxiety that should be treated?

In looking at the results of any test, several things must be considered. The test must be valid, meaning it is testing an idea or construct and has been shown to measure that construct. The test must be reliable, meaning that the results can be replicated over and over with the same results. Tests are given in a standard way described in a manual and are always conducted according the protocol. The word "standardized" in a test means that it is always conducted in the same way with all subjects. An important point is that the test is practical and reasonable to administer.

Intelligence and Achievement Tests

The Wechsler Intelligence Scale for Children (WISC) is an IQ test that is simple to administer and can help clinicians determine cognitive factors that may contribute to inattention and academic underachievement. Intelligence tests are set up to measure short-term or working memory, facility with numbers, visual-spatial skills, and arithmetic calculation. On the other hand, achievement tests are designed to determine academic performance based on information or skills in various subject areas, such as math, language, spelling, etc. Tests such as the Stanford Achievement Test (SAT), California Test of Basic Skills (CTBS), the Iowa Test of Basic Skills (ITBS) are achievement tests. These tests are norm-referenced tests, meaning they have been given to numbers of students and then calculated on a normal curve. Tests that are given in the classroom or state tests that are based on standards test the student's knowledge of information relating to standards or a specific body of information. These tests are called criterion-referenced tests in that they have specific facts or skills that should have been taught and all students should be able to perform. Most state tests that have developed from the No Child Left Behind Act are criterion-referenced tests based on state adopted standards.

Generally in relating to ADHD, these tests are hard to interpret, especially for children who are impulsive. The meaning of a low test score is unclear if the youngster has spent a lot of time grabbing test materials, hiding under the table, or running to the bathroom. For highly active children, it would be expected that the gulf between competence and performance is large. Thus, for a child with ADHD symptoms, tests for cognitive abilities and achievement may be more accurate if administered while the child is on therapeutic medication.

Neuropsychological Measures

Several individual tests may have a role in the evaluative process. The relationship of ADHD to executive function may be determined from some of these tests. The following are individual measures that are most often used:

- Wisconsin Card Sort test. The most common measure of adult frontal lobe or executive function.
- Stroop Word-Color test. A timed test measuring the ability to suppress or inhibit automatic responses. Children must read the names of colors, although the names are printed in a different-colored ink from the color of the word.

These results relate to frontal lobe functioning in adults but cannot be used to accurately diagnose children as having ADHD.

- Rey-Osterrieth Complex Figure Drawing. A paper-and-pencil test requiring planning and visual-spatial abilities and is sensitive to frontal lobe injuries.
- Trail Making test (parts A and B). Part A: a test requiring the subject to connect a series of numbered circles distributed at random on a page; in part B: the subject alternates connecting letters and numbers. This test is not recommended for diagnosing children with ADHD.
- Continuous Performance test. This test is widely used for evaluation in ADHD. The subject observes a screen while individual letters or numbers are projected onto it at a rapid pace, typically one per second. The child is told to press a button when a certain stimulus or pair appears in sequence. This test looks at sustained attention and impulse control.
- Motor inhibition tasks. A task called go/no-go responds with a button for one class or stimuli but should not respond when another stimuli is presented.
- Matching familiar figures test. A picture is presented and the subject must match it from an array of six similar variants.
- Gordon Diagnostic System Delay task. This test measures response inhibition using a computer and large blue button.

Observational Measures

The diagnosis of ADHD requires subjective input from a variety of people. One way to acquire this information is to use behavior rating scales. Although no reliable objective tests exist for ADHD, several scales have been developed for diagnosis.

One rating scale that is used widely is called the Conner's Teacher's Rating Scale (CTRS) developed in 1969. In use for more than 25 years, CTRS is important because of its wide acceptance. CTRS uses a four-point scale that includes the following ratings of an observed behavior: not at all present, just a little present, pretty much present, and very must present. There are 28 items in the scale, and then several items that collect demographic information from both parent and teacher. Then the two respondents are compared and a score of the different responses called a discrepancy score is calculated. The determination is then made if the child is exhibiting symptoms that are consistent with ADHD.

Another rating scale is the Conner's Abbreviated Symptoms Questionnaire (ASQ), which is often referred to as the Hyperactivity Index. This 10-item scale is used to screen hyperactivity in children and is often used to assess conduct problems before and after interventions such as stimulant therapy. Criticisms of ASQ are that it perhaps overidentifies normal children, disproportionately identifies children who are hyperactive and aggressive, and underidentifies distractible children.

One type of ADHD called predominantly inattentive type (formerly called attention-deficit disorder or just ADD) is especially difficult to diagnose. According to a study by Epstein (1991), this subtype is diagnosed correctly only about 50 percent of the time. Barkley (1990) developed the BAADS as a diagnostic tool T. E. Brown uses the BAADS in combination with a careful clinical history of the individual and family, school reports, and an analysis of WISC/WAIS subtest scores. The WISC/WAIS are intelligence tests. In considering assessment, the evaluator considers that it is only a tool and that multiple assessments must be used to effectively diagnose ADHD (Table 1).

For adults several tests have been developed:

- The Adult ADHD Clinical Diagnostic Scales v. 1.2 (ACSD)
- The Conner's Adult ADHD Diagnostic Interview for the DSM-IV (CAADID)
- The Adult ADHD Investigator Symptom Rating Scale (AISRS)

Table 1   Scales for Rating Children with ADHD

Scale	Author	Description	Advantages
Conners Rating Scale Revised CRS-R (3–17 years)	Multihealth systems, (Connors 1997)	Popular scale with a long history of evaluation of ADHD. Assesses a variety of common behaviors such as sleep, peer relations, and eating. Revised scale updates age- and gender-normed data. Available in short and long forms and teacher, parent, and self-report versions.	DSM-IV based; large normative base; multiple observer forms that correlate; shorter forms allow easier monitoring; available in French
Brown Attention Deficit Disorder Scale (BADDS) for children and adolescents 3–12 years, parents, teachers; self-report for 8–12 years	Psychological Corp. (Brown 2001)	BADDS is DSM-IV based and measures executive functioning associated with ADHD. Also measures developmental impairments; separate rating scales for 3–7 years, 8–12 years, and 12–18 years. Scales should be administered in an interview formal especially for parent and youth self-report	Measures inattentive ADHD, accounts for inattentive behavior as a function of age; strong psychometrics
Vanderbilt ADHD rating scale (6–12 years); parents and teacher forms	Association for Academic Psychiatry and NICRQ	2002. Newer DSM-IV rating scale; parent and teacher forms; similar to CRS-R and SNAP-IV; assesses for comorbidity and school functioning	Measures OCD, anxiety, and depression; Spanish and German version; strong psychometric scales
Swanson, Nolan, and Pelham; Version IV (SNAP-IV); 5–11 years; parent and teacher rating scale		One of first scales based on DSM-IV criteria; frequently used in ADHD research	Scoring available on Web site; same scale used for both parent and teacher; measures comorbidity

- The Attention-Deficit Hyperactive Disorder Rating Scale (ADHD-RS)
- Adult ADHD Self-Report Scale (ARSC)
- Conner's Adult ADHD Rating Scale-Short (CAARS-S:S)
- Achenbach Child Behavior Checklist (CBCL)
- Copeland Symptoms Checklist for Adult ADHD
- Brown Adult Attention Deficit Disorder Scales

Further Readings: Barkley, R. A. et al. 1990. Comprehensive evaluation of ADD with and without hyperactivity as defined by research criteria. *Journal of Consulting and Clinical Psychology* 58:775–89; Brown, T. E. et al. 1992. Attention-Activation Disorder in Hi-IQ Underachievers. Abstract. Proceedings of American Psychiatric Association 145th Annual Meeting, Washington, D.C., May 1992; Epstein, M. A. et al. 1991. Boundaries of attention deficit disorder. *Journal of Learning Disabilities* 24:110–20.

Attention Deficit Disorder Association (ADDA)

According to its mission statement, "the Attention Deficit Disorder Association (ADDA) is a 501c3 nonprofit international organization that has been in existence since 1989. The mission of ADDA is to provide information, resources, and networking to adults with ADHD and to the professionals who work with them. In so doing, the organization generates hope, awareness, empowerment, and connection worldwide in the field of ADHD. The groups brings together scientific perspective and the human experience, the information and resources provided to individuals and families affected by ADHD, and professionals in the filed to focus on diagnosis, treatment, strategies, and techniques for helping adults with the condition lead better lives."

ADDA provides the following resources to it members: an annual national conference; *FOCUS*, a quarterly publication; a Web site; written tools for helping adults with ADHD; ADHD teleclasses; networking opportunities for adults with ADHD; and most importantly advocacy for those with the disorder. Members also provide expert information for media resources. The address of the organization is 15000 Commerce Parkway, Suite C, Mount Laurel, New Jersey.

Further Readings: Attention Deficit Disorder Association. http:www.//add.org. Accessed 5/19/2009; The HealthCentral Network. http://www.thehealthcentralnetwork.com/news/20080312.html. Accessed 5/19/2009.

Auricular Medicine

The Latin root *auris* meaning "ear" gives its name to things pertaining to the ear. Auricular medicine is a subspecialty of acupuncture that uses the human ear as a means of diagnosis. This type of medicine considers the ear an indication that certain parts or systems of the body are not functioning properly. By stimulating certain points on the ear with a mild electrical pulse the practitioner will treat symptoms of ADHD. They believe that when treated with auricular medicine, the symptoms will disappear after 1 to 4 months of weekly treatment sessions. *See also* Acupuncture.

Further Reading: "Medical Acupuncture Treats ADD without Drugs." http://www.medicalacupuncture.org/acu_info/pressrelease/adhd.html. Accessed 5/19/2009.

Autism

Some scientists have called autism an epidemic, which has erupted over the last couple of decades. The number of children diagnosed with autism has leapt in recent years from 1 child in 2000 to 1 child in 166. Researchers "have not found the reasons for and causes of autism, although they have proposed several ideas for the escalating rates of the condition. Considerable controversy surrounds the issue as to why this condition has developed so rapidly.

Various degrees of severity exist, so the term autism spectrum or autism spectrum disorder (ASD) or autism spectrum condition (ASC) sometimes replaces just the single word autism. ASD is used to describe a spectrum of psychological conditions. According to DSM-IV-TR, the symptoms are characterized by widespread abnormalities of social interactions, communication, and behavioral development that include severely restricted interests and highly repetitive behaviors. There are four main forms of ASD:

- Autism
- Asperger syndrome
- Pervasive developmental disorder not otherwise specified (PDD-NOS)
- High-functioning autism

Autism and ADHD are often diagnosed together, are commonly found in children, and are first observed in the child's early years, but some symptoms may persist into adulthood. Diane Kennedy, author of *The ADHD Autism Connection*, makes a strong case for the distinct similarities between the symptoms of ADHD and autism. She notes that both are developmental disorders, share similar features, and affect children in the same three central areas: communication, social interaction, and behavior. Both conditions arise from a similar place, a deficit in the executive functions of the frontal lobe. Both groups share the difficulties in gross and fine motor skills.

Table 2 illustrates the behavioral similarities between autism and ADHD.

Although some of the behaviors are similar, there are still distinct differences in the person who has autism and one with ADHD.

The WHO *Statistical Classification of Diseases and Related Health Problems*, 10th ed. (ICD-10) suggests a possible genetic and behavioral connection between ADHD and autism. A study published in the *American Journal of Human Genetics* (2002) found the two may be caused in part by the same gene. Several studies have found that a region on chromosome 16 is likely to contain a gene contributing to the development of autism. Dr. Susan Smiley and researchers at the University of California Los Angeles performed a genetic scan on 277 pairs of siblings, both of whom had been diagnosed with ADHD. The scan looked at the specific chromosome that was associated with ADHD. They found the same area of chromosome 16 that had been implicated in autism. Some scientists think a gene on this chromosome causes the behaviors that are similar in each disorder. Others believe that certain genes in the genome simply predispose people to develop any of a variety of mental disorders. Other genes and environmental influences may determine which disorder the person develops.

Table 2   Behavioral Similarities between Autism and ADHD

ADHD Behaviors	Autism Behaviors
Difficulty playing with other children	Cannot talk or play quietly; disrupts others with talk or actions
No real fear of danger	Engages in potentially dangerous activities; is impulsive
Tantrums; expresses distress for no apparent reason	May have temper tantrums if things do not go his or her way
Inappropriate laughing or giggling	Plays without normal cautions or consideration or consequences
May not want cuddling or act cuddly	When younger, may have difficulty accepting soothing or holding
Noticeable physical overactivity or extreme underactivity	Interrupts, disrupts, talks, or acts inappropriately
Little or no eye contact	Difficulty in awaiting turn at games or in school activities
Works impulsively making careless mistakes with sloppy work	May appear overactive even during sleep
	Does not appear to listen when directly spoken to

Most likely the combined effects of many genes and the effects of unknown environmental factors cause both ADHD and autism. It is highly unlikely that one gene of chromosome 16 will decide either of these disorders. The role of the gene has not yet been confirmed, and additional study is needed to follow through on this idea.

A study released by researchers at the University of Rochester found that children who have both autism and attention-deficit hyperactivity disorders are four times more likely to bully other children than children in the general population. Writing in *Ambulatory Pediatrics*, Dr. Guillermo Montes said that the study pulled data from the 2003 National Survey of Children's Health that included 53,219 children ages 6 to 17. The researchers asked whether children with autism actually bully other children more often. The researchers did not find that children with autism had a higher rate of bullying, unless they had ADD or ADHD. Those with both disorders showed a rate four times higher than children with just autism and for children overall. They also had a higher rate than children with ADD or ADHD and no autism. About half the children in the autism spectrum have ADHD. Depending on the severity of the symptoms, these children could benefit from additional support services, such as a behavioral or mental health specialist.

Goldstein and Schwebach (2004) studied 57 clinic-referred cases involving PDD-NOS, autism, or ADHD. They found that 26 percent of the children with PDD-NOS met criteria for a diagnosis of ADHD-C and 33 percent met criteria for ADHD, predominantly inattentive type. This study suggests that the majority or 59 percent of those with PDD-NOS or autism had comorbid ADHD. Although the likelihood that those with ADHD have comorbid autism spectrum disorder is low, the inverse is true: those children with ASDs may also have ADHD.

Several specialists have proposed that early treatment for autism and ADHD can capitalize on the brain's neuroplasticity with regulated sensory stimulation. The combination of movement and therapeutic music can enhance handwriting. Music engages many areas throughout the brain, which are normally involved in other kinds of cognition. These strategies believe the brain can be retrained to overcome learning disabilities, cognitive impairments, and ADHD. Proponents of a multisensory program called "Train the Brain to Pay Attention" report that using this type of training influences individual impulse control and progress in children with ASD and ADHD.

Although no single treatment protocol exists for all children with ASD and ADHD, most children respond best to highly structured behavioral programs. The nonprofit organization Autism Speaks lists the following programs specifically for children with autism:

- Applied Behavioral Analysis (ABA). Behavioral modification has been used for many types of therapy. It began in the 1930s and uses positive reinforcement to encourage desired behaviors. This techniques is probably one of the favorites and most preferred methods of dealing with autism.
- Floortime. Stanley Greenspan developed a treatment called floortime as a method of interacting with autistic children. The child moves through six basic developmental milestones that the individual must master for intellectual and emotional growth. For example, the individual must master crawling before beginning to walk.
- Gluten-free, casein-free diet (GFCF). The parent removes gluten (protein found in barley, rye, oats, and wheat) and casein (protein found in dairy products) from the diet. Some nutritionists believe that children with autism process these proteins differently from other children and that causes false opiate-like chemicals in the brain. This reaction to gluten is not an allergy but has to do with processing chemicals in the brain.
- Occupational therapy (OT). OT introduces skills such as coping, motor, play, self-help, and socialization to improve the quality of life of the individual.
- Picture exchange cards (PECS). PECS is a type of alternative communication technique where individuals with little or no verbal ability learn to relate using picture cards. The children use the pictures to vocalize a need, desire, observation, or feeling.
- Relationship Development Intervention (RDI). Steven Gutstein, a noted psychologist, developed RDI, a system that focuses on improving the long-term quality of life for children with autism. This intense training program helps parents show children how to become friends, feel for others, show love, and share with others. RDI consists of a series of core modules.
- The SCERTS Model. This model is a comprehensive, team-based, approach that uses a multidisciplinary model for enhancing abilities in social communication, emotional regulation and transactional supports. This model was developed by several clinicians and is an adaptation of ABA.
- Sensory Integration Therapy. Children with autism often have symptoms of sensory integration dysfunction that make processing information and

communication difficult. The goal of this therapy is use the senses to assist children in processing input in a more normal way.

- Speech Therapy. Communication problems of autistic children vary and may depend on intellectual development. Therapists work on language development, attention, and social initiation.
- Training and Education of Autistic and Related Communication Handicapped Children (TEACCH). This program builds on the fact that autistic children are visual learners. The process clarifies the learning process to build receptiveness, understanding, organization, and independence. Structure is important in this program.
- Verbal Behavior Intervention (VIB). VIB seeks to capture a child's motivation to develop a connection between the value of a word and the word itself. VIB bridges some of the gaps left in ABA.

Further Readings: Autism Speaks. http://www.autismspeaks.org. Accessed 5/19/2009; "Children with Both Autism and ADHD Often Bully, Parents Say." http://www.medical newstoday.com/articles/71296.php. Accessed 2/8/2008; Cohen, Don, and Fred Volmar. 2005. *The handbook of autism and pervasive development disorders.* 3rd ed. New York: Wiley; Farmer, Jeannette. "Train the Brain to Pay Attention." http://www.retrainthebrain.com/index.html. Accessed 5/19/2008; Goldstein, S., and Schwebach, A. J. 2004. The comorbidity of pervasive developmental disorder and attention deficit hyperactive disorder: Results of a retrospective chart review. *Journal of Autism and Developmental Disorders* 34:328–39; Kennedy, Diane. 2002. *The ADHD autism connection.* Colorado Springs, CO: Waterbrook Press; Kutscher, Martin. 2006. *Kids in the syndrome mix of ADHD, LD, Asperger's, Tourette's, bipolar, and more: The one stop guide for parents, teachers, and other professionals.* Philadelphia: Jessica Kingsley, 2006; Montes, G., and Halterman, J. S. Bullying among children with autism and the influence of comorbidity with ADHD: A population-based study. 2007. *Ambulatory Pediatrics* 7:253–57; Smalley, S. L. et al. 2002. Genetic linkage of attention-deficit/hyper activity disorder on chromosome 16p13 in a region implicated in autism. *American Journal of Human Genetics* 71:959–63; "Treatments for Autism." http://www.autismspeaks.org/whattodo/index.php. Accessed 5/18/2008; World Health Organization. 2006. F84 Pervasive development disorders. *International statistical classification of diseases and related health problems.* 10th ed. (ICD-10). Geneva, Switzerland: WHO.

B

Bach Flower Therapy

For centuries, folk healers used flowers and plants as therapy for different ailments. Many modern medications, such as digitalis used by heart patients, come from plants. In the early 1930s, Dr. Edward Bach, a bacteriologist and homeopathic physician, became disillusioned with the limitations of modern medicine at that time. He turned to answers in nature to meet the needs of mankind and developed a system of treatment using the essences of flowers for healing.

Bach believed that disease had roots in the mental and emotional condition of the individual. According to Bach, our brains are powerhouses of energy and nerves conduct electrical energy. A magnetic field called an aura is around the body and certain energies interact. Learning to improve attitude and outlook and eliminating negative emotions like anger, fear, and sorrow lead to positive energy and good health. His search for medications that could heal the soul and create positive energy led him to flowers, plants, and shrubs. Using himself as the model, he placed flower petals or leaves under his tongue and observed changes in mood the flowers produced. Through a process of trial and error, he found 38 remedies prepared from wild flowers, which he believed balanced energy in the body.

He created the 38 flower essences by placing flowers in spring water in the sun so that the sun energy would fill the solution. To present the flower essences, he used a small amount of brandy. Today the essences are preserved in ethyl alcohol, although the remedies are available in vinegar. The essences are placed under the tongue or applied to the skin.

Bach identified useful flower remedies for children showing symptoms of ADHD as follows:

- Aspen for the person whose fears and worries are of unknown origin; calms nervous and anxious symptoms
- Cherry plum for the child who is losing it, and who is about to throw things or scream
- Chestnut bud for those who fail to learn by experience and repeatedly make the same mistakes

- Chicory for those who are overprotective, possessive, and selfish
- Crab apple for poor self-image, feelings of shame, sense of uncleanliness
- Heather for those who are egocentric and think the world revolves around them
- Holly for a child who is jealous, envious, suspicious, or revengeful
- Impatiens for a baby who screams for attention; this treatment may abort an early stage of development of ADHD
- Vervain for those who are high strung, tense, frustrated or hyperactive; this remedy is the most frequently given for ADHD
- Willow for a child who is resentful or bitter

Rescue is a composite of five or remedies for the hyperactive child. Bach remedies do not change the person but help them acquire equilibrium to allow the positive aspects of character to emerge.

Further Readings: "Bach Flower Essences and Therapy." http://www.healing-arts.org/children/ADHD.bachflower.htm. Accessed 5/29/2008; Cooper, Paul, and Katherine Bilton. 1999. *ADHD: Research, practice and opinion.* London: Whurr Publishers.

Barkley, Russell A.

Russell A. Barkley, Ph.D., a researcher, clinical scientist, educator, and practitioner, is a professor in the department of psychiatry at the Medical University of South Carolina (MUSC). He received his B.A. in psychology from the University of North Carolina at Chapel Hill and his M.A. and Ph.D. from Bowling Green University in Ohio. After an internship at Oregon Health Sciences University, he joined the Department of Neurology at the Medical College of Wisconsin, where he founded the neuropsychology service and served as its chief until 1985. He then moved to the University of Massachusetts Medical School, where he was director of psychology for 15 years until moving to MUSC in 2002.

Barkley has authored, coauthored, or coedited 20 books and clinical manuals and published more than 200 scientific articles related to the treatment of ADHD and related disorders. His books include *Attention-Deficit Hyperactivity Disorder: A Handbook for Diagnosis and Treatment, Taking Charge of ADHD: The Complete Authoritative Guide for Parents, Defiant Children: A Clinician's Manual for Assessment and Parent Training,* and *Child Psychopathology.* He has created five professional videotapes on ADHD. In 1993 he established a newsletter for the clinical professional, *The ADHD Report,* and serves as editor. Barkley serves on the editorial boards of five scientific journals and as a reviewer for numerous journals.

Barkley has won numerous awards form the American Academy of Pediatrics for his research career in child development and from the American Psychological Association for his contributions to research in ADHD, to clinical practice, and for the dissemination of science. He resides near Charleston, South Carolina.

Barkley and Reconceptualization of ADHD

In 1997 Dr. Russell Barkley proposed a change in thinking about ADHD. This reconceptualization emphasizes that ADHD is a neurological disorder and that the response inhibition or impulsive behavior in people with ADHD is linked to executive function. There are three types of response inhibition:

1. The ability to inhibit a prepotent response or the urge to act before it happens
2. The ability to stop an ongoing response or action that is ineffective, maladaptive, or detrimental and shift to one that you can stop quickly
3. The ability to protect the delay in response from outside interference

Barkley and several Australian practitioners describe the attention part of ADHD as referring to the allocation of mental resources. The person with ADHD does not have a problem knowing what to do: they have difficulty doing what they know. Barkley's reconceptualization as an issue of executive function has clinical and legal implications and has been used extensively in current studies.

Further Readings: Barkley, Russell A. "Biography." WebMD. http://www.webmd.com/russell-a-barkley. Accessed 5/29/2008; Barkley, Russell. 2006. *Attention-deficit hyperactivity disorder: A handbook for diagnosis and treatment.* 3rd ed. New York: Guilford Press.

Bedwetting

Enuresis, or bedwetting, and ADHD are both common conditions that affect children and adolescents. Although no evidence exists that one causes the other, children with ADHD appear to have a higher incidence of enuresis. In early studies, bedwetting, especially at nighttime, was noted in hyperactive children. Stewart et al. in a 1966 study found that as many as 43 percent of hyperactive children had bedwetting problems compared to 28 percent of children in the control group. Also, Hartsough and Lambert in a 1985 study reported that children with ADHD were more likely to have bowel difficulties, a condition known as encompresis.

However, Barkley et al. in a 1990 study were not able to replicate any of these studies that related either enuresis or encompresis to ADHD any more than with controls. According to Barkley, the study and evidence to date are not conclusive that children with ADHD have more problems than other children. However, a 1997 article in the *Southern Medical Journal* found children with ADHD had a 2.7 times higher incidence of enuresis and a 4.5 times higher incidence of daytime enuresis.

The clinical definition of a bedwetter is one who is 5 years old or older who has had at least one episode of urinating while asleep in bed at night, and there do not have to be repeated episodes. Bedwetting is not supposed to happen at all in 5 year olds. However, with the high correlation there is some reason for concern. Bedwetting is devastating to children because it may hinder social activities such as sleepovers, causing children to feel left out. For most children, the exact cause is never known; however, the following may be present:

- The condition tends to run in families and may be hereditary.
- The development of the neurological system may be delayed.
- The person may have a small bladder or increased production of urine during the night.

- There may be a urinary tract infection.
- The person may have a sleep disorder, having a hard time rousing from a deep sleep, and may not be aware of the full bladder; difficulty waking at night is a difficulty similar to waking in the morning, which is present in 91 percent of those with ADHD, according to Dr. Monroe Gross (2007).
- There may be emotional trauma or high stress situations.
- Physical problems, such as diabetes or congenital deformities of the urinary tract, may be present.

Sometimes bedwetting may be more upsetting for a child with ADHD than for the child without ADHD, who may find it easier to cooperate with behavioral interventions. His inattention and disorganization may make it more difficult to cooperate with efforts to correct the situation. Although most children with enuresis experience remission by age 18, people with adult ADHD, who experience inattention and impulsivity, may have enuresis well into adulthood.

Dr. Gross states there are several treatments for bedwetting. The one approach that does not work is the "no-no" treatment. Scolding, punishment, and attempts to shame young people cause pain, embarrassment, and loss of self-esteem. Parents should not be harsh or judgmental. The following are some of the treatments for bedwetting:

- Behavior modification. Reminding the child to urinate before going to bed and eliminating liquid intake at least 2 hours before bedtime. He is taught to wakeup regularly at night to void. Bedwetting alarms are available.
- Hypnosis. Some practitioners have used hypnosis to help children become dry by themselves.
- Psychotherapy. When a child shows anxiety in relating to bedwetting, counseling may help deal with stress and trauma.
- Allergies. Rare allergies may be related to bedwetting.
- Medication. Two medications are used for bedwetting. One is desmopressin acetate (DDAVP), a nasal spray similar to the hormone that regulates urine production. Children who do not respond may be given a tricyclic antidepressant such as imipramine (Tofranil).

Further Readings: Barkley, R. A. et al. 1990. The adolescent outcome of hyperactive children diagnosed by research criteria: An 8-year follow-up study. *Journal of the American Academy of Child and Adolescent Psychiatry* 29:546–57; Gross, Monroe. 2007. "A History of Bedwetting Is a Very Strong Clue to the Diagnosis of ADD/ADHD." http://www.addmtc.com/bedwet. Accessed 5/19/2009; Hartsough, C. S., and N. M. Lambert. 1985. Medical factors in hyperactive and normal children: Prenatal, developmental, and health history findings. *American Journal of Orthopsychiatry* 55:190–210; Stewart, M. A. et al. 1966. The hyperactive child syndrome. *American Journal of Orthopsychiatry* 36:861–67; Watkins, Carol. 2000. "ADHD and Enuresis (Bedwetting)." http://www.addforums.com/forums/archive/index.php/t-12270.html. Accessed 6/17/2009.

Behavioral Treatments

Behavioral therapy is an important nonmedical approach used in treating children with ADHD. Much of behavior therapy or behavior modification is an expansion of the work of psychologist and educator B. F. Skinner. Many behavior therapists seek to avoid use of drugs for treatment and propose that although stimulant therapy may be effective for some cases of ADHD, medication is no panacea and that some children with ADHD should not receive it.

David Rabiner, Ph.D., senior research scientist at Duke University, lists reasons why people should not just depend on medication:

- As many as 20 percent of children receive no benefit from the medication.
- Some children experience side effects that prevent taking medication for an extended period of time.
- Many children who take medication still have difficulty with the core behavioral symptoms of ADHD.
- Some people have strong objections to taking medications; trying to force it may create more problems than it solves.

Behavior therapy or behavior management is based on four simple and common sense principles in dealing with children:

1. Children generally want to please their parents and feel good about themselves when parents are proud of them.
2. When the relationship between the two is positive, motivation is strong. Children behave appropriately to obtain positive consequences such as rewards or privileges.
3. Children will behave appropriately to avoid negative consequences that follow inappropriate behavior.

When children have ADHD/ADD symptoms, the relationships between parents and children often become fraught with conflict. The child's desire to please parents disappears because the child loses interest in pleasing the ones that they argue constantly with. Then parents often resort to threats and punishment, resulting in ongoing conflict and struggle. Thus the first step in behavioral therapy is to enhance the amount of positive feelings between parent and child. For example, the parent sets aside a certain amount of time each day (usually 30 minutes is sufficient) as a child's special time. The parent's only focus is to have a good time with the child, focusing on what the child is interested in.

Behavior control of children with ADHD is extremely important. Russell Barkley developed a specific format for training families of children with ADHD in 1981 and revised it in 1997. This was a major development for child behavior skills based on substantial research literature, demonstrating the efficacy of time-out procedures and differential interventions. The focus here is to counsel parents to conceptualize ADHD as a developmentally disabling condition and to teach children using home token economies to reinforce behavior.

The second focus is to provide the child with positive consequences for behaving in appropriate ways. The idea here is to give praise for something good that the child does, although it may be such a simple task as putting toys away. Think about the behaviors you want to encourage, make sure they understand what you want, and then let them know that good behavior is appreciated.

In behavior therapy the parent is encouraged to develop a game plan and is encouraged to keep the following things in mind:

- Be very specific about what you want the child to do. Something like listening to what I say is very vague, but picking up your toys the first time I tell you is specific and measurable and can be easily rewarded.
- Make sure your expectations are reasonable. A 5-year-old cannot be expected to sit quietly at the dinner table for an hour and listen to adults talk. If the child has ADHD, the situation worsens.
- Do not work on too many things at one time. The parent is encouraged to pick battles that are most important.
- Let the child choose the types of rewards.
- Design the program so that the child has a chance to experience success.
- Provide social rewards such as praise but also have more tangible rewards that can be earned.
- Be consistent. Behavioral therapy does not work if the parent applies the rules one day and then does not the next.

Three types of behavioral therapies are being used today for children with ADHD:

1. Special classroom or summer camps with regular sets of rewards and punishment can be highly effecting in creating a supporting learning environment; such programs are costly and may be limited to the special setting or camp. The programs may not carry over into other areas.
2. Cognitive behavioral therapy. The therapist works directly with the child to manage behavior. This approach appears to be effective in depression, but for children with ADHD, self-management may be a distant goal.
3. Clinical behavioral therapy. This treatment is the best current nondrug intervention. The therapist consults with parents and teachers to train them to change the learning environment for the child. The goal is to teach parents and teachers to use rewards and punishment consistently and change the learning environment at home and school. The therapist, parents, and teachers find rewards that will motivate the child to work.

Families learn how to set clear limits and negative consequences and also how to respond to difficult behavior. The parent will not shout but will explain how the behavior is unacceptable. Parents can apply these skills outside the home to places such as restaurants and other public places. Some parents have used the timeout strategy very effectively.

Teachers can assist with interventions, ranging from seating a child with ADHD up in front, calling a child's name to get attention, or helping the child break down tasks into small steps. Teachers can complete a daily report card for parents to see. Such strategies help the parents and teachers follow through on goals. For adolescents, creating contracts or negotiations may work instead of rewards. Parents who implement changes at home and teachers who are more regular and consistent in their demands will see improved behavior and enhanced learning.

Mastering Timeout

Dr. Daniel Amen suggests that parents can master the time out for children. This strategy can work for children ages 2 to 12 years of age.

- Be sure that your commands are clear and simple. For example, Joshua, please take out the trash now. Then count to 5 or 10 seconds to yourself. Do not count out loud as the child will cue from your voice.
- Expect compliance immediately. A parent who repeats the command ten times is teaching the child not to listen. Expect them to obey the first time. When the child complies, let him or her know how much you appreciate listening the first time.
- When they do not comply, warn them once and give them a choice to comply or not. Using the illustration: Josh, (spoken in a firm but not hostile tone) I told you to take out the trash now. You have a choice. You may take it out now or you can spend 10 minutes in timeout and then you can do it. It's up to you.
- If he does not comply, put him in timeout immediately. The timeout area should be a neutral, boring corner of a room. Do not sent him to the bedroom. Use a specific timeout chair. Also establish the rule that both buttocks need to be on the seat of the chair.
- A good rule of thumb is to have the time in timeout to be twice the child's age. It is good to get a timer.
- The timer starts when he or she is quiet. It is a time for kids to think about their behavior. Some kids may cry, whine, or nag. Simply reset the timer but say very little. Some kids may try to engage you in a fight, but do not take the bait.
- Don't give in to protests. If a child leaves timeout, you have some choices. Take away token points or ground him or her from an activity that he or she enjoys.
- For this behavior modification to work, the parent must be very firm and give the child the message that you are serious and mean what you say.

Source: Amen, Daniel. 2001. *Healing ADD: The breakthrough program that allows you to see and heal the 6 types of ADD.* New York: Berkley Books.

A major message here is to reduce blame and guilt. Because ADHD has a genetic component, there is one-in-three chance that a parent may have the condition. Clinical behavior therapy aims to remove this guilt or shame for difficulties that the family is experiencing. Responsibility is one of the major themes for both parent and child.

Using both behavior and pharmaceuticals may help. The foundation belief here is that medication improves brain chemistry and sets the stage for better learning. If the medication modifies brain chemistry, the child may be more amenable to regular rewards and expectations to optimize learning. Using combination therapy may help lower doses of medication, an important consideration to lower side effects of drugs. However, constant monitoring of medications and behavior may lead to burnout of both parents and teachers. *See also* Behavior Modification (B-mod).

Further Readings: Amen, Daniel. 2001. *Healing ADD: The breakthrough program that allows you to see and heal the 6 types of ADD.* New York: Berkley Books; Barkley, Russell. 2006. *Attention-deficit hyperactivity disorder: A handbook for diagnosis and treatment.* 3rd ed. New York: Guilford Press; Barkley, R. 1997. *ADHD and the nature of self-control.* New York: Guilford Press; Barkley, R. A. 1990. ADHD adolescents: Family conflicts and their management. Grant from National Institute of Mental Health, MH41583.

Behavior Disorders

Disruptive behavior disorders are highly correlated with ADHD. According to a study by Wilens et al. (2002), from 30 to 50 percent of children with ADHD in a community sample and 50 percent in a clinically referred sample are likely to have some other type of disruptive behavior disorder. The most common disorder related to ADHD is oppositional defiant disorder (ODD). Children with ADHD are more likely to develop conduct disorder (CD) than those who do not have ADHD. Presence of ODD/CD in ADHD is associated with more aggression and delinquency, greater academic underachievement, greater risk of substance abuse, increased social maladjustment, and lower self-esteem. The severity of conduct problems in children with ADHD predicts antisocial personality in adulthood.

Children with ADHD are often considered to have behavioral problems as a result of ADHD and are not likely to be diagnosed as having the comorbid conditions of ODD/CD. Because the correlation is high, the possibility should be considered. The presence of the following symptoms indicate possible behavioral disorders:

- Consistent negativity
- Defiance
- Disobedience in numerous situations
- Hostile behavior toward authority
- Repetitive and persistent behavior that varies from age-related social norm and threatens the rights of others.

Diagnosing behavior disorders may be difficult because extreme, irritable aggression may be a sign of mood disorder; those children with ADHD with severe aggression should be also evaluated for bipolar disorder.

The presence of ODD/CD complicates the presentation of ADHD and is associated with overall impairment, a greater risk for substance abuse, and worse overall long-term prognosis. Considering the negative predictions, early identification and treatment of conduct problems in ADHD is imperative.

According to Kunwar et al. (2007), medications used for ADHD such as stimulants and atomoxetine are effective and used as the first line for treatment of ADHD and comorbid ODD/CD. If the symptoms of ADHD appear to respond but ODD/CD symptoms persist, psychosocial treatment should be added. If symptoms are extreme, multimodal treatment is often needed from the beginning. In clinical practice, atypical antipsychotics are needed in selected cases.

According to a study by Dr. Nigel Mellor (2008), teachers and parents need to be aware of confusing children who are attention seeking with those who suffer from ADHD. Mellor, an educational psychologist, presented research at a January 2008 meeting of the British Psychological Society's Division of Child and Educational Psychology Annual Conference. He emphasized that researchers have largely neglected children who are seeking attention; the two problems can appear very similar. His research focused on fifteen schools over a period of time. Mellor determined that it is possible to distinguish between the two. Children who were acting up were doing so to gain attention of nearby adults and were able to relate well to older or younger people, not just their peers. They also have good language skills. He believes that attention seekers can be corrected with as little as two to five sessions. *See also* Conduct Disorder (CD); Oppositional Defiant Disorder (ODD).

Further Readings: "Attention Seeking Confused with ADHD." http://www.medical-newstoday.com/articles/93732.php. Accessed 1/22/2008; Kunwar, A. et al. 2007. Treating common psychiatric disorders associated with attention-deficit/hyperactive disorder. *Expert Opinion Pharmacotherapy* 8:555–62; Mellor, Nigel; Wilens, T. E. et al. 2002. Psychiatric comorbidity and functioning in clinically referred preschool children and school-age youths with ADHD. *Journal of American Academy of Child Adolescent Psychiatry* 41:262–68.

Behavior Modification (B-Mod)

Behavior specialists in many school districts are recommending the use of the technique of behavior modification for students with ADHD in special and regular classes; however, many teachers have adopted the principles of this technique a part of a consistent management plan. The inclusion of former special education students in the regular classroom has evoked great interest in utilizing discipline plans.

Behavior modification is based on the work of Harvard researcher B. F. Skinner (1902–1990), who spent most of his academic career conducting experiments in learning. He challenged traditional views of freedom and dignity and instead claimed that environmental conditions under which we live and what has happened to us determine our choices. The application of this to education uses reinforcement and punishment to shape behavior. The distinguishing features of behavior modification include the idea that behavior is shaped by consequences that happen immediately afterwards, the systematic use of reinforcers or rewards to shape the desired behavior, and that behavior becomes weaker if it is not followed by reinforcement.

Behavior modification is applied in the classroom in two ways: when teachers reward students after a desired act, students tend to repeat the act and when students perform an undesired act, teachers ignore the student or punish the student. The misbehaving student then becomes less likely to repeat the act. Several types of reinforcers can be used:

- Edible reinforcers, such as candy, cookie, gum, nuts or other snacks (These currently are not suggested to be used but are still used in many class rooms.)

The Last Normal Child: An Ethical Perspective

Lawrence H. Diller, M.D., in his 2006 book *The Last Normal Child: Essays on the Intersection of Kids, Culture, and Psychiatric Drugs,* believes that people are taking the easy way in giving medication as a quick fix and ignoring the difficult path of psychosocial interventions. He cites more than a hundred studies that demonstrate how parent- and teacher-training programs improve compliance, reduce disruptive behaviors, and improve adult child interactions. The idea that medication should be the first line of treatment derives from two short-term studies: the MTA study of 600 children and the Klein series of articles that reviewed the MTA study of 103 children over a period of 3 years.

Diller believes that the discussion about ADHD has rarely focused on moral and ethical issues as we decide the best course of action for children with developmental disorders. He is concerned that the use of medication as the first and only treatment for the vast majority of cases of ADHD exists without convincing data that this is the best treatment in the long term. According to Diller, pills are no substitute for skills; symptom relief is not the equivalent as helping the child self-regulate in the long term. Handicaps should not define human beings, but their conditions should be understood within the broader context of the forces that shape their lives. Advocating for psychosocial treatments for ADHD is simply not a matter of political correctness; it is an ethical recognition of a moral reality.

Source: Diller, Lawrence H. 2006. *The last normal child: Essays on the intersection of kids, culture, and psychiatric drugs.* Westport, CT: Praeger.

- Social reinforcers, such as words, gestures, stickers, certificates, and other facial and bodily expression of approval
- Material or tangible reinforcers, which are real objects that students can earn for good behavior
- Token reinforcers, such as stars, points, buttons, or other items that can be accumulated for desired behavior and then "cashed in" for other materials or tangible reinforcers
- Activity reinforcers, which include activities that students prefer in school.

Behavior modifications works best when used in an organized, systematic, and consistent ways. Five categories of items may be involved:

1. The "catch them being good" approach involves making positive statement to students who are doing what is expected of them. For example, a teacher may thank a student for having his materials out ready for class.
2. The rule–ignore–praise approach involves establishing a set of classroom rules, ignoring inappropriate behavior, and praising appropriate behavior. This works well in an elementary setting.

3. The rule–reward–punishment approach involves establishing classroom rules, rewarding appropriate behavior, and punishing inappropriate behavior. This is more appropriate for older students.
4. The contingency management approach is a system of tangible reinforcers where students earn token for appropriate behavior that can be exchanged for a larger tangible reward.
5. Contracting involves preparing a contract for an individual student who has chronic problems or is hard to manage.

The management plans using behavior modification are receiving lots of attention in colleges of education. Parents may also find applying these principles effective. *See also* Behavioral Treatments.

Further Readings: Burden, Paul. 2006. *Classroom management: Creating a successful K-12 learning community.* New York: John Wiley & Sons; Diller, Lawrence H. 2006. *The last normal child: Essays on the intersection of kids, culture, and psychiatric drugs.* Westport, CT: Praeger.

Beta-Hemolytic Streptococcus (Strep)

Strep is the common name for beta-hemolytic streptococcus. This bacteria is normally associated with strep throat or a strep skin infection. However, left untreated, strep can wreak havoc with the heart, causing rheumatic fever and a movement disorder called Sydenham's chorea.

More recently, poststreptococcal infections have caused a spectrum of disorders that have been associated with anti-basal ganglia antibodies. Many of the problems indicate movement disorders. For example, an encephalitis illness may follow a strep infection; unusual adult-onset movement disorders have been documented. Also, some susceptible children have a group of symptoms known as PANDAS (pediatric autoimmune neuropsychiatric disorders). Some symptoms of PANDAS include hyperactivity, obsessive-compulsive behavior, cognitive problems, fidgeting, and Tourette's syndrome.

Bipolar Disorder

ADHD and bipolar disorder (BPD) in children and adolescents are comorbid disorders. Studies have found estimated rates of BPD of 10 to 22 percent in children with ADHD, and rates of ADHD ranging from 57 to 98 percent in children with BPD. The symptoms of ADHD and BPD may overlap:

- Inattention
- Distractibility
- Impulsivity
- Psychomotor agitation
- Poor sleep

However, although a mild level of irritability and aggression can be present in ADHD, severe uncontrollable aggression is not common and should arouse suspicion for the possibility of BPD.

At one time BPD was not considered to exist in children but has become a topic of debate in current thought. One of the reasons for the question is the

Diagnostic and Statistical Manual of Mental Disorder (DSM-IV) criteria for mania were developed for adults and are not clear for adolescents and children.

Children with BPD present a mixed picture characterized by frequent short periods of intense moodiness and irritability rather than the classic euphoric mania. The course tends to be chronic or constant, rather than episodic, which is characteristic of the disorder in adults.

Differences between ADHD and BPD relate to the age of onset, quality of the disturbed moods, and the course of each disorder. The following are some of the symptoms that are more specific in children with BPD:

- Depression cycling with grandiosely elated moods
- Racing thoughts
- Severe separation anxiety
- Hypersexuality
- Extreme irritability
- Extreme rages that last for hours
- Gory dreams
- Extreme fear of death
- Extreme sensitivity to stimuli
- Often oppositional or obsessive traits
- Heat intolerance
- Craving for sweets
- Bedwetting
- Hallucinations
- Less need for sleep

Children with ADHD demonstrate an onset of symptoms before the age of 7 years, and these symptoms tend to remain constant over a long period of time. Onset of BPD is generally uncommon before the age of 7, and symptoms are likely to fluctuate over time.

According to Kunwar et al. (2007), if a child has ADHD/BPD, the recommendation is to treat the bipolar symptoms first and then if the ADHD symptoms persist, treat the ADHD. Stimulants should be considered the first line for treating ADHD symptoms in comorbid ADHD/BPD after treatment with mood stabilizers. However, clinicians need to be aware that stimulant treatment may aggravate manic symptoms in some patients.

Medical treatment for BPD and ADHD may include the following:

- Valproate (Depakote)
- Carbamazepine (Tegretol). Clearly helps bipolar and aggressive symptoms in adults but there are no controlled studies in children
- Lithium. Although it is not clear that it works in children who cycle so rapidly; does not help ADHD
- Cautious use of stimulants or antidepressants for ADHD symptoms. Because they may trigger mania
- Risperidone (Risperdal). For psychotic symptoms and aggression

Further Readings: Kunwar, A. et al. 2007. Treating common psychiatric disorders associated with attention-deficit/hyperactive disorder. *Expert Opinion Pharmacotherapy* 8:555–62; Kutscher, Martin L. 2002. "The ADHD e Book." http://www.booklocker.com/p/books/952.html?s=pdf. Accessed 5/19/2009.

Biofeedback

Biofeedback is a treatment technique that utilizes instruments to measure a person's physiological responses, such as hand temperature, sweat gland activity, breathing rates, blood pressure, and brainwave patterns. The instruments then feed the information back to the patient who focuses on changing certain patterns. As a behavior therapy, biofeedback uses stress-reduction techniques to help people learn to control certain body responses, such as heart rate and muscle tension. It may help teach adults and children with ADHD to change their brain wave patterns to move toward more normal ones.

A variation of biofeedback is called neurofeedback, designed to help people control brain wave patterns using electroencephalography (EEG) feedback. By placing electrodes on the scalp, the EEG measures the waves of electrical activity and the brain wave pattern of the brain. Five types of brainwave patterns are recognized:

1. Delta waves. A very slow wave of one to four cycles per second seen mostly during sleep
2. Theta waves. Slow brain waves of five to seven cycles per second, seen during daydreaming and twilight states
3. Alpha waves. Eight to twelve cycles per second seen during relaxed states
4. Sensorimotor rhythm wave (SMR). Twelve to fifteen cycles per second seen during focused relaxation
5. Beta waves. Fast waves of thirteen to twenty-four waves per second seen during concentration or mental work states

Dr. Joel Lubar of the University of Tennessee and others have reported effective of neurofeedback in the treatment of people with ADHD. In studying more than 1,200 children, Lubar found that the basic issue for these people is the inability to maintain beta concentration states for sustained periods of time. He also found these children have excessive theta daydreaming feedback. Through the use of neurofeedback, the patients were taught to increase the amount of beta waves and decrease the amount of theta waves. In other words, they learned to make their brains more active.

The format of the neurofeedback is like a game. The patient's brain is hooked up to the equipment with electrodes, and the computer feeds back the activity of the brain to the person. Sitting in front of the computer monitor, patients watch their brainwave activity as they respond to games. Many are able to gradually shape brainwaves to appear normal. NASA has developed a technique that blends biofeedback with video games.

Neurofeedback gives the patient control over the process, and some have reported success. However, it is still considered controversial and long-term effective needs to be established. *See also* Neurofeedback.

Further Readings: Amen, Daniel. 2001. *Healing ADD: The breakthrough program that allows you to see and heal the 6 types of ADD.* New York: Berkley Books; Lubar, Joel. "Neurofeedback Training for ADHD." http://www.eegfeedback.org/pdf/o_donnell.pdf. Accessed 6/17/2009; Rabiner, David. "The Role of Neurofeedback in the Treatment of ADHD." http://www.attention.com/library/articles/article.jsp?id=744&parentCatId=4&

categoryID=20. Accessed 5/29/2008; "The Role of Neurofeedback in ADHD Treatment." http://www.addadhdadvances.com/neurofeedback.htm. Accessed 5/29/2008.

Bowen Therapy

Bowen Therapy is an alternative or complementary procedure that is occasionally used for people with ADHD. Bowen Therapy is a noninvasive therapeutic bodywork system that employs cross-fiber muscle movements throughout the body. The person lies on a treatment table and remains clothed as the "moves" are carried out for about 45 to 60 minutes. Short waiting periods are interspersed into the session so that the brain will have time to assimilate and create a positive response to send back to the area being treated. Similar to acupressure, Bowen Technique uses a rolling manipulation of key body points to stimulate energy flow; the difference is in the use of light touch through light clothing. The practitioner uses thumbs and fingers on precise points at once, identifying areas of built-up stress in the muscles. The moves create a sense of relaxation, relieving pain and stress from many ailments.

Tom Bowen (1916–1982), an Australian osteopath, originated the technique in the 1950s while watching sports trainers. The technique was limited to Australia until after Bowen's death in 1982 when his followers named the procedure after him and spread the use to other countries. Milton Albrecht brought Bowen Therapy to the United States in 1989.

Further Readings: Amethyst Natural Healing. "The Bowen Technique." http://www. amethystnaturalhealing.co.uk/bowen.html. Accessed 5/19/2009; "Bowen Technique." http://www.inspirationalfriends.co.uk/bowen.php. Accessed 6/2/2009.

Brain and ADHD

To understand research about ADHD and how it implicates specific areas of the brain, it is essential to know about the structure of the brain. The brain has basically three main parts:

1. The cerebrum or thinking part of the brain, characterized by folds and wrinkles
2. The cerebellum or part that controls some motor functions and looks like a small head of cauliflower at the base of the cerebellum
3. The brain stem, a structure that connects the brain to the spinal cord and controls automatic systems such as breathing and digestion.

Each one of these three parts is made of multiple regions. The brain has two halves called hemispheres, which are joined by a tough band of fibers called the corpus callosum. The brain weighs about 3 pounds and has the consistency of thick custard.

Some scientists trace the impairments of ADHD to deficits in the brain. One area of interest is called the frontal lobe of the cerebrum. This area, located to the front and upper part of the brain, allows people to solve problems, plan ahead, understand the behavior of other, and restrain impulses.

A second area of interest is the basal ganglia, interconnected gray masses deep in the cerebrum, which connect the cerebrum and the cerebellum. The cerebellum is responsible for motor coordination and is divided into three parts. The middle part is called the vermis.

Scientists use imaging to look inside the brain. These methods include functional magnetic imaging (fMRI), positron emission tomography (PET), and single-photon emission computed tomography (SPECT). Imaging has allowed scientists to link certain parts of the brain with certain behaviors related to ADHD. Although imaging tools are important for studying the brain, they cannot be used for diagnosis.

Weighing about 3 pounds, the human brain is composed of about 100 billion neurons, the building blocks of the brain. Electrical messages progress from neuron to neuron across a gap called the synapse and are assisted by chemicals called neurotransmitters. Several centers in the brain process, organize, and regulate this constant flow of electrical communication.

Three basic types of areas operate to control this communication between the neurons: local centers, regional centers, and integrative centers.

- Local centers. Located in the rear of the brain, local centers process specific types of information, such as perceptions from the senses, seeing, smelling, taste, and touch. The sense organs pick up the stimuli and transmit it to the appropriate area of the brain. These bits of information are only fragmented.
- Regional centers. Regional centers pull all the fragment bits of information to create more complex informational maps. An example is when the visual area of the brain receives the fragmented images of objects from the retina. The visual association cortex assembles the fragments into a more coherent and recognizable picture of what is being looked at during each moment.
- Integrative centers. The integrative centers are not just located in one area like the sensory receptors but are linked throughout the brain to allow for the flow of information from one network to another. These areas assemble data from vision, smell, and hearing, to create a multimedia experience with the outside world.

The networks operate also on both the left and right sides or hemispheres of the brain. Traditional thinking recognized the left hemisphere as dealing with language data, whereas the right hemisphere dealt primarily with visual and spatial operations. Robert Ornstein in 1997 presented research that suggests that the right hemisphere tends to deal more with getting the "big picture," whereas the left side works with details and focuses information. The corpus callosum mediates these messages. Thus, the brain works not only from local and regional centers but also from circuits that crisscross hemispheres.

With all the complex flow of information, a managerial system is essential. Some networks monitor, coordinate, and manage other networks. These systems stop, start, and put everything together and are the networks that are most implicated in ADHD. Areas of the brain include the prefrontal cortex, where working memory circuits are located; the hippocampus, which is responsible for long-term memories; the amygdala; and the cerebellum. The circuits from these areas interact with many others.

The prefrontal cortex, a relatively small area, is located just behind the forehead and takes up slightly less than one-third of the brain's total volume. This area controls working memory circuits and is the only segment fully connected with every functional unit of the brain. Working memory is the ability to take the active thoughts of the moment and link them with stored memories, allowing the person to string together experiences that make sense of what is perceived and to act on those thoughts. Working memory allows the person not only to live in the present but to make sense of the streams from the past. In 1987, Richard Levy and Patricia Goldman-Rakic found specific cells in the prefrontal cortex for spatial working memory in a tiny area of the prefrontal cortex.

Although working memory functions like RAM on a computer, files are not saved unless the command is given to save them. In the brain the hippocampus processes working memory into long-term memory. The brain produces specific proteins that make the connections in a process called long-term potentiation (LTP). If the hippocampus is damaged, the individual does not hold new memories.

However, not all information that is in short-term memory is stored permanently. What determines which information will be stored and held onto and what will fade out? What can be called into conscious attention when it is needed? What drives the "file manager" and "search engines" of the brain so the information will be there when needed? One of the key elements is emotion.

Circuits in the limbic region, a center beneath the cortex of the brain, are critical in assigning emotional importance and priorities to incoming perceptions. For example, the area tells the brain to act quickly on conditions that are threatening. The amygdala, a tiny structure in the midbrain, screens incoming perceptions for any sign of danger. The danger is not from physical danger like that of an oncoming car but from other situations that might cause pain such as ridicule, disgust, or rejection from others. These experiences are highly individualized. Although some fear reactions are based on instinct, many are based on memories. However, the amygdala not only scans for dangers but also indications that something will be particularly rewarding. The brain uses the neurotransmitter dopamine to highlight important stimuli.

At the back of the brain are centers that regulate alertness and fine-tune cognitive processes. Two structures at the back of the brain regulate stages of sleep and alertness, or vigilance:

- The reticular formation in the middle of the brain stem that has widespread connections throughout the brain and spinal cord
- The locus coeruleus that is important in the regulation of sleep and wakefulness

The primary neurotransmitter chemical in the reticular system and locus coeruleus is norepinephrine. Lack of such firing and reduced norepinephrine is associated with inattention, increased drowsiness, and sleep.

The cerebellum, another structure at the back of the brain, makes up about 10 percent of the total brain volume and has extensive loops to every part of the brain. The cerebellum has such wide functions as correlating which verbs go with certain nouns and may be involved in adjusting social behaviors, such as laughing or crying, to specific occasions.

All the circuits that are involved in brain management do not work in isolation and are interactive. Multiple circuits integrate perceptions, assign importance, facilitate memories, regulate alertness, and control emotion. They interact continuously to maintain the activities of daily life.

Neuroimaging of ADHD Youth

Magnetic resonance imaging (MRI) evaluates what is happening in the brains of children with ADHD. The studies reveal that the entire cerebrum is involved, as well as several specific brain regions. Some research groups have shown a 5 percent reduction in total cerebral volumes, as well as a difference in the ventricle areas. The ventricles are space-like areas in the brain that are found in both hemispheres. Other researchers report 8.3 percent reductions in total cerebral volume in boys with ADHD compared with controls. One of the most consistent findings shows abnormalities in the frontostriatal brain regions. Also, right-sided abnormalities are reported as more common than left-sided differences. One of the first MRI studies reported a narrower width measurement in the front part of the brain when compared with healthy controls. This study later correlated with another study of the connection between response on inhibition tasks and the measurements of the prefrontal cortex and caudate nuclei on the right hemisphere. These findings support the idea that the right frontostriatal circuitry plays a role in response inhibition.

The basal ganglia are located at the base of the brain in the subcortical region. The areas include the caudate, putamen, and globus pallidus and are connected to various circuitries responsible for control of a wide range of activities including motor and executive functioning. Several studies have found that these areas are reduced in volume in the brains of people with ADHD. However, many of the studies are contradictory, and conclusions about the role of this area are not clear.

The corpus callosum has been speculated to be involved in ADHD. As one of the most recognized structures in MRI studies, a smaller cross-sectional area has been correlated with teacher and parent ratings of ADHD symptoms.

fMRI is a technique in which the person does an actual task while the scanner looks at the workings of the brain. Usually, the study uses a go/no-go response as illustrated in the following study. Dr. Stephen Pliszka of San Antonio, Texas, used fMRI with software to pick up changes in oxygen and blood activity when a particular part of the brain is used. Working with a control group of non-ADHD teens and teens with ADHD, Pliszka asked them to perform a stop-go task while brain scans were taken. An overhead screen inside the machine displayed letters, and teens reacted to them by pressing the left button for the letter "A" and the right button for "B."

About 25 percent of the time, the letter "S" flashed on the screen right after the "B." Subjects were told not to press the button when this happened. For children with ADHD who lack impulse control, this type of task is very difficult. When teens were actively trying not to push the button, the right frontal lobe of the brain lit up and showed strong activity in the non-ADHD group, but those with ADHD showed an absence of activity in that same part of the brain. The researchers were surprised that the frontal lobes on the right side played such an important part in the inhibitory process.

2007 Brain Mapping Studies

A 2007 study by Stewart H. Mostofsky and colleagues in the journal *Human Brain Mapping* revealed an association between ADHD and three physical characteristics of the brain: decrease in the cortical volume, decrease in surface area of the brain, and folding throughout the brain. As reported in the November 23, 2007, press release "Research Identifies New Features of Brain Structure That May Lead to ADHD," the researchers, who are from the Kennedy Krieger Institute in Baltimore, studied children ages 8 to 12. Twenty-one children diagnosed with ADHD were compared to a control group of thirty-five. The developing children were matched typically in age and gender. The study found children with ADHD showed decreased total brain volume and decreased volume throughout the cortex of the brain or outer gray matter regions comprise of neurons. They also found that this reduction in cortical volume may be attributed to decreased folding in the cortex, suggesting that folding is the key brain feature associated with ADHD. This study is the first to examine cortical folding and ADHD and suggests that biological causes may begin early in development, during gestation through infancy.

Prior studies that have been conducted have examined the brains of children with ADHD with imaging studies that measure the size and volume of various brain regions. However, this study used computer-generated images or brain maps for each subject that allowed them to measure and examine additional important structural features, including surface area and thickness, and to following activity throughout the brain, as well as within specific regions. These areas of the frontal lobe of the brain are associated with control of attention and behavior.

Cortical folding appears to be an important element in the development of ADHD. Results of the study found that children with ADHD showed a greater than 7 percent reduction in total cerebral volume (TCV) compared to the control group of typically developing children. In addition, children with ADHD showed reduced cortical volumes and surface area of the brain compared to typically developing children, with a reduction of more than 8 percent in each brain hemisphere. Because the study looked beyond volume, additional measures of brain structure revealed that children with ADHD showed a significant decrease in cortical folding across the entire cerebral cortex, even after accounting for the decrease in TCV. Because no significant difference was found in the thickness of the brain, the results indicated that cortical folding is an important factor to the reduced cortical volume observed in ADHD. Cortical folding begins in early development of the fetus at about 16 weeks' gestation and reaches its peak at about 18 months of age. It is then followed by a gradual leveling out to adult levels at about 23 years of age. During development when the brain can no longer expand because of the size of the skill, the only way to increase in surface area is if the cortex becomes more folded. Thus, cortical folding is critical to increasing the structural and functional capacity of the brain.

A 2007 report by Shaw et al. in the *Proceedings of the National Academy of Sciences USA* found that crucial parts of brains of children with ADHD develop more slowly than other youngster's brains. Earlier studies of brain imaging research missed this happening. According to Dr. Shaw, National Institute of Mental Health, the lag can be as much as 3 years in brain regions that suppress inappropriate actions and thoughts, focus attention, and assist in remembering things from moment to moment. The study did find a normal pattern of cortex maturation, although it was delayed in children with ADHD. This could explain why many youths eventually seem to grow out of the disorder. However, some children do not appear to grow out of the disorder, and researchers are working to determine the differences between those that have a good outcome and those who do not.

As an organ, the brain is very complex in its functioning. Although scientists are hard at work trying to identify how basic structure affects function, conclusions are still sketchy. Exploring the deep mysteries of the inner space of the brain is still as much of a challenge as studying the unknowns of outer space. *See also* Cognitive Research.

Further Readings: Barkley, Russell. 2006. *Attention-deficit hyperactive disorder: A handbook for diagnosis and treatment.* 3rd ed. New York: Guilford Press; Brown, Thomas E. 2005. *Attention deficit disorder: The unfocused mind in children and adults.* New Haven: Yale University Press; Levy, R., and Goldman-Rakic, P. S. 1999. Association of storage and processing functions in the dorsolateral prefrontal cortext of the nonhuman primate. *Journal of* Neuroscience, 19:5149–58. http://www.jneurosci.org/cgi/reprint/19/12/5149.pdf. Accessed 6/17/2009; Ornstein, Robert. 1997. *The right mind: Making sense of hemispheres.* New York: Harcourt Brace; Piano, Marina. 2003. Scientists Use MRIs to study ADHD, depression in children. *San Antonio Express-News* (Texas), May 19:F1; Pliszka; "Research Identifies New Feature of Brain Structure that May Lead to ADHD." http://www.medicalnewstoday.com/articles/89793.php. Accessed 5/19/2009; Shaw, Philip et al. 2007. Attention-deficit/hyperactivity disorder is characterized by a delay in cortical maturation. *Proceedings of the National Academy of Sciences USA* 104:19649–54.

Bupropion

Bupropion is an antidepressant medicine that works in the brain and is approved for the treatment of major depressive disorder (MDD), seasonal affective disorder (SAD), and to help people quit smoking. It is sometimes used for ADHD combined with these disorders. Bupropion is an aminoketone and is not chemically related to other antidepressant agents such as tricyclic, tetracyclic, or selective serotonin reuptake inhibitors (SSRIs). Bupropion is a relatively weak inhibitor of the neuronal uptake of norepinephrine, serotonin, and dopamine and not inhibit monamine oxidase. Although the mechanism of action of bupropion is unknown, it is presumed that his action is mediated by noradrenergic and/or dopaminergic mechanisms.

Brand names include the following:

- Wellbutrin, WellbutrinSR, and Wellbutrin XL
- Zyban

- Budeprion
- Buproban

All the above come in immediate release tablets, 75 and 100 mg; sustained release tablets, 100, 150, and 200 mg; and extended release tablets, 150 and 300 mg. The drug is also available as the generic bupropion.

Side effects are usually mild and most commonly are weight loss, nausea, loss of appetite, fast heart beat, trouble sleeping, dizziness, headache, and sore throat.

Bupropion should not be taken within 2 weeks of taking monamine oxidase inhibitors (MAOIs). Certain medication may increase the risk of a seizure when combined with bupropion. These include other antidepressants, antipsychotics, theophylline, isonizid, certain antibiotics such as Cipro, anticonvulsive medications, or the stomach medication cimetidine (Tagamet).

Warning: People should be aware that WellbutrinSR contains the same active ingredient found in Zyban, used as an aid to stop smoking. The two should not be used in combination.

FDA Alert 9/2007 Suicidality and Antidepressant Drugs

Antidepressants increased the risk compared to placebo of suicidal thinking and behavior in children, adolescents, and young adults in short-term studies of major depression disorder and other psychiatric disorders. Anyone considering the use of Wellbutrin or any other antidepressant in a child, adolescent, or young adult must balance this risk with the clinical need. Short-term studies did not show an increase in the risk of suicide with antidepressants compared to placebo in adults beyond age 24; there was a reduction in risk with antidepressants compared to placebo in adults aged 65 and older. Depression and certain other psychiatric disorders are themselves associated with increases in the risk of suicide. Patients of all ages who are started on antidepressant therapy should be monitored appropriately and observed closely for worsening of symptoms, thoughts of suicide, or unusual changes in behavior. Families and caregivers should be advised of the need for close observation and communication with the prescriber. Wellbutrin is not approved for use in pediatric patients.

Further Readings: National Alliance on Mental Illness. http://www.nami.org. Accessed 5/19/2009; "Wellbutrin (bupropion)." GlaxoSmithKline. http://www.gsk.com/products/prescription_medicines/us/wellbutrin.htm. Accessed 5/19/2009.

C

Caffeine

Caffeine, an herbal stimulant, has been proposed as an alternative to stimulant drugs for treating ADHD. The active part of caffeine is methyxanthine, a mild stimulant that activates noradrenaline neurons and appears to affect the release of the neurotransmitter dopamine. In several studies researchers have found that caffeine may benefit people with ADHD; however, side effects may also be present. Drinks with caffeine fail to match or exceed those derived from conventional medications. Garfinkel (1981) treated six children with ADHD with different stimulant medications. In the double-blind, cross-over study, the children received caffeine in a low dose or in a high dose. Methyphenidate was added to both dosages. Results indicated that caffeine in low dosage with methyphenidate was superior to all other treatments. High-dosage caffeine was not different from placebo. However, other studies of caffeine therapy for ADHD have failed to show clear benefits compared to stimulant drugs or even placebo.

Caffeine also appears to reduce blood flow in the brain, an effect similar to that of stimulant medications. Cognitive effects of caffeine are similar to stimulants, making rapidly processing information and paying attention more efficient.

Dalby (1985) suggests that many ADHD children who go into remission as adults have self-medicated with regular coffee consumption. If coffee is eliminated from their diets, the condition appears. Coffee may mask the underlying ADHD condition. The health risks for long-term caffeine use are better understood than those of Ritalin. Mild levels are considered safe. However, evidence exists that withdrawal from those individuals who are heavy users of caffeine may result in headaches; very large amounts can induce heart attacks and is associated with hand tremors. However, the user is advised to be aware that hidden amounts of caffeine are in soft drinks, sweets, and cold medicines and may increase the amount of caffeine intake.

Further Readings: "Caffeine and ADHD." http://www.myomancy.com/2006/07/caffeine_and_ad. Accessed 5/19/2009; Dalby, J. T. 1985. Will population decreases in caffeine consumption unveil attention deficit disorder in adults *Medical Hypotheses* 18(2):163–67; Garfinkel, B. D. et al. 1981. Responses to methylphenidate and varied doses of caffeine in children with attention deficit disorder. *Canadian Journal of Psychiatry* 25(6):395–401.

CAM

CAM is the term used to describe complementary medicine and alternative medicine. These practices are not part of standard care medicine performed by doctors of medicine, doctors of osteopathy, registered nurses, and other allied health professionals. Complementary or integrative medicine may be used in conjunction with standard care; alternative medicine is used in place of standard care. Many CAM treatments have been used for people with ADHD. *See also* Alternative Medicine; Complementary Medicine.

Candidiasis. *See* Yeast Infections.

Carbamazepine

Carbamezepine (Tegretol) or CBZ is first generation anticonvulsive medication that has been used to control epilepsy. As an anticonvulsive, CBZ is believed to work by enhancing the actions of a natural brain neurotransmitter, gamma aminobutyric acid (GABA), which carries messages between neurons. GABA inhibits the transmission of nerve signals and reduces nervous excitation.

Although CBZ is not considered a first-time treatment, some studies have suggested that it may be useful to treat ADHD in some people. It is also used in Europe to treat ADHD combined with conduct disorder.

In 1996 a metaanalysis of ten reports from the world literature found in seven open studies, for children with ADHD responses to the drug were significant. In three double-blind placebo-controlled studies, treatment effects for CBZ were superior to placebo. CBZ has generally not been given much attention as a treatment for ADHD, but there is evidence that it is an effective alternative.

In 2006, a small 2-month open pilot study of oxcarbazepine was conducted for eight adults who met the DSM-IV criteria for ADHD. The study found that a significantly high proportion of subjects who were receiving this drug were considered improved. The treatment was generally well tolerated, with dizziness, sedation, and nausea the most frequently reported side effects. The small study indicated that this drug may be effective in treating ADHD but to provide conclusive evidence, placebo-controlled, randomized trials are needed.

Further Readings: "Carbazepine Use in Children and Adolescent with Features of Attention-Deficit Hyperactivity Disorder: A Meta-analysis." http://www.ncbi.nlm.gov/pubmed/8714324. Accessed 5/29/2008; "Tegretol (Carbamazepine) for ADHD." http://www.revolutionhealth.com/blogs/earthling/tegretol-etc-carbam-4851. Accessed 5/20/2008.

Carbon Monoxide (CO) Poisoning

Carbon monoxide poisoning has long been known as the Great Imitator in medicine including mimicking the behaviors of ADHD. Other disorders include Alzheimer's disease, Addison's, anemia, asthma, autism, chronic fatigue syndrome, depression, fibromyalgia, irritable bowel syndrome, lupus, migraine, multiple chemical sensitivity, panic disorder, Parkinson's, psychosis, and stress. Note how many of these diseases are similar in symptoms and behaviors. Research into many of these disorders suggests that CO poisoning caused them and treatment for CO may help the conditions.

For more than 100 years CO has been the most common cause of both accidental poisoning and death in the United States. CO is an odorless, colorless, nonirritant gas from incomplete combustion or burning of any fuel. The CO combines with the hemoglobin in the red blood cells and prevents the hemoglobin from carrying oxygen, the substance essential for life. When gas, oil, kerosene, wood, or charcoal are burned, CO is produced. If household equipment is properly installed and used, it is a rare problem, but gas appliances, oil-burning furnaces, kerosene heaters, or wood-burning fireplaces can cause problems if the area is not properly vented. CO is also present in cigarette smoke. The CO poisoning can be chronic, with long-term effects on health, or it can be acute.

Thousands of children each year are exposed to toxic levels of this gas from heaters and improperly working home appliances. A problem with CO poisoning is that most people are not aware of the sources and how to avoid it. The symptoms of the poisoning are similar to many disorders, but CO poisoning should be considered if a majority of the symptoms are present, especially if gas or wood has been burning in the house:

- Headache
- Fatigue, weakness
- Muscle pain, cramps

Edgar Allen Poe: Victim of CO Poisoning or ADHD?

Edgar Allen Poe, the famous mystery writer, most likely suffered CO poisoning from the coal gas that was used in the 1800s for heat and light. In Poe's 1839 tale, *The Fall of the House of Usher*, he describes many of his symptoms. He had complete nervous agitation and was alternately alive and then sullen. He had great indecision. His skin was a ghastly pallor, and his complexion was cadaver-like. He was very sensitive to odors of all flowers, and his eyes were tortured by light. He had intense concentration only in particular moments and roamed from chamber to chamber with objectless steps.

Poe has become the poster child for information about carbon monoxide poisoning, and the poster "Ten Tell-Tale Signs of Carbon Monoxide Poisoning" features his face and information about the symptoms, sources, effects, and populations that are at risk. A free poster can be ordered from http://www.mcsrr.org.

Source: Multiple Chemical Sensitivity. "Edgar Allen Poe and the tell-tale signs of carbon monoxide poisoning." http://www.mcsrr.org/poe/index.html. Accessed 5/20/09.

- Nausea, vomiting
- Upset stomach, diarrhea
- Confusion, memory loss
- Dizziness, poor coordination
- Chest pain, rapid heartbeat
- Difficult or shallow breathing
- Changes in sensitivity of hearing, vision, smell, taste, or touch

Further Readings: Donnay, Albert. 2006. "Background of Sources, Symptoms, Bio-markers, and Treatment of Chronic Carbon Monoxide Poisoning." http://www.mcsrr.org/resources/articles/P11.html. Accessed 8/8/2008; Rutherford, Dan. "Carbon Monoxide Poisoning." (2005) http://www.netdoctor.co.uk/health_advice/facts/carbonmonxide.htm. Accessed 8/8/2008; Zimney, Ed. "Dr. Z's Medical Report: Carbon Monoxide Poisoning." (2006) http://www.blog.healthtalk.com/zimney/carbon-monoxide-poisoning/. Accessed 5/18/2009.

Causes of ADHD

What causes ADHD is unknown, and the knowledge about its origin is quite incomplete. In the history of ADHD, the condition was referred to a minimal brain damage or MBD because it was first described in children who had suffered some type of injury or infection. ADHD has been the focus for much high-quality research and has been extensively reported in international and highly respected peer-reviewed journals. The use of the term "brain damage" is inaccurate and understandably is upsetting to parents. Researchers now know that brain damage is not the cause of ADHD.

Three major theoretical areas of investigation into the causes of ADHD include cognitive research, neurobiological research, and genetic research. Cognitive research focuses on the mechanisms that underlie traits such as impulsivity, which have been traced to the frontal lobes of the brain and possibly other areas. Neurobiological research is based on new technology to locate the sources of ADHD in the functioning brain. The genetic approach seeks to study the occurrence in families.

Studies have shown a possible correlation between certain environmental agents and ADHD. Michael Lyon in the book *Healing the Hyperactive Brain* has established a functional model of the causes ADHD that include the antecedents, triggers, mediators, signs and symptoms, and results. He sets these factors up as a pyramid with the foundation or antecedents as underlying risk factors:

1. Antecedents or underlying risk factors include environmental toxins, genetic predisposition, nutritional deficiencies, abuse, neglect, or family stresses
2. Triggers or resulting physical problems include leaky gut, environmental allergies, food allergies or intolerance, chronic or recurrent infections, less of normal gut flora, immune system impairment leading to impaired digestive function
3. Mediators or the biochemical effect include brain neurotransmitter dysfunction, immune modifiers, neuropeptides, and neurotoxins leading to brain structural problems and critical nutrient deficiencies
4. Signs and symptoms include impulsivity, inattention, hyperactivity

This pyramid's apex results in problems that include a long list of difficulties including, extreme moodiness, trouble with the law, difficulty starting projects, diminished self-esteem, forgetfulness, tardiness, taking on too many projects, addictions, personality problems, aggression, many unfinished projects, self-medication, antisocial behaviors, risk taking factors, chronic anxiety, procrastination, psychological disorders, troubled relationships, self-destructive behaviors. *See also* Cognitive Research; Genetics.

Further Readings: Lyon, M. 2000. *Healing the hyperactive brain: Through the new science of functional medicine.* Calgary, AB, Canada: Focused Publishing; Wender, Paul. 1987. *The hyperactive child, adolescent, and adult: Attention deficit disorder through the lifespan.* New York: Oxford University Press.

Center for Science in the Public Interest (CSPI)

Some physicians have associated ADHD and nutrition and food additives since the 1970s. Organizations such as the Feingold Association are convinced that what goes in the mouth is responsible for much of the behavior associated with hyperactivity. Since 1971 another organization, the Center for Science in the Public Interest (CSPI), has also been a strong advocate for promoting the link between diet and public health. Studies by CSPI have also questioned the wisdom of certain additives and foods.

CSPI has been active in winning passage of laws requiring Nutrition Facts on packaged foods and later to include trans fats on these labels. The group has been active in removing sodas and junk foods from some schools. Other initiatives include getting junk food out of schools nationwide, getting rid of partially hydrogenated oil (source of trans fat), reducing sodium in processed foods, and improving food safety laws.

CSPI has a newsletter *Nutrition Action Healthletter* and a strong action network. It has dual goals of education and advocacy.

Further Reading: "About CSPI." http://www.cspinet.org/about/index.html. Accessed 7/13/2008.

Central Auditory Processing Disorder (CAPD)

Many children are being diagnosed with ADHD when they have other health problems. Perth (Australia) audiologist Brad Hutchinson said the overlap between ADHD and a condition known as central auditory processing disorder or CAPD. Children with CAPD struggle to make sense of verbal instructions, especially in noisy classrooms. They complain and appear fidgety, symptoms that are like ADHD. He believes that at least 50 percent of children with behavioral and learning problems have some type of auditory processing problem. The condition leads to problems such as dyslexia and learning delays of being able to distinguish between sounds such as "pat" or "bat." Deafness does not cause CAPD, but the child's brain cannot process what it heard. CAPD is not picked up in normal hearing screens but is diagnosed using an extended test that requires children to identify words in noisy circumstances.

Further Reading: "Deaf Ear to ADD." 2007. http://www.news.com.au/perthnow/story/0,21598,21596450-948,00.html. Accessed 8/9/2008.

Children and Adults with ADHD (CHADD)

Children and Adults with Attention-Deficit/Hyperactive Disorder (CHADD) was founded in 1987 by a small group of parents of children with ADHD and two treating psychologists in Plantation, Florida (near Miami). The parents came together because they felt frustrated and isolated, and they had few places to turn for support and information about ADHD.

CHADD, a nonprofit organization, describes its mission in the following terms:

- To provide a support network for parents and caregivers
- To provide a forum for continuing education
- To be a community resources and disseminate accurate, evidence-based information about ADHD to parents, educators, adults, professionals, and the media
- To promote ongoing research
- To be an advocate of the behalf of the ADHD community

Specific programs include those to improve lives of people affected by ADHD through collaborative leadership, advocacy, research, education, and support. CHADD publishes a variety of printed materials to keep members abreast of current research advances, medications, and treatments affecting individuals with ADHD. These materials also include *Attention!* magazine, the CHADD Information and Resource Guide to ADHD, news from CHADD, a free electronically mailed current newsletter, as well as many publications of interest to educators, professionals, and parents.

CHADD has 20,000 members, mostly children and adults with CHADD, and about 2,000 professionals. The organization does not endorse, recommend, or make representations with respect to the research, services, medication, treatments, or products.

Further Reading: CHADD Web site. http://www.chadd.org. Accessed 5/19/2009.

Chiropractic

Chiropractic is a form of medicine of alternative or complementary medicine that may be considered for treatment for ADHD. The term chiropractic comes from the Greek *chiro* meaning "hand" and *practikos* meaning "concerned with action." The practice focuses on diagnosis, treatment, and prevention of mechanical disorders of the musculoskeletal system and their effects on the nervous system and general health with special emphasis on the spine. D. D. Palmer founded chiropractic in the 1890s; the idea expanded in the early 20th century and is now well established in the United States, Canada, and Australia.

Doctors of Chiropractic (D.C.) or Chiropractic Neurologists, who support the term integrative medicine, believe that nondrug treatments that focus on posture, muscles, nutrition, and lifestyle changes can help students with ADHD. They believe that motor activity especially development of the postural muscles is the baseline function of brain activity. According to their beliefs, musculoskeletal imbalance will create imbalance in brain activity, and another part of the brain of the brain will develop faster than the other; this is basically what happens in ADHD.

Utilizing this basic principle, the doctors admit that the cause of ADHD is unknown but they believe that major contributors to ADHD include adverse responses to food additives, intolerances to foods, sensitivities to environmental chemicals, molds, and fungi, and exposures to neurodevelopmental toxins, such as heavy metals or organophosphates. The holistic/integrative management program includes supplementation, dietary modification, detoxification, and removal of environmental toxins and toxic cleaners from the home.

According to Dr. Frederick Carrick, American Chiropractic Association (ACA) Council on Neurology, Chiropractic neurologists are identify the underfunctioning part of the brain and find treatments to correct the problem that will help the hemisphere grow. The diagnosis includes a thorough brain function exam such as testing visual acuity by flashing light in the eyes or auditory acuity by asking patients to listen to music in one or the other ear. The treatments are then prescribed that can be done at home. Patients may be asked to smell certain things several times a day or wear special glasses. The treatment may focus on individual problems such as planning, organization, and coordination. Children may be asked to clap their hands, tap to a metronome, or practice balancing activities. Although no studies compared the chiropractic neurology treatment program to standard medical treatment, they are compiling data and believe that their treatments are more long term compared to short-term changes that lasts only as long as medication is taken.

A pilot study published in the *Journal of Vertebral Subluxation Research* suggests that adults with concentration and attention deficit problems may benefit from chiropractic. Yannick Pauli, D.C., Lausanne, Switzerland, specializes in wellness neurology. He is convinced that the spine is as much about neurology as it is biomechanics and that each time the practitioner works with the spine, he or she activates neurological circuits in the direction of the brain and bring the nerve system into balance. If the cerebellum or motor area of the brain does not function, then the rest of the brain becomes clumsy. By activating the spinal receptors and balancing the cerebellum, the chiropractor helps the brain function better, according to Pauli.

According to the ACA, the following program should be followed to treat ADHD:

- Remove as many food dyes, sugar, preservative, and additives from the diet as possible.
- Focus on natural, mostly on organic food with as few pesticides or herbicides as possible.
- Determine if there is an allergy, usually starting with dairy and gluten or things made from flour.
- Use no pesticide sprays in the house.
- If adult ADHD is suspected, try to relaxation and stress reduction.

Although a wide diversity of belief exists among chiropractors, they share the principle that the spine and health are related in fundamental ways.

Further Readings: American Chiropractic Association. "Research." http://www.chiro. org/pediatrics/ADD.shtml. Accessed 7/23/2008; "Attention Deficit Disorder (ADD)." http://www.chiro.org/pediatrics/ADD.shtml. Accessed 7/23/2008; "Chiropractic Care May Help Adult ADHD." 2007. http://www.newsmax.com/health/adult_ADHD_chiroprac tic/2007/09/06/30292.html. Accessed 5/19/2009; Pauli, Yannick. 2005. The drugging of our children's minds . . . and what chiropractors can do about it. *Journal of Vertebral Subluxation Research*, Feb. 7. http://www.jvsr.com/researchupdate/detail.asp?ID=885. Accessed 6/17/2009.

Clinical Trials and Medical Approval

All pharmaceuticals in the United States must go through an approval process by the Food and Drug Administration (FDA) through its Center for Biologics Evaluation and Research. Drugs for ADHD and related comorbid conditions are no exceptions. To have a drug approved, it must go through a long, rigorous period of development and testing and then close scrutiny once it gets on the market. It may take 10 to 15 years for a new formulation to come to the market.

Table 3 shows the various trials that a drug must go through before approval.

Table 3   Trials Required before a Drug Is Approved

Research State and Phase	What Happens during the Trials
Preclinical state	This stage includes informal experiments on animals, rats, and primates. This phase is known as basic research, during which experiments are carried out on a new formulation.
Phase I	If preclinical research is favorable, applications are made to the FDA for an investigative new drug designation (IND). Phase I trials are very small and are usually from 2 to 20 adults who are healthy and have given informed consent. Informed consent means the person is told in detail about the drug and what may happen. This phase is to test the safety of the formulation.
Phase II	With some safety issues resolved, the investigators use a larger number of subjects (from 100 to 300) to continue looking at safety but now to study efficacy (i.e., how well the drug works).
Phase III	If Phase II is effective and toxicity is low, investigators recruit thousands of patients at a variety of research centers. This phase is very expensive and time consuming. The investigators gather and assess all the data and, if the drug looks promising, they will submit a New Drug Application (NDA). After a long period of study and scrutiny from a committee, the FDA may approve the drug for marketing.
Phase IV	After approval, the drug's performance is monitored for long-term effect, and the follow up may extend from 10 to 20 years. The FDA may pull the drug from the market if a problem is discovered.

Drugs are tested using controls. The control may be a standard treatment or a placebo. A placebo is an inert compound identical in appearance to the material being tested, which may or may not be known to the investigator and/or patient. For example, in a controlled clinical trial, a control group might receive a sugar pill (the placebo) instead of an actual formulation. If neither the person giving the pill nor the person receiving the pill knows whether it is a drug or a placebo, the study is called "double-blinded."

Terms for Understanding Clinical Trials

Phases I, II, III, and IV: *See* Table 3.

Subject: The person who is involved in the study

Informed consent: The person in the study must be fully aware of the nature of the study, the conditions, what is expected, and what might happen; the informed consent document must be written in language that the person can understand; the recipient of the treatment must sign the document.

Institutional Review Board (IRB): This is a review board of experts that consider the details of the study to make sure that it is viable, accurate, and one that will not violate the interests of the subjects in the study.

Efficacy: How well does the drug work; is it doing what it is supposed to do?

Safety: How are the subjects responding to the drug as far as side effects?

Adverse event: Have any problems been detected? These problems must be reported to the FDA, and they may stop the study; these problems are considered red flags.

Randomized: Subjects are chosen and placed into groups for testing drugs according to chance.

Double-blinded: Neither those people who are conducting the research nor those who are taking the treatment do know if they are receiving a drug or a placebo.

Placebo: A substance that is an inert compound identical in appearance to the material being tested, which may or may not be known to the investigator and/or the patient.

Placebo-controlled study: Subjects are randomly assigned to the treatment of interest or to an inactive pill that looks just like the study pill.

Parallel study: The study has two variables that are being conducted at the same time.

Black box: A warning that is placed on the package insert that tells of certain adverse events that may take place with the drug. For example, amphetamines have a black box label that adverse heart conditions may be occur. Certain antidepressants such as Wellbutrin have the warning that the risk of suicidal behavior may be increased.

Open-label: The subjects continues in the trial but know they are taking the drug.

Safety concerns may arise at any stage of animal investigations or clinical trials. If this happens, the FDA may request that more information be provided. If the data show consistent adverse events (AEs), the manufacturer or FDA may suspend the trials. Common AEs are determined by comparing the number of cases in those receiving the treatment with those receiving the placebo. If more AEs occur in the drug recipients, the drug may be the cause of the reaction.

AEs and side effects are different. An AE is something that occurs at the same time as the drug trial and may or may not be caused by the administration of the drug. A side effect is a reaction that is caused after the drug is administered. A rare side effect, such as 1 in 10,000, may not be detected because the numbers of participants in the trials are not large enough to spot these rare conditions. In addition, Phase IV trials or postlicensing studies may be conducted after the approval.

Various words and expression are used in the scientific community but have a completely different meaning for the public. The following are some examples:

- To the scientist an AE is something that occurred at about the same time as the trial and may or may not be related to the trial; the public thinks an AE or side effect is something caused by the drug.
- Naive means the person or animal has not previously been exposed to a particular infection, drug, or vaccine; the layperson thinks the term means unsophisticated and lacking experience or training.
- Significant means that the results may not be due to chance; the public understands the meaning as "important."
- Safe means there is a remote or insignificant risk; the public thinks that it means that there is no risk or zero risk.

Further Readings: U.S. Food and Drug Administration. http://www.fda.gov. Accessed 5/19/2009; Myers, Martin, and Diego Pineda. 2008. *Do vaccines cause that?* Galveston, TX: I4ph Press.

Clonicel. *See* Clonidine.

Clonidine

Clonidine (Catapres) has been FDA-approved for use in hypertension since the early 1970s. Because of its well-recognized ability to down-regulate noradrenergic output from the CNS, it is possible to use it in psychiatric disorders characterized by excessive autonomic nervous system arousal, such as hyperactivity and impulsivity. The FDA does not presently label clonidine for any indication in child and adolescent psychiatry; however, some clinicians continue to use clonidine in a variety of early-onset psychiatric conditions. It is considered a third-line medication for overarousal, impulsivity, excessive hyperactivity, and explosive outbursts of aggression in children and adolescents with ADHD who have not responded to stimulants, atomoxetine, or antidepressants. It may also be used in combination therapy with stimulants to decrease overarousal and to treat sleep disturbances.

In June 2008, Sciele Pharma, a pharmaceutical company specializing in therapeutic agents for the well being of children, announced they have completed patient enrollment for its first Phase III clinical trial in the United States for Clonicel as treatment of ADHD disorder. Clonicel is a sustained-release formulation of clonidine hydrochloride for the treatment if ADHD and hypertension. The drug is a combination of stimulants such as methylphenidate and dextro-amphetamine/amphetamine. In earlier phase test Clonicel has shown to alleviate debilitating symptoms associated with ADHD, especially hyperactivity, impulsivity, and aggression. The goal of this formulation is to provide an option for patients who need an alternative to stimulants or who may benefit from combination therapy using Clonicel with other approved ADHD medications.

Further Readings: "Sciele Pharma Announces That Addrenex Has Completed Enrollment of Pivotal Phase III trial for Clonicel for ADHD." http://www.medicalnewstoday.com/articles/109952.php. Accessed 5/19/2009.

Cognitive Research

Several theories about the cognitive function of the brain of the person with ADHD exist. Increasingly the focus has been on impulsiveness as the central feature of ADHD and the possibility that a dysfunctional inhibition system is the underlying cause of the problem. The mechanism is located in the frontal lobes of the brain. According to these researchers, children with ADHD have greater problems than most people in stopping or delaying a behavioral response. Two happenings appear to be related here:

- Underactivity in which the inhibitory control system has a tendency not to be activated.
- Extreme slowness of the inhibitory control system, causing the individual to respond to he impulse before the system is fully activated.

Russell E. Barkley (1997) proposes a different model that suggests that the neurological problems are directly connected to four major executive functions of the brain: working memory, internalized speech, motivational appraisal, and the ability to synthesize behavior.

Sonuga-Barke in 1992 proposed another cognitive theory that suggests problems with inhibiting responses are situation-specific and are characterized by the individual's hesitance to delay. One of the differences between this model and that of Barkley is that there is a much greater role for socialization in the development of the problem.

Almost every cognitive model relates to the hyperactive/impulsivity subtypes of ADHD. Impairments in individual speed of processing information and the ability to focus or select the object for attention, the foundation of these models, are believed to cause ADD or inattentive subtypes. *See also* Barkley, Russell A. Executive Function.

Further Readings: Barkley, R. 1997. *ADHD and the nature of self-control.* New York: Guilford Press; Cooper, Paul, and Katherine Bilton. 1999. *ADHD: Research, practice and opinion.* London: Whurr Publishers.

Color Therapy

Color therapy is sometimes referred to as chromotherapy and is a complementary or alternative medicine technique. A person who is trained as a color therapist uses color and light to balance physical, emotional, mental, or spiritual energy that may be out of sync in the body. Color therapy is based on the idea that color brings out emotional reactions in people.

Healers have used color and light since the beginning of recorded time. The technique probably has its beginnings in ancient forms of Indian medicine called Ayurveda. Ancient Egyptian medical practitioners linked color to healing and built solariums or sunrooms fitted with colored panes of glass. When the sun struck the panes, the colors flooded the patient. Traditional Chinese medicine (TCM) associated each organ with a color.

Color therapists apply color and light to specific areas of the body. According to their beliefs, colors are associated with both positive and negative effects; therefore, specific and exact amounts of the color must be used in the healing process. Too much color or color that is applied improperly may cause adverse effects. Tools for color therapy include candles, wands, prisms, colored fabric, gemstones, bath treatments, colored glass or lenses, and colored lights. Although the therapy may be administered in several ways, aromatherapy or hydrotherapy may accompany the treatment to heighten the effect.

Alternative medicine practitioners relate the seven colors of the spectrum to specific body areas called charkas. The practice is similar to yoga, which locates specific spiritual energy centers at different spots of the human body. The colors that correspond to specific charkas are the following:

- Red. The first chakra, to the base of the spine
- Orange. To the pelvic area
- Yellow. To the solar plexus just above the navel
- Green. To the heart
- Blue. To the throat
- Indigo. To the lower part of the forehead
- Violet. To the top of the head

In the early 1900s Dr. Max Luscher created a diagnostic test that measures a person's psychophysical state and the ability to withstand stress. The diagnostic is used to uncover the cause of psychological stress and therefore the application of color to remedy the situation.

Theo Gimbel developed the idea of color therapy as useful in treating ADHD. Like sound and radio waves, color is an energy that vibrates at a much higher frequency. Color is made when white light splits into the colors of the rainbow as it reaches the visibility of the spectrum between ultraviolet and infrared. According to Gimbel, color influences the focusing of the eye. Blue is the kindest color for the eye as it focuses in front of the retina.

Cells on the retina receive light and transmit nerve impulse to the brain, where they perceive vision. On the retina are rods and cones. The rods relate to night visions; the cones are used in bright light and to distinguish color. The eye can distinguish about 7,500,000 hues. According to Gimbel, children with ADHD, autism, and dyslexia may use specially selected filters as spectacle lenses or placed directly on reading material. Color therapy uses one the positive aspects of colors, which usually mean only the brighter colors are used. For example, red is the symbol of life and vitality and energizes and stimulates.

Further Readings: Little, Nan? "What is Color Therapy?" http://www.anxiety-and-depression-solutions.com/articles/complementary_alternative_medicine/color_therapy/color_therapy.php Accessed 5/20/2009; Wills, P. 1993. *Color Therapy: The Use of Color for Health and Healing.* Shaftsbury Dorset: Element Books.

Comorbidities of ADHD

A comorbidity is a condition that often accompanies a certain disorder. Several disorders are often associated with ADHD, and a number of mental and physical conditions may be present. Major depression, bipolar disorder (manic depression), anxiety disorders, oppositional defiant disorder (ODD), and Tourette's syndrome (tic disorder) are commonly found in both children and adults with ADHD. Brain researchers are beginning to explore the connection between additions and ADHD. They may likely experience "reward deficiency syndrome" as their brains crave adequate levels of daily pleasure through simple daily activities. Thus, those with ADHD may be described as "sitting ducks" for addiction.

Oppositional defiant disorder (ODD) occurs when a person seems to always defy others, whether an authority figure or not. Of all the comorbid conditions, ODD appears to have the highest correlation with ADHD, between 35 and 50 percent. A person dealing with this condition may ask the following questions:

- Does the person openly defy you or a teacher by simply saying "no" or ignoring you?
- Does the person appear to be annoyed easily and bothered by trivial things?
- Does the person appear to annoy other people on purpose? When and where does this happen?
- Does the person appear angry, hot-tempered, resentful, or full of spite?

ADHD and conduct disorder (CD) are also closely related. The person may appear impulsive and aggressive. The following questions may relate to these two conditions:

- Does the person lie a lot, and about what?
- Does the person get into physical fights and possibly use a weapon?
- Does the person try to hurt or intimidate people?
- Has the person ever stolen or damaged other people's property?

Anxiety disorders, such as obsessive compulsive disorder and unusual fears, are characterized by extreme nervousness and worries. There is a high correlation between ADHD and anxiety disorders, and the following are some questions to ask:

- Does the person appear nervous or anxious?
- Are there times when the person appears panic stricken or frozen by anxiety?
- Does the person appear very shy, compared to others of his same age?
- Does the person repeat certain actions over and over again like a ritual?

Depression or extreme sadness may sometimes appear in people with ADHD. The following are some questions that may help determine this relationship:

- Does the person appear sad, blue, or down, and how can you tell?
- Is the person irritable, cranky, or moody?
- What does the person do in his/her spare time? Has the person abandoned activities once enjoyed?
- Does the person talk about suicide or about the uselessness of life?
- Has the person attempted suicide?

The relationship between ADHD and bipolar disorder is unclear. The questions that one may ask include the following:

- Are there times when the person thinks he or she may do or is able to do anything?
- Does the person appear unusually energetic at times or almost high without drugs?
- Does the person miss lots of sleep at night but is hardly affected by it the next day?
- Does the person appear to have thoughts that appear so fast that it is impossible to keep up with them?

Correlation of ADHD with learning disability (LD) and cognitive delay is common. Here are some questions that may relate this condition with ADHD:

- Even when the person is paying attention, is learning difficult?
- Are there certain subjects that the person has extreme difficulty with?
- How does the person do in reading, writing, and arithmetic?
- Has the person ever been tested for an LD?

Tourette's disorder is characterized by tics or movements that are not planned but appear to come from nowhere. The following questions may help in analyzing the connection with ADHD:

- Does the person have movements, such as blinking, making an odd face, shrugging, or moving an arm a lot, that are not intentional?
- Does the person may noises without meaning to, such as grunting, sniffling, or saying certain words?

Substance abuse may vary by age, but is highly correlated with persons with ADHD. Here are some relevant questions? Do you suspect that the person smokes, uses drugs or drink alcohol? Why do you suspect this?

In addition to psychological disorders, the person with ADHD may experience physical problems. Recurrent headaches, muscle aches and pains, abdominal pain may result from bacterial infections, intestinal parasites, food allergies, and neurotoxins, environmental toxicity, severe fatigue, allergic disorders such as asthma and eczema, respiratory infections, and ear infections. Many adults may suffer from fibromyalgia or chronic fatigue syndrome.

A problem may arise with medications. Those medicines that are given for comorbid conditions may have an undesirable effect on ADHD and vice versa. *See also* Behavior Disorders; Depression.

Further Readings: Kirley, Aileen. 2005. Scanning the Genome for Attention Deficit Hyperactive Disorder. In *Attention deficit hyperactive disorder: From gene to patients,* edited by David Gozal and Dennis Molfese. Totawa, NJ: Humana Press; Lyon, M. 2000. *Healing the hyperactive brain: Through the new science of functional medicine.* Calgary, AB, Canada: Focused Publishing.

Complementary Medicine

The term "complementary" medicine is used to describe practices that are not part of standard medical care but may be used with medical care. Standard care is carried out by health professionals such as medical doctors, osteopathic physicians, registered nurses, and physical therapists. Complementary medicine is also referred to as integrative medicine. Complementary medicine differs from alternative medicine that is used instead of standard practices. The two are grouped together and designated as CAM. The National Institutes of Health has established a National Center for Complementary and Alternative Medicine (NCCAM) to gather information about complementary medicine.

NCCAM divides the therapies into five major groups:

1. Whole medical systems that cut across many groups, such as Traditional Chinese Medicine and Ayurveda)
2. Mind-body medicine that focuses on holistic health and explores the interconnection between mind, body, and spirit
3. Biologically based practices that use substances found in natures such as herbs, vitamins, and other natural substances
4. Manipulative and body-based practices that are based on movement of body parts, such as chiropractic and osteopathic manipulation
5. Energy medicine are of two kinds: energy fields that purportedly surround and penetrate the bodies and bioeletromagnetic based therapies that use the magnetic energy fields that supposedly surround and penetrate the body

Several studies have considered CAM, but most of these studies are not evidence based and have not used double-blind, placebo-controlled, peer-reviewed methods. Ramirez (2001) studied EEG biofeedback for the treatment of ADD. He found one of the more promising EEG treatments involved theta/beta training. However, these treatment approached have been marred by inadequate methods and lack of follow-up studies, an essential for establishing evidence-based medicine.

Arnold (2001) identified 24 alternative therapies that have been studied in adults with ADHD. Few food dies do not appear promising for adults. However, some tests have show efficacy with biofeedback, relaxation, iron supplementation, magnesium supplementation, Chinese herbals, massage, meditation, mirror feedback, and vestibular stimulation. Laser acupuncture is more promising for adults than children. Megadose multivitamins are probably ineffective for most patients and are possibly dangerous. Possibly sugar restriction seems ineffective. The study determined that a few of the treatments have been effective in certain patients, but have not proven helpful in controlled trials. Most need research to determine both safety and effectiveness.

Further Readings: Arnold, L. E. 2001. "Alternative Treatments for Adults with Attention-Deficit Hyperactivity Disorder (ADHD). *Annals of New York Academy of Science* 931: 310341; "Complementary and Alternative Medicine." http://www.nlm.nih.gov/medline plus/complementaryandalternativemedicine.html. Accessed 7/20/2008; Ramirez, P. M. et al. 2001. EEG biofeedback treatment of ADD. A viable alternative to traditional medical intervention? *Annals of the New York Academy of Science* 931:342–58.

Computerized Tomography (CT)

Pronounced "cat" scan, computerized tomography or CT is a technology tool to examine the brain in cross sections. The word "tomography" is derived from the Greek *tomos* meaning "slice" and *graphein* meaning "to write." CT employs digital geometry to generate a three-dimensional (3-D) image of the internals of an object from a large series of 2-D x-ray images taken around a single axis of rotation. As multidimensional views of multiple axial slices are captured from various angles, x-rays on various paths through the CNS create contrast, which creates lighter or darker areas seen on the image. CT produces a volume of data that can be manipulated through a process known as windowing. Modern scanners allow this volume of data to be reformatted in various planes or as 3-D representations of structures. The trained reader can then read various anatomical sites.

The British scientist Sir Godfrey Newbold Hounsfield first conceived the idea in 1967 at the research branch of Electric and Musical Industries. The first machine was called an EMI scanner. An American Allan McLeod Cormack of Tufts University in Massachusetts independently invented a similar process. Together the two shared the 1979 Nobel Prize in Medicine for the invention.

CT has been used for over 30 years to look into the central nervous system (CNS) and other body systems. In medicine CT has been used to evaluate CNS lesions, tumors, or structural change, as well as areas when the blood-brain barrier has broken down. Early studies of ADHD using CT were useful in establishing some of the foundation information about brain structure. However, recently use has been limited because there is a risk of allergic reaction to the iodine-based contrast dyes that are commonly used. Although it is less expensive that MRI, it does expose the subject to ionizing radiation creating ethical concerns when used solely for research purposes. *See also* Neuroimaging.

Further Readings: Gozal, David, and Dennis L. Molfese, eds. 2005. *Attention deficit hyperactive disorder: From genes to patients.* Totowa, NJ: Humana Press; "Computed Tomography." http://www.en.wikipedia.org/wiki/Computed_tomography. Accessed 5/19/2009.

Concerta

Concerta is a central nervous system stimulant prescription medicine used in the treatment for ADHD. The drug may increase attention and decrease impulsiveness and hyperactivity in patients with ADHD. Concerta, a methylphenidate compound, is the registered trademark of Alza Corporation, Mountain View, California, and is a federally controlled substance (CII) because it can be abused or lead to dependence. Selling or giving away the drug may harm other and is against the law. Concerta should be used as a total treatment program for ADHD that may include counseling or other therapies.

What Are the Kinds of Counseling Therapies?

Keith Londrie reminds people with ADHD that any kind of counseling is better than none. Just talking to someone may help. However, several of the following types of professional counseling are available:

- Psychotherapy. Talking with a psychiatrist or psychologist may help older children and adults with ADHD to talk about issues that bother them and learn ways to deal with symptoms. It is important that one get help from a doctor who is familiar with ADHD. All doctors are not familiar with the nuances of dealing with people with ADD and ADHD.
- Behavior therapy. This type of therapy helps teachers and parents learn strategies or contingency management procedures for dealing with children's behavior. These strategies may include token reward systems and timeouts. *See* Teaching Children with ADHD. Behavior modification using contingency management techniques has proved especially beneficial for people with ADHD.
- Family therapy. Family therapy can help parents and siblings deal with the stress of living with a child who has ADHD.
- Group therapy. Support groups can offer adults and children with ADHD and their parents a network of social support, information, and education. People with ADHD thrive on the idea of belonging and that someone understands and has similar problems.
- Parenting skills training. This counseling helps parents develop ways to understand and guide their child's behavior.

Source: Adapted from Londrie, Keith. "Counseling in ADHD." http://www.ezinearticles.com/?Counseling-and-ADHD&id=217187. Accessed 5/19/2009.

Because it is a stimulant medication, it is important to know there are two major risks associated with Concerta:

1. Heart-related problems such as sudden death in patients who have heart problems or heart defects; stroke and heart attack in adults; increased blood pressure and heart rate. The physician should be informed if these conditions are present or if there is a family history of the conditions.
2. Mental or psychiatric problems. If there are new or worse behavior and thought problems or new or worse bipolar illness, new or worse aggressive behavior or hostility. If children and teenagers experience new psychotic symptoms such as hearing voices, believing things that are not true or that are suspicious or if there are new manic symptoms.

Concerta should not be taken if you or your child has the following symptoms:

- Have heart disease or hardening of the arteries
- Have moderate to severe high blood pressure
- Have hyperthyroidism
- Have glaucoma, an eye condition
- Are anxious, tense, or agitated
- Have a history of drug abuse
- Are taking or have taken within the past 14 days an antidepression medicine that is a monoamine oxidase inhibitor (MAOI)
- Is sensitive or allergic to or has had a reaction to other stimulant medicine.
- Have tics or Tourette's syndrome
- Have liver or kidney problems
- Have a history of seizures or abnormal brain wave tests (EEG)

Possible side effects of Concerta include the following:

- Slowing of growth both height and weight in children
- Seizures, mainly in patients with a history of seizures
- Eyesight changes or blurred vision
- Blockages of the esophagus, stomach, or small or large intestine in patients who already have a narrowing in any of these organs
- Upper belly pain
- Headache
- Dizziness
- Irritability
- Nausea
- Decreased appetite
- Dry mouth
- Trouble sleeping

This list may not be complete, and other side effects may occur. Check with the health professional if any unusual changes happen when taking Concerta. *See also* Methylphenidate (MPH).

   Further Reading: "Medication Guide." Concerta, http://www.concerta.net Accessed 5/19/2009.

Conduct Disorder (CD)

Conduct disorders (CD) show up early in life but take on a new life when the child enters a group setting, such as preschool or school. Conduct disorders are characterized by both overt and covert antisocial behavior. The most common types of conduct problems found in studies are lying, stealing, truancy, and to a lesser degree physical aggression. Conduct disorders differ from oppositional defiant disorders (ODD) in which children display significant problems with stubbornness, defiance and refusal to obey, temper tantrums, and to some degree antisocial behavior. Studies have shown that more than 65 percent of those who are referred to clinics may have ODD, and 45 to 84 percent of those with ADHD may meet the full diagnostic criteria for ODD either alone or with CD. ODD may occur by itself in the absence of CD; CD rarely occurs alone in children with ADHD and almost always occurs being seen in the context of ODD.

Bird et al. (1988) found that 93 percent of their Puerto Rican children with ADHD also had either ODD or CD. The most common types of conduct problems found in these studies are lying, stealing, truancy, and to a lesser degree physical aggression. Children with comorbid ADHD and CD/ODD have higher levels of impulsivity than children with only ADHD. This implies that the presence of ODD/CD implies a more serious form of ADHD. However, in the United States, the difference between ADHD and ODD are defined. Symptoms of hyperactivity do not mean the child is defiant. ODD by itself appears to decline significantly with age, whereas CD increases with age.

Barkley et al. (1990) studied behaviors in a group of hyperactive children compared to a normal group. Several of the differences were not significant: ran away from home overnight, broken into places, forced someone into sexual activity, used a weapon in a fight, fights, stolen with confrontation. The prevalence of these behaviors in CD is reflected in the Table 4.

Disrupted parenting correlates more with CD than ODD and may reflect antisocial characteristics of the parents. One form of CD may be genetic existing in spite of family environment. CD is highly associated with later substance abuse disorders.

Further Readings: Barkley, Russell. (2006) *Attention-deficit hyperactivity disorder: A handbook for diagnosis and treatment,* 3rd ed. New York: Guilford Press; Barkley, Russell et al. 1990. Does the treatment of ADHD with stimulant medication contribute to illicit drug and abuse in adulthood: Results from a 15-year prospective study. *Pediatrics* 111:109–21; Bird, H. R. et al. 1988. Estimates of the prevalence of childhood maladjustments in a community survey in Puerto Rico. *Archives of General Psychiatry* 32:361–68.

Conner's Rating Scales

The Conner's Rating Scales are a collection of scales for assessing ADHD.

The Conner's Rating Scales-Revised (CRS-R) is an assessment instrument that uses observer ratings and self-report ratings to help determine ADHD and problem behavior in children and adolescents. Three versions are available: parent, teacher, and adolescent self-report. Each has a short and a long form available. Also, three screening tools offer the option of administering

Table 4   Prevalence of Conduct Disorder Bhaviors in ADHD

Behavior	In Hyperactive Subjects, %	In Normal Subjects, %
Stole without confrontation	49.6	7.6
Runs away from home overnight two or more times	4.9	3.0
Lies	48.8	4.5
Deliberately sets fires	27.6	0.0
Truant	21.1	3.0
Broke into a home, building, or car	9.8	1.5
Deliberately destroyed other's property	21.1	4.5
Physically cruel to animals	15.4	0.0
Forced someone into sexual activity	5.7	0.0
Used a weapon in fight	7.3	0.0
Physically fights	13.8	0.0
Stole with confrontation	0.8	0.0
Physically cruel to people	14.6	0.0

Source: Barkley, Russell et al. 1990. Does the treatment of ADHD with stimulant medication contribute to illicit drug and abuse in adulthood: Results from a 15-year prospective study. *Pediatrics* 111:109–21.

a 12-item ADHD Index or the 18-item DSM-IV Symptoms Checklist or both. The various versions offer flexible administration options and gather the observations of parents, teachers, caregivers, and the child or adolescent.

According to C. Keith Conners, originator of the scales, the CRS-R has many advantages, including the following:

- A large normative data base helps support the validity (accuracy) and reliability (consistency) of the test; to establish validity and reliability, the test has been administered to more than 8,000 plus students/people. Data have been collected and evaluated. Standardized data are based on the means and standard deviations of groups of children with ADHD and children without psychological problems.
- Multidimensional scales help assess ADHD and the presence of comorbid conditions with links to DSM-IV categories.
- Teacher, parent, and self-report scales are in long and short formats.
- Applicability to managed-care situations quantifies the measurement of a variety of behavior problems.

The tests are used for routine screening in schools, mental health clinics, residential treatment centers, pediatric offices, juvenile detention facilities, child protective agencies, and outpatient settings. They can be used to measure hyperactivity in children through routine screening, provide a look at the child's behavior from those who interact on a daily basis, establish a base point in beginning therapy, and provide normed information to support conclusions, diagnoses, and treatment decisions.

The test is recommended for parents and teachers of children ages 3–17 and self-reports from adolescents ages 12–17. The reading level is 6th through 9th grade, varying with the version. The long version takes about 15–20 minutes to take and the short version about 5–10 minutes. Paper and pencil scores are hand scored.

The following are versions of the Conner's scales, as described in the Conner's manual:

- Conner's Parent Rating Scales Long Version (CPRS-R:L) contains 80 items and is used when parents and caregivers must give comprehensive information for DSM-IV consideration, such as ODD, cognitive/inattention, hyperactivity, anxious, perfectionism, social problems, psychosomatic, Conner's Global Index, DSM symptoms subscales, and ADHD index.
- Conner's Parent Rating Scale Short Version (CPRS-R:S) contains 27 items and covers a subset of scales and items on the long parent form, such as ODD, cognitive/inattention, hyperactivity, and ADHD index.
- Conner's Teacher Rating Scales Revised (CTRS-R:L), the long form, contains 59 items and includes oppositional, cognitive problems/inattention, hyperactivity, anxious-shy, perfectionism, social problems, Conner's global index, ADHD Index, DSM-IV symptom subscales.
- Conner's Teacher Rating Scale (CTRS-R:S) is a quick score test of 28 items and can be used when time is important. Scales include oppositional, cognitive problems/inattention, hyperactivity, ADHD index.
- Conner-Wells' Adolescent Self-Report Scale (CASS-L) contains 87 items and is appropriate for adolescents between the ages of 12 and 17. The scales include family problems, emotional problems, conduct problems, cognitive problems/inattention, anger control problems, hyperactivity, ADHD index, DSM-IV Symptom subscales. The CASS-L includes a Treatment Progress Color-Plot Form for proper age and gender profiling of scale scores.
- Conner Wells' Self-Report Short Form (CASS:S) has 27 items and is designs for adolescents between ages of 12 and 17 and scales for conduct problems, cognitive problems/inattention, hyperactivity, ADHD index.
- Conner's ADHD/DSM-IV Scales includes the following forms: Parents (CAD-P), 26 items; Teacher (CADS-T), a quick-score form of the scale; and Adolescent (CAD-A).
- When the profile forms are completed, an easy-to-interpret graphical display of results helps present results to parents, teachers, or other relevant parties.

Further Reading: Conners, C. Keith. "CRS-R (Conner's Rating Scales-Revised)." (2008) http://www.pearsonassessments.com/test/crs-r.htm. Accessed 7/4/2008

Controlled Substance—Class II (CII)

Some drugs including many of those prescribed for ADHD have a high potential for abuse. Realizing that several drugs have that potential, in 1970, Congress passed the Comprehensive Drug Abuse Prevention and Control Act. Dextroamphetamines and other drugs were classified as schedule II, the most restrictive category possible for a drug with recognized medical uses. The drugs are commonly designated as Class II or CII.

Further Reading: U.S. Department of Justice. "Controlled Substance schedules." http://www.deadiversion.usdoj.gov/schedules/schedules.htm. Accessed 5/19/2009.

Costs of ADHD

The burden of illness associated with ADHD is high for affected individuals, their families, and society at large. The costs associated with the condition makes safe, effective, and economical treatments a public health priority.

Howard Birnbaum et al. (2005) performed a comprehensive study of the cost of ADHD by considering healthcare and work loss costs of persons with ADHD, as well as the costs associated with family members. The study included excess per capita medical and prescription drug expenses and work loss from disability and work absences. Using administrative data from a single large company, the researchers studied patients, ages 7 years through 44 years and family members under 65. Excess costs are the additional costs of patients and their family members over and above those of comparable control individuals. The study found that in 2000 the total excess cost of ADHD was $31.6 billion. Of this total, $1.6 billion was for the ADHD treatment of patients, $12.1 billion was for all lost costs of adults with ADHD and family members of persons with ADHD. They concluded the economic burdens for ADHD were substantial.

In September 2004 Biederman presented a study to the American Medical Association of an April-May 2003 survey of 500 adults with ADHD and 501 who did not have ADHD. The survey showed that on average people with ADHD have household incomes that are $10,791 lower for high school graduates and $4,334 lower for college graduates, compared with those who do not have the disorder. The study also suggests that adult ADHD is responsible for an estimated $77 billion in lost household incomes in the United States each year.

G. T. Ray et al. (2006) determined the excess costs for children in the years surrounding initial diagnosis of ADHD. Costs were compared with those for children without ADHD, adjusted for age, sex, ethnicity, pharmacy co-pay, estimated family income, coexisting mental health disorders, and chronic medical conditions. Compared with children without ADHD, the mean costs for children with ADHD were $488 more in the second year prior to ADHD diagnosis, $678 more in the first year before diagnosis, $1,328 more in the year after diagnosis, and $1,040 more in the second year after diagnosis.

ADHD appears to be global problem. De Graaf and colleagues (2008) reported in the *British Medical Journal* of screening 18- to 44-year-old respondents in ten national surveys in the World Health Organization (WHO). The WHO World Mental Health Survey Initiative interviewed 7,075 people in paid or self-employment situations and asked questions about ADHD treatment. An average of 3.5 percent of workers in the 10 countries was estimated to meet DSM-IV criteria for adult ADHD. ADHD was associated with a statistically significant 22.1 annual days of excess lost role performance compared to those without ADHD. The effect was most pronounced in Colombia, Italy, Lebanon, and the United States. Only a small minority of workers with ADHD received treatment for the condition.

Further Readings: Birnbaum, Howard et al. 2005. "Costs of attention deficit-hyperactive disorder (ADHD) in the US: Excess Costs of persons with ADHD and their family members in 2000. *Current Medical Opinion* 21(2) 195–205; De Graaf, Ron et al. 2008. The prevalence and effects of adult attention-deficit/hyperactivity disorder (ADHD) on the performance of workers: Results from the WHO Mental Health Survey Initiative. *Occupational Environmental Medicine* 65 (Dec 2008): 835–42. http://oem.bmj.com/cgi/content/abstract/65/12/835?maxtoshow=&HITS=10&hits=10&RESULTFORMAT=&fulltext=WHO+Mental+Health+Survey+Initiative&searchid=1&FIRSTINDEX=0&sortspec=relevance&resourcetype=HWCIT. Accessed 5/18/2008; Ray, G. T. et al. 2006. Attention deficit/hyperactive disorder in children: excess costs before and after initial diagnosis and treatment cost differences by ethnicity. *Archives of Pediatric Adolescent Medicine* 160:1063–69.

Craniosacral Therapy

Several alternative, complementary therapies or nontraditional therapies have been tried for ADHD. According to Dr. John Upledger, D.O., the craniosacral system (CSS) is a newly acknowledge physiological system composed of the tough waterproof membrane, the dura matter, which lines the skull, the spinal column, and other delicate membranes. A semi-closed hydraulic system controls the flow of fluid into and out of the membrane and is responsible for the production, circulation, and reabsorption of the cerebrospinal fluid. This system maintains the environment in which the brain and nervous system develop and function. Craniosacral therapy is a light touch, hands-on therapy that focuses on bringing the CSS into balance. The procedure seeks to create an effective form of treatment for a wide range of illnesses, including ADHD. The therapy is based on a whole-person approach to healing, acknowledging the inter-connections of mind, body, and spirit.

More than 100 years ago, Dr. William Sutherland (1873–1954), an osteopath, discovered that while examining the sutures of the cranial bones, that these bones that were supposedly locked expressed small degrees of motion. He undertook many years of research to show this existence of this motion and concluded that is essentially was produced by the body's inherent force. He referred to this force as the "Breath of Life." The Breath of Life produces a series of subtle rhythms that may be adapted in the body to make three tides.

The emphasis in Biodynamic Craniosacral therapy is to help resolve the trapped forces that underlie and govern patterns of disease and fragmentation in both body and mind. The practitioner listens through the hands to the body's subtle rhythms and any patterns of inertia or congestion. The practitioner reads the story of the body and then follows the natural priorities for healing as directed by the patient's own physiology.

Craniosacral therapy is claimed to be particularly beneficial in children. The procedure is used by message therapists, naturopaths, chiropractors, and osteopaths. However, critics both inside and the osteopathic profession level say there is lack of evidence for the existence of cranial bone movement, the existence of cranial rhythm, and its link to disease.

Further Readings: Upledger, John. "Craniosacral Therapy and the Central Nervous System." http://www.latitudes.org/articles/cranio_upledger_ld.html. Accessed 5/19/2009; The Biodynamic Craniosacral Therapy Association of North America. http://www.cranio sacraltherapy.org. Accessed 7/7/2008.

Creativity and ADHD

Many gifts accompany ADHD. Some people with ADHD possess the gift of creativity; however, sometimes social demands may restrict the natural creativity and the thinking process by putting labels of value judgments, such as right or wrong, good or bad, proper or improper. Many famous creative people such as Robert Frost, Frank Lloyd Wright, Samuel Taylor Coleridge, Virginia Woolf, Thomas Edison, and Nikola Tesla had behaviors of inattention and hyperactivity that got them in trouble with their family and peers.

Dr. Calvin Taylor, a pioneer in education for the gifted and talented, believes that small children have no conception of these values and interact without these limitations. Expressing creativity gradually drops off as children learn to accept other's opinions. E. Paul Torrance, another expert in the field of creativity, thinks that curiosity of creative children is killed when questions are brushed aside as silly, and their thinking outside the box is not accepted.

As early as 1960 Dabrowski formulated the "Theory of Disintegration" that says the persons born with overexcitabilities have greater developmental potential than others (Ackerman 1997). This theory says that these individuals are hyperactive to the environment in the following areas:

- Psychomotor
- Sensuality
- Imagination
- Intellectual behavior
- Emotionally

Creative People with Attention Problems

Creative people may have a broad range of interests and tend to play with ideas, thus jumping from one project to another.

- The famous painter Leonardo da Vinci created only seventeen paintings in his 67 years as an artist, and some of them are incomplete. It is reported that Pope Leo X became so exasperated with him that he said that the man would never accomplish anything because he thinks of the end before he thinks of the beginning.
- Nikola Tesla, a famous inventor who worked with electricity, had so many ideas that he did not follow up on many of them. He never wrote an idea down until he had completely thought it through. Other inventors then finished his projects and got credit for them. For example, he claimed that Marconi got credit for his idea about the telegraph.
- Frank Lloyd Wright, the architect, would be so lost in his thoughts that his uncle would have to shout at him to get his attention.
- Robert Frost was expelled from school for daydreaming, probably creating word pictures of a poem in his mind.

Source: Cramond, Bonnie. 1995. "The Coincidence of Attention Dificit Hyperactive Disorder and Creativity." http://www.borntoexplore.org/adhd.htm.

Hallowell and Ratey in a 1994 study pointed out how several elements of the ADHD mind favor creativity. Creativity is defined as the ability to see elements in a new way and to combine personal experiences into new forms and give new shapes to ideas. There are four attributes of ADHD that may fit the creative mind:

1. Tolerance for chaos. The person with ADD may be able to endure chaotic conditions that others find intolerable. Although chaos may cause problems for some individuals, the tension of the unknown may bring about new conditions or ideas. People with ADHD react to most stimuli with uncertainty and that allows for messages to change before the items solidify in the mind. This tendency to get things confused can enhance creativity.
2. Impulsivity. Most people with ADHD live in a world where thoughts appear out of nowhere. Creative thoughts appear to happen unscheduled or at unusual times. Creativity is the attribute of impulsivity that has gone in the right direction.
3. Hyperfocus. One of the attributes of ADHD is often overlooked. A person with ADHD may focus on a project for hours if it is something that they are interested in. This characteristic often disturbs educators because the person is focusing on projects that they do not see advancing an educational purpose. Such focus, however, may lead to creative moments for a detail that will solve a problem.
4. Hyperreactivity of the ADHD mind. People with ADHD are always reacting, even when they look calm on the outside, they are churning on the inside. They move pieces of data and put ideas in new perspectives. Such activity causes creativity in the brain.

Others add that sensation seeking, not finishing boring projects, enthusiasm and playfulness, difficult temperament, deficient social skills, academic underachieve, mood swings, and the use of imagery in problem solving. Some of these attributes have been seen in creative artists, writers, and even scientists.

Bonnie Cramond (1995) studied the coincidence of ADHD and creativity and produced a document funded by the United States Department of Education. She relates some possible common etiologies of the coincidence:

- Brain structure or brain anomalies are reported in the literature, especially the predominance of the right hemisphere in spatial orientation, emotional expression, and attention.
- Cognitive processing that results in ideation and demands on attention was noted in several studies with students with ADHD.
- Temperament and mood may result in sensation seeking, sensitivity to stimulation, and depression.

People with ADHD are a fit for certain types of jobs that require high energy. Many individuals who distinguish themselves in advertising, sports, selling, and the performing arts have ADHD. In fact, the condition is common among people with Type A personalities who work in high energy and

Is the Ritalin Revolution Affecting Creative Productivity?

The Ritalin Revolution may affect the behavior of those who at one time mixed chemicals in the science lab to see what would happen or stare blankly out the window during English class, but some researchers think the use of such drugs for ADHD may stymie creative thinking. Dr. William Pollack, Harvard Medical School, has researched boyhood and found that stimulants may render some kids less interested in pursuing creative opportunities. Whether the use of such drugs will have repercussions in corporations, comedy clubs, or research labs remains to be seen.

Laura Honos-Webb, a psychologist at Santa Clara University, in her book *The Gift of ADHD* (2005) identifies gifts that accompany the disorder, including creativity, exuberant, and intuition. She states that a person taking Ritalin is like a horse with blinders, plodding along, maybe moving forward and maybe get things done, but being less open to inspiration.

In the 1970s, in seventh grade Erich Muller was such a creative class clown that he spent more days in detention than there were days in the school year. He was put in a cubicle-like enclosure built atop his desk to keep his eyes from wandering. He stated that as a kid he saw a thousand different things in every cloud. Teachers told his parents he was too creative and should be on medication; they refused. Later, he became one of the nation's highest paid radio personalities.

Honos-Webb believes that ADHD drugs are good for patching up weaknesses but not enhancing strengths. Spaciness may be a path to inspiration. What if Einstein had taken Ritalin?

Source: Honos-Webb, Laura. 2008. *The gift of ADHD: How to transform your child's problems into strengths.* Oakland, CA: New Harbinger.

high stimulus fields. The trick is for the person to harness these processes productively. The challenge is to manage them in positive ways and encourage them to use their assets and strengths to their advantage.

Dr. Torrance suggests ways that parents and teachers may encourage creativity and nurture the creative spark:

- Never discourage the imagination of a child. A great quality of a creative person is the ability to move freely from the world of fantasy to a world of reason.
- Let the child make mistakes and learn from them. Sometimes creative children will take on more than they can handle; let them learn from their mistakes.
- Avoid gender stereotypes. Do not belittle boys as "sissy" if they are interested in color, art, or ideas. Likewise, if girls are interested in exploring and experimenting, let them do so.
- Do not criticize the child's writing or reading. Often creative children lag behind the group in verbal abilities. However, they may score high in creativity tests.

- Assist the child in working through their social relations. Help them learn to get along with others but still keep the qualities that make them different. They can learn to assert themselves without being domineering or hostile and work with others without criticizing.

See also Giftedness; Hyperactivity.

Further Readings: Ackerman, Cheryl. 1997. Identifying gifted adolescents using personality characteristics: Dabrowski's overexcitabilties. *Roeper Review—A Journal on Gifted Education* 19(3):229-36; Cramond, Bonnie. "The Coincidence of Attention Deficit Hyperactive Disorder and Creativity." 1995. http://www.borntoexplore.org/adhd.htm Accessed 6/29/2008; Hallowell, Edward M., and John J. Ratey. 1994. *Driven to distraction: Recognizing and coping with attention deficit disorder from childhood through adulthood*. New York: Touchstone Press; Low, Keith. "Understanding and Nurturing Your Child's Creativity." http://add.about.com/od/childrenandteens/a/creativity2.htm. Accessed 6/29/2008; Taylor, Calvin. "Human Intelligence." www.indiana.edu/~intell/taylor.shtml. Accessed 6/18/2009; Torrance, E. Paul. "Obituary." www.highbeam.com/doc/1G1-105451164.html. Accessed 6/18/2009.

Cylert

Cylert, or pemoline, is a central nervous system stimulant but is not similar to amphetamines and methyphenidate. It is an oxazolidine compound that is chemically identified as 2-amino-5-pheny-2-oxazolin-4-one. Cylert has an action on the central nervous system similar to that of other stimulants. Although its effect on dopamine levels in animals is ascertained, the exact mechanism of action in humans has not been determined.

Cylert is supplied as tablets containing 18.75, 37.5, or 75 mg for oral administration. It is also available in 37.5-mg chewable tablets.

Because of the association with threatening hepatic or liver failure, Cylert has been withdrawn from the market. Since the marketing began in 1975, fifteen cases of acute hepatic failure have been reported to the FDA. Although the absolute number of reported cases is not large, the rate of reporting ranges from four to seventeen times the rate expected in the general population. This estimate may be conservation because of under reporting and because the long latency between initiation of Cylert treatment and the occurrence of the liver failure may limit recognition of the association. If only a portion of actual cases were recognized and reported, the risk could be substantially higher.

Of the fifteen cases reported as of December 1998, twelve resulted in death or liver transplantation, usually within four weeks of the onset of signs and symptoms of liver failure. The earliest onset of hepatic abnormalities occurred 6 months after initiation of Cylert. Although some reports describe dark urine and nonspecific prodromal or preoccurring symptoms, such as anorexia, malaise, and intestinal symptoms, in other reports it was not clear if any prodomal preceded the onset of jaundice. Pemoline was removed from the Canadian market in 1999 because of safety consideration; the U.S. FDA removed it from the market in 2005 because of liver toxicity.

Further Reading: Cylert Official FDA information. "Side Effects and Uses." http://www.drugs.com/pro/cylert.html. Accessed 7/4/2004.

D

Daytrana: Patch for ADHD

Daytrana is the registered trademark of the methylphenidate (MPH) patch developed by the Shire Corporation. It is unlike other compounds in that it is applied directly to the skin. Daytrana was approved in 2005 to treat ADHD in children between the ages of 6 and 12 and is applied to the child's hip 2 hours before symptom relief begins.

According to the Daytrana prescribing information, the most common side effects of Daytrana include decreased appetite, sleeplessness, sadness or crying, twitching, weight loss, nausea, vomiting, nasal congestion, inflammation of the nasal passages, and irritation of redness or itching at the site of application. If the person develops contact sensitization from Daytrana, it is possible that he or she would have the symptoms from any form of MPH, including Concerta and Ritalin LA, and could not take any of these drugs again. Other side effects seen with MPH, the active ingredient of Daytrana include dizziness, headache, fever, drowsiness, nervousness, allergic reactions, increased blood pressure, and psychosis such as abnormal thinking or hallucinations.

People who have a hypersensitivity to MPH, glaucoma, tics, or a family history of Tourette's or who are taking or recently took a monoamine oxidase inhibitor (a drug for depression) should not use Daytrana. Like other stimulant medications, Daytrana should not be used in children with structural cardiac abnormalities, and it should be used cautiously in people with hypertension.

The patch may be beneficial for those who have difficulty taking pills or medication that can be sprinkled on food. Another benefit is that the patch gives more flexibility in that it can be taken off if the person does not need the symptom control for the full 9 hours.

Other important facts about the patch include:

- Heat can increase the release of MPH from the Daytrana patch, and the person wearing the patch should avoid exposing it to a heating pad or electric blanket.

- Daytrana should not be applied under tight clothing.
- The site of application should be alternated each day.
- Daytrana should stay on even if the person is swimming, bathing, or exercising.

In May 2008, Shire Pharmaceuticals released the results of a new data analysis examining the differences between boys and girls ages 6 to 12 years. The study found that Daytrana had an established safety profile and effectively controlled ADHD symptoms in both boys and girls for the duration of the study. The study is important because only a modest amount of work has been done to examine the effect of ADHD treatment by gender. Shire reported figures from the CDC that 11 percent of boys have been diagnosed with ADHD, in contrast to 4.4 percent of girls. This discrepancy may exist because girls tend to be less disruptive and inattentive, whereas boys exhibit more hyperactivity and impulsivity. The 12-month study included 326 children who were divided into groups assigned to OROS, Daytrana, or placebo. Rating on an accepted scale showed a 78 percent improvement in both boys and girls. The study only used the placebo for 7 weeks. This patch is the first and only nonoral medication for treating ADHD in children for up to 12 months. *See also* Drug Interventions; Methylphenidate (MPH).

Further Readings: Shire Pharmaceuticals. "Daytrana Prescribing Information." (Rev. 4/2006) http://www.fda.gov/watch/SAFETY/2008/Feb_plp. Accessed 7/7/2008; FDA News Release. "FDA Approves Methyphenidate Patch to Treat Attention Deficit Hyperactivity Disorder in Children." April 10, 2006; "New Analysis in Boys and Girls Shows the ADHD Patch Daytrana offered ADHD symptom control for 12 months." http://www.medicalnewstoday.com/articles/106735.php. Accessed 5/8/2008.

Depression

Early studies noted a connection between ADHD and depression. Several studies have now shown this connection. R. C. Kessler (2005) presented this data from the National Comorbidity Survey-Replication, which shows that a lifetime prevalence for major depression disorder (MDD) is more than 16 percent greater in women than men; the same survey found clinically significant ADHD in adults in 4.4 percent of the same population, with a higher prevalence in men than in women. Dysthymia, a mild form of depression, related 22 percent in those who met the criteria for ADHD. These data suggest that if individuals have ADHD, they are likely to have MDD, and those with dysthymia were more likely to have ADHD. Table 5 shows the prevalence rates of ADHD within psychiatric populations. ADHD and major depressive disorder (MDD) are the most common psychiatric disorders occurring in adulthood.

Also, a two-way connection between ADHD and depressive disorders in many generations has shown a possible genetic link. Several studies have suggest that the incidence of ADHD in offspring of adults with recurrent depression is higher than in the general population and that first-degree relatives of juveniles with ADHD show higher rates of MDD. Scientists also know mood disorders are highly heritable In a 2004 twin study,

Table 5 Rates of ADHD within Psychiatric Populations

DSM-IV Diagnosis	Prevalence Rates in Psychiatric Populations, %
Bipolar depression	21.2
Major depression	9.4
Dysthymia	22.6
Generalized anxiety disorder	11.9
PTSD	13.4
Panic disorder	11.1

Source: Kessler, R. C. et al. 2005. Lifetime prevalence and age-of-onset distributions of DSM-IV disorders in the National Comorbidity Survey Replication. *Archive General Psychiatry* 62:593–802.

M. J. Rietveld and colleagues found that ADHD is one of the most heritable psychiatric disorders, estimated at 80 percent. Thus the connection between ADHD and mood disorders indicates a genetic component.

The problem of which comes first—ADHD or depressive disorder—is difficult to determine. J. D. Burke (2004) assessed adolescent boys for a period of years up to age 18 and found that ADHD predicted a later diagnosis of oppositional defiant disorder (ODD), which later predicted anxiety and depression. This study suggests that children with ADHD begin school with difficulty in conforming to social and scholastic norms, which causes them to use undesirable behaviors. The cycle of further social isolation and school difficulties then leads to anxiety, anger, and depression. These findings shed light on many of the comorbidity of ADHD and MDD occurring in adults.

Diagnosis of ADHD and MDD is difficult because no reliable objective tests are available to evaluate them. The symptoms are similar and may overlap: inattention, memory difficulties, poor motivation, irritability, restlessness, and procrastination. Even an experienced clinician may have difficulty in making the assessment. However, the major factor in establishing the presence of chronic adult ADHD symptoms is the presence of these symptoms in childhood and looking for absence of a major depressive episode. Several rating forms are available.

Treatment of both MDD and ADHD is accepted as effective. The treatments fall in four categories: antidepressants and ADHD, psychostiumlants and depression, psychostimulants+antidepressants, and psychotherapy:

- Antidepressants and ADHD. More than a dozen FDA approved medications are available for depression, and several have moderate effect for treating ADHD. Bupropion, a norepinephrine reuptake inhibitor (NRI) has treated both conditions. The class of serotonin-norepinephrine reuptake inhibitors (SNRI) includes venlafaxine and duloxetine. A new norepinephrine reuptake inhibitor, atomoxitine entered the market as a treatment for ADHD. No studies have shown that purely serotonergic drugs affect the core symptoms of ADHD.
- Psychostimulants and depression. The most common treatment for ADHD has long been the stimulants, which are used in children. For adults studies

Table 6 Results of the Multimodal Treatment Study (MTA)

Treatment	Subjects Achieving Excellent Responses, %
Community-based treatment as usual	25
Behavioral therapies alone	35
Methylphenidate alone	55
Behavior therapies plus methylphenidate	65

Source: Jensen, P. S. et al. 2001. Findings from the NIMH multimodal treatment study of ADHD (MTA): Implications and applications for primary care providers. *Journal of Behavior Pediatrics* 22:60–72.

are just now appearing that include several formulations of methylphenidate (MPH), including the most recently approved transdermal patch and dextro-amphetamine. In adults use of mixed amphetamine salts extended release (MAS-XR) and dexmethylphenidate XR has been approved.

- Psychostimulants+antidepressants. Combining psychostimulants and selective seretonin reuptake inhibitor (SSRI) antidepressants can be safe and effective, with little potential for drug-drug interaction. Combining psychostimulants with SNRIs or NRIs can be successful, monitoring for possible side effects.
- Psychotherapy. The use of cognitive-behavior therapy (CBT) and interpersonal therapy has been effective in treating MDD and is comparable to use of drugs. S. A. Safren et al. in a 2005 study found that combining CBT and medication showed promising results in adults with ADHD. Psychotherapeutic interventions for ADHD have been successful in children. One study, the Multimodal Treatment of ADHD (Jensen 2001), found excellent responses using a combination of treatments.

Table 6 shows the results of the NIMH Multimodal Treatment Study (MTA).

Patient Education

Education is the heart of any therapeutic intervention. For the adult who has long attempted to overcome the personal shortcoming of ADHD, understanding that there is a neurological basis can be valuable. Personal coaching can provide strategies and encouragement and help the person set goals. According to Kessler (2005), MDD costs the economy nearly $40 billion annually in lost economic productivity and is estimated to be responsible for loss of thousands of lives a year through suicide. Adults who have the problems of executive function as seen in ADHD have a lower socioeconomic status than adults without these deficits. The outlook for treatment is good and comes at a relatively low cost; helping people to see the value of treatment is invaluable.

Further Readings: Amen, Daniel. 2001. *Healing ADD: The breakthrough program that allows you to see and heal the 6 types of ADD.* New York: Berkley Books; Burke, J. D. et al. 2005. Developmental transitions among affective and behavioral disorders in adolescent boys. *Journal of Child Psychology and Psychiatry* 45:577–88; Jensen, P. S.

et al. 2001. Findings from the NIMH multimodal treatment study of ADHD (MTA): Implications and applications for primary care providers. *Journal of Behavior Pediatrics* 22:60–72; Kessler, R. C. et al. 2005. Lifetime prevalence and age-of-onset distributions of DSM-IV disorders in the National Comorbidity Survey Replication. *Archive General Psychiatry* 62:793–802; Rietveld, M. J. et al. 2004. Heritability of attention problems in children: Longitudinal results from a study of twins, age 3 to 12. *Journal of Child Psychology and Psychiatry* 45:577–88; Safren, S. A. et al. 2005. Cognitive-behavioral therapy for ADHD in medication-treated adults with continued symptoms. *Behavior Research Therapy* 43:831–42.

Dexedrine

Dexedrine is the registered brand name of GlaxoSmithKline Pharmaceuticals for dextroamphetamine sulfate. Available in tablets or sustained release spansules, Dexedrine is a central nervous system (CNS) stimulant drug used for the treatment of ADHD. Dexedrine may help increase attention and decrease impulsiveness and should be used as part of a total treatment program for ADHD that may include counseling and other therapies. It is also used to treat narcolepsy, a sleep condition in which the person may fall asleep suddenly during normal activities. Dexedrine comes in 5-mg tablets and 5-, 10-, and 15-mg spansules.

People who have certain health conditions or a family history of the following conditions should not take Dexedrine:

- Heart disease or hardening of the arteries
- Moderate to severe high blood pressure
- Hyperthyroidism
- Glaucoma
- Are very anxious, tense, or agitated
- Have a history of drug abuse
- Are taking or have taken within the past 14 days an antidepression medicine called a monoamine oxidase inhibitor (MAOI).
- Is sensitive or allergic to other stimulant medications
- Has mental problems such as psychosis, mania, bipolar illness, or depression
- Has tics or Tourette's syndrome
- Has thyroid problems
- Has seizures or an abnormal brain wave test (EEG).

It is not recommended for children less than 3 years old.

Common side effects include fast heartbeat, tremors, trouble sleeping, decreased appetite, headache, dizziness, upset stomach, weight loss, and dry mouth. Dexedrine may affect the person's ability to drive or do other dangerous activity.

Dexedrine is a federally controlled substance (CII) because it can be abused or can lead to dependence. Keep Dexedrine in a safe place to prevent misuses and abuses. Selling or giving away Dexedrine may harm others and is against the law. *See also* Dextroamphetamine Drug Interventions Ritalin.

Further Readings: "Dexedrine Medication Guide." GlaxoSmithKline, 2007. http://www.gsk.com. Accessed 5/20/2008.

Dexmethylphenidate. *See* Methylphenidate (MPH); Dexedrine; Dextrostat.

Dextroamphetamine

Dextroamphetamine, a central nervous system (CNS) stimulant drug, is the generic name for Dexedrine (GlaxoSmithKline) and Dextrostat (Shire). One may also see it written as D-amphetamine or dexamphetamine.

Amphetamine may take many forms, and D-amphetamine is a dextrorotary (D) stereoisomer of the amphetamine molecule. Dextroamphetamine is a powerful psychostimulant or "go Pill," which produces increased wakefulness, energy, and self-confidence in association with decreased fatigue and appetite. Primarily, dextroamphetamine is used to treat ADHD. Some physicians use it in place of methylphenidate or Ritalin as the first-choice medication for ADHD. It is also used to treat narcolepsy and was one time given as a diet pill for weight control. The U.S. Air Force may give dextroamphetamines to pilots on long missions to help them remain focused and alert. Other branches of the U.S. military have commonly used or dispensed dextroamphetamine to troops to prevent fatigue in combat situations.

In Berlin in 1887, the Romanian chemist Lazar Edeleaou became the first scientist to synthesize amphetamine. It was Smith, Kline, and French (now GlaxoSmithKline), however, that popularized the drug when it introduced the benzedrine inhaler as a treatment for cold symptoms. It was not until 1935 that the medical community realized dextroamphetamine's stimulant properties, prompting Smith, Kline, and French to market Dexedrine tablets beginning in 1937 as a treatment for narcolepsy, attention disorders, and obesity. Though it became readily apparent that the drug could be abused, it was not until 1970, when Congress passed the Comprehensive Drug Abuse Prevention and Control Act, that they became closely controlled.

Today, these drugs are widely abused on college campuses, particularly as study aids but also for recreational use. Four percent of American college students reported nonprescription stimulant use in 2004, according to the National Institute on Drug Abuse.

Further Readings: "Dextroamphetamine Molecule: Dexadrine, Dextrostat, D-Amphetamine, and Dexamphetamine." http://www.3dchem.com/molecules.asp?ID=401. Accessed 5/18/2009; "Dexedrine Medication Guide." GlaxoSmithKline. 2007. http://www.gsk.com. Accessed 5/18/2009.

Dextrostat

Dextrostat is the trade name of Shire Pharmaceuticals form of the generic dextroamphetamine sulfate. Dextrostat is used as an integral part of a total treatment program for ADHD that includes other remedial measures in stabilizes children ages 3 to 16. For specific information about the effects and cautions for the drug, *See* Dextroamphetamine.

Further Reading: Drug Information Online. "DextroStat." http://www.drugs.com/cdi/dextrostat.html. Accessed 5/20/2009.

Diagnosis of ADHD

Diagnosis of ADHD is not an all-or-nothing concept. If one has food poisoning or measles, the diagnostician can point to an absolute cause based on symptoms and behavior. However, there are no concrete medical tests to diagnose ADHD, which therefore makes the diagnosis of ADHD subjective.

Although the diagnosis is not like other medical conditions, several strategies for determining ADHD are in play. These strategies lie in careful observation and analysis of the behaviors of the individual from many sources. Because many conditions can mimic ADHD, a thorough physical examination is essential. ADHD may be diagnosed by excluding many other possible conditions.

There are four important reasons for the proper diagnosis of ADHD:

1. Diagnosis gives information regarding treatment planning and the long-term course.
2. Diagnosis is necessary to obtain special services.
3. It is necessary for medical and legal reasons.
4. Diagnosis guidelines are important for consensus on who is included and how many are treated in research projects.

To the physician or psychologist, diagnosing ADHD is much more like trying to determine if the person has clinical depression. Everyone feels sad from time to time, but clinical depression will significantly impair the function of the person over a sustained period of time. Thus, the ADD/ADHD diagnosis is not for people who have occasional symptoms but for those whose function over a period of time is affected.

Making the problem even more perplexing is that some people will demonstrate proficiency at times. For example, a high school student is the star of the football team; he can remember and execute complex plays to perfection and concentrate to catch the ball with efficiency. He is bright, with an IQ in the superior range, but is in constant trouble with his teachers for not doing work, not paying attention in class, and making inappropriate comments in class. His teachers might ask, "If you can pay such attention on the football field, why can't you pay attention in class?" It may not just be the field where the person may concentrate; some may be involved in playing video games, drawing, building with Legos, or completing mechanical tasks. Yet, these same people may have trouble preparing for a major exam.

To diagnose ADHD, several types of professionals are involved: pediatricians, clinical psychologists, educational psychologists, teachers and school staff, and neurologists. Guidelines in the United States are provided in a manual known as the Diagnostic and Statistical Manual, 4th ed., revised, usually referred to as DSM-IV-R and gives direction for diagnosis of recognized mental illnesses. To begin the diagnosis of ADHD, DSM-IV-R lists six essential steps:

1. The parent interview. This should include discussing problems, developmental history, and family history. Parents are encouraged to recount

Table 7   Doctors Qualified to Supervise ADHD Treatment

Specialty	Can Diagnose ADHD	Can Prescribe Medications	Can Provide Counseling or Training
Psychiatrists	Yes	Yes	Yes
Psychologists	Yes	No	Yes
Pediatricians or family physicians	Yes	Yes	Usually no
Neurologists	Yes	Yes	No
Clinical social workers	Yes	No	Yes

specific situations and instances and try not to make general statements about behavior, such as "he is bad" or "he just won't pay attention."

2. Interviewing the child about home, school, and social functioning.
3. Teachers and parent complete behavior-rating scales describing home and school functioning.
4. Obtaining data from the school. The data should include grades, achievement test scores, current placement, and other pertinent information.
5. The psychological testing for IQ and screening for a learning disability. This step may have been completed previously but is pertinent here for completing the picture of ADHD.
6. Physical and/or neurological exams.

DSM-IV states that these steps are only suggested and are not universally followed. The diagnosing professional should always consider other possibilities and rule them out before making a diagnosis of ADHD. *See also* Assessment Tools.

Table 7 from the National Institute of Mental Health lists the types of doctors who are qualified to diagnose and supervise treatment for ADHD. However, not all may have specific training in the disorder. It is important to look for a professional who does have special interest and training for the disorder.

Knowing the differences in the qualifications and services may help the family choose the health care provider who can best meet their needs. Child psychiatrists are doctors who specialize in diagnosing and treating childhood mental and behavioral disorders. Pediatricians and psychiatrists can provide therapy and prescribe medications. Child psychologists can diagnose and help the family in many ways with the disorder, but they are not medical doctors and must rely on the child's physician to do medical exams and prescribe medication. Neurologists are medical doctors who work with disorders of the brain and nervous system; they can diagnose ADHD and prescribe medicine. However, unlike psychiatrists and psychologists, neurologists usually do not provide therapy for the emotional aspects of the disorder.

What are the Subtypes of ADHD?

Although DSM-III used the term Attention Deficit Disorder (ADD), DSM-IV uses only the term Attention Deficit/Hyperactivity Disorder (ADHD) but classifies it into three different subtypes: ADHD predominantly hyperactive, ADHD inattentive, and a combined type.

Dr. Thomas Brown of Yale University has championed the recognition of children who have ADHD without hyperactivity. He believes these children are underdiagnosed because they are not the restless, intrusive, driven as if by a motor, Dennis-the-Menace stereotype. He notes these children are more like the stereotypes of "space cadet" or "couch potato" rather than the "whirling dervish" that one depicts as being the person with ADHD. Brown believes that even publications about ADHD offer little guidance about this disorder without hyperactivity.

Adults tend to overlook three specific groups of people with ADHD:

- Bright students. Adults think these people who underachieve are lazy and choosing not to do their work. However, individuals with ADD are found at all IQ levels.
- Females. Girls with ADD do not tend to stand out in the crowd and usually do not draw attention to themselves with dramatic disruptive behavior.
- Students under stress. When a student is daydreaming, the adult may explain away such behavior with family circumstances, such as divorce, unemployment, poverty, or multiple moves. What may be forgotten is that ADD is common in families under psychosocial distress.

Dr. Daniel G. Amen, a child, adolescent, and adult psychiatrist, uses neuroimagery to establish diagnosis of six types of ADHD. In his book *Healing ADD: The Breakthrough Program That Allows You to See and Heal the 6 Types of ADD*, he describes differences in the six types—not the three that are currently believed—according to brain structure, as follows:

1. Type 1. Classic ADD. People are inattentive, distractible, disorganized, hyperactive, restless, and impulsive. This type is usually evident early in life. As babies, they tend to be very restless, active, and hard to soothe and hold. They may wiggle a lot. According to Amen, it appears that type 1 is caused by a deficiency of the neurotransmitter dopamine. Neuroimaging shows low activity in the prefrontal cortex of the brain and in the basal ganglia activity.
2. Type 2. Inattentive ADD. Individuals are inattentive, sluggish, and slow-moving; have low motivation; and are often described as space cadets, day-dreamers, or couch potatoes. As in type 1, dopamine is generally considered the neurotransmitter involved, but its imbalance is felt in another area of the brain. Single-photon emission computed tomography (SPECT) analysis shows markedly decreased overall brain activity, especially in the prefrontal and temporal lobes, the areas involved with concentration and memory.
3. Type 3. Overfocused ADD. Individuals have trouble shifting attention and frequently get stuck in loops of negative thought or behaviors. They may be obsessive, inflexible, argumentative, and defiant and worry constantly. Amen found excessive activity in the anterior cingulated gyrus, the brain's gearshift, which allows a person to shift from thought to thought or idea to idea. When it is overactive, people tend to get "stuck" or locked into

negative thoughts and behaviors. It is a common trait among children and grandchildren of alcoholics.

4. Type 4. Temporal Lobe ADD. Individuals are inattentive, irritable, and aggressive; have dark thoughts and mood instability; and are severely impulsive. These children are usually those with severe behavior problems and mood disorders. The temporal lobes, located between the temples and the eyes, show increased activity in this type, along with reduced blood flow to the prefrontal cortex during concentration tasks.

5. Type 5. Limbic ADD. People are inattentive, experience chronic low-grade depression, are negative, have low energy, and frequently have feelings of hopeless and worthlessness. SPECT analysis shows that the prefrontal cortex activity at rest is decreased and too much activity in the deep limbic or emotional center of the brain. Depression looks similar to ADD on SPECT.

6. Type 6. Ring of Fire ADD. Individuals are inattentive, extremely distractible, angry, irritable, overly sensitive to the environment, hyperverbal or overtalkative, extremely oppositional, and experience cyclic moodiness. A brain scan shows that these individuals have a lot of brain activity across the whole cerebral cortex, especially in the cingulated gyrus, parietal lobes, and prefrontal cortex. A brain scan looks like a ring of hyperactivity around the brain.

Dr. Amen believes that each group has specific biological treatments that respond to individualized diet, exercise, herbs and supplements, medications, and biofeedback. Some believe his organization of types describes other conditions such as oppositional defiant disorder (ODD), which is defined in more recent diagnostic manuals.

How is ADHD Diagnosed Formally?

Formal diagnostic criteria of ADHD differ depending on what country one resides in. The criteria used most in North and South America is the American Psychiatric Association's Diagnostic and Statistical Manual, 4th ed.(DSM-IV). There is also an updated version designated as DSM-IV-TR (Text Revision). Europe, Asia, and Africa use the *International Statistical Classification of Diseases and Related Health Problems* (ICD-10, 2006). The American Academy of Pediatrics also issues certain clinical guidelines for diagnosis. Each of these tools organizes the diagnosis in a slightly different manner, but in each there are three major categories of symptoms: (1) hyperactivity, (2) inattention, and (3) problems with conduct.

A child who has six or more of the symptoms in either of two categories—inattention or hyperactivity impulsivity—may be determined to have ADHD (Table 8). According to DSM-IV, the physician will ascertain if the symptoms have persisted for at least 6 months to a degree that it varies with the development level of the child or adolescent, and if six or more of the following symptoms have been present to the point that the symptom is disruptive and is not appropriate for the developmental level. The diagnosis includes criterion items A, B, C, D, and E:

- Criterion A. Symptoms can be from category 1 or 2.
- Criterion B. The person had some of the symptoms present before age 7. The hyperactive-impulsive or inattentive symptoms were noted to be a problem.

Table 8 Two Categories of Diagnostic Criteria Used for Diagnosis of ADHD According to DSM-IV

Inattention	Hyperactivity and Impulsivity
Does not pay attention to details and makes careless mistakes in school work or other activities	Plays with hands or feet and squirms often
Has trouble staying on tasks such as play activities	Gets up from seat and runs around the room when staying seated is expected
Does not appear to listen when spoken to	Runs or climbs when it is not appropriate
Does not follow directions and instructions and does not follow through on school or work, chores, or duties in the workplace or appears not to understand the directions	Has trouble playing quietly
Has trouble organizing activities	Is often on the go and acts like being driven by a motor
Has trouble doing things that take a lot of mental activity	Talks a lot
Loses things such as pencils or books needed to accomplish tasks	Blurts out answers before questions have been finished
Is easily distracted by things nearby or by outside things	Has trouble taking turns
Is often forgetful in daily activities	Interrupts others or interferes in games or conversations

Source: American Psychiatric Association. 2004. *Diagnostic and Statistical Manual of the American Psychiatric Association.* 4th ed. Arlington, VA: American Psychiatric Association.

- Criterion C. The person has the symptoms in two or more settings, for example, at school, at home, or at work.
- Criterion D. The person must show significant impairment in social, school, or work settings.
- Criterion E. The symptoms are not related to another mental disorder, such as mood disorder, anxiety disorder, dissociative disorder, or a personality disorder. Also, the symptoms are not part of a pervasive developmental disorder, schizophrenia, or other psychotic disorder.

Based on the above criteria, DSM-IV identifies three types of ADHD that are coded as follows:

- 314.01. Attention-Deficit/Hyperactive Disorder, Combined Type, if both criteria A1 and A2 are met in the past six months
- 314-0. Attention-Deficit/Hyperactive Disorder, Predominantly Inattentive Type, if Criterion A1 is met but not Criterion A2 in the past 6 months
- 314-1. Attention-Deficit/Hyperactive Disorder, Predominantly Hyperactive/ Impulsive Type, if criterion A2 is met but not criterion A1 in the past 6 months

International Classification of Diseases and Related Health Problems (ICD-10 Used in Europe and United Kingdom)

The World Health Organization publishes the *International Statistical Classification of Diseases and Related Health Problems*. The tenth version of the ICD was published in 2006 and is known as ICD-10. The original *International Statistical Classification of Diseases and Related Health Problems* was adopted in Geneva, Switzerland in 1992. The naming of conditions relating to ADHD is somewhat different from the DSM-IV.

A conduct order is referred to as a "hyperkinetic conduct disorder." Otherwise the disorder is classified as the following:

- Disturbance of activity and attention
- Other hyperkinetic disorders
- Hyperkinetic disorders (HKDs), unspecified or sometimes called hyperkinetic syndrome

The writers of the ICD believe that a person must be hyperactive to be diagnosed with a hyperkinetic disorder. Inattention is considered a separate disorder. According to ICD classification, the prevalence with HKD is 1 to 3 percent.

American Academy of Pediatrics

According to the American Academy of Pediatrics clinical practice guidelines (2001), constitutes the following criteria constitute a reliable diagnosis:

- Using the explicit criteria of DSM-IV. A scale called the Conner's Rating Scale may be used to determine these criteria.
- Obtaining information about the child's symptoms in more than one setting. Parents, teachers, or even the person may provide this history.
- Searching for coexisting conditions that may make this diagnosis more difficult. Use of intelligence and psychological testing may rule out other complicating factors.

Generally concerns about a child's inattention and activity levels are first noted in the context of the school where greater demands for attention and self-discipline are placed on the child. Recognition of ADHD as a disability to be served under existing education laws (Individuals with Disabilities Education Act) and Section 504 of the Rehabilitation Act of 1973 has demanded that schools generate protocols for evaluation. The school has a legal responsibility to provide assessment for students who are suspected of having ADHD.

The Professional Group on Attention and Related Disorders (PGARD) has developed a two-tier approach to evaluate children who appear to have ADHD. The guiding principle is to have many sources of information that can shed light on whether the behavior is affecting educational perform-ance. The two tiers are as follows:

1. Confirm the presence of important characteristics; confirm early onset and duration; rule out other conditions.
2. Determine adverse impact on educational performance; determine impair-ment of academic performance.

See sources for information about PGARD.

Because some groups accused ADHD of being a fraudulent or benign diag-nosis, the American Academy of Pediatrics convened a Committee of Quality Improvement and Subcommittee on Attention-Deficit/Hyperactive Disorder and spurred the development of an International Consensus Statement pub-lished in 2002. Researchers and scientists came together to address the valid-ity of this condition and to discuss the importance of diagnosis and treatment to prevent serious harm. In addition, numerous associations have supported its existence. *See also* International Consensus Statement on ADHD.

Centers for Disease Control and Prevention

The **Centers for Disease Control and Prevention** (CDC) believes that only trained health care professionals should make a diagnosis of ADHD. This position is held because the symptoms may be part of other physical conditions, such as hyperthyroidism. Some normal individuals may exhibit some of these conditions from time to time. It is the pervasiveness of the symptoms that keep the person from functioning in school, work, and social relationships that form the strength of the factors in diagnosis.

Neurological diagnosis may also be done by imaging. SPECT scans may investigate areas of underfunction and overfunction. Because there are no lesions in ADHD, the use of EEG, CAT, and MRI and ineffective because they detect abnormalities in the superficial layers or cortex of the brain and do not tap into the deeper layers of the brain. In the late 1980s SPECT and PET scans looked at blood flow and glucose metabolism of different parts of the brain. In 1990 Dr. Alan Zametkin published a landmark study in the *New England Journal of Medicine* that found individuals with ADHD metabolized glucose at rate 8 percent lower than the control group when taking continuous performance tests that were designed to measure atten-tion and vigilance to stimuli. The decrease in metabolic activity was noticed in the prefrontal and premotor regions of the brain. Also, decreased blood flow was indicated in the frontal lobes and posterior periventricular region of the right hemisphere. The caudate nuclei/striatum were the most consist-ent areas of under functioning in ADHD individuals. However, presently neuroimaging is not commonly used as a tool for diagnosis because it is very expensive and criteria are not established for diagnosis. It is useful in research and may be developed in the future.

The striatum, frontal lobes, and posterior periventricular regions suppos-edly underlie aspects of response inhibition, inattention, and incentive learn-ing or sensitivity to reinforcement. These regions are also interconnected with sensory centers. The continuous bombardment shows up in SPECT scans as increased blood flow in regions that receive sight and sound stimuli. *See also* Brain and ADHD; Single-Photon Emission Computed Tomography (SPECT).

Nash Butros et al. (2005) has proposed a four-step approach for developing diagnostic tests in psychiatry using the electroencephalograph or EEG in ADHD as a test case. The EEG is comprised of four classical frequencies: delta, theta, alpha, and beta. The power of these ranges can be calculated and the relative power in each of the four ranges can be determined. The researchers found a promising increase in EEG theta in ADHD. A metaanalysis for the effect size was conducted and the majority of articles supported the findings that EEG theta had the increased activity. The researchers recommend developing the EEG as a definitive diagnostic test—something that has not been done in the past.

Sattler and Barkley have published some lists for general background questioning that can help with diagnostic assessment. Table 9 is a composite of several lists.

S. K. Katusic et al. (2005) suggests a multistep procedure for case definition and identification in population-based epidemiologic studies of ADHD, which includes the use of school and medical records, a computerized diagnostic index, private psychiatric records, and an combination of DSM-IV-TR questionnaire and clinical records. Because no gold standard for diagnosis of ADHD exists, data from multiple sources and procedures are usually collected in clinical practice.

The diagnosis and evaluation of ADHD actually currently has no reliable objective tests. Because several of the symptoms overlap with other conditions, even a skilled clinician can have difficulty in determining differences. An astute clinician must perform a thorough medical and psychiatric evaluation. Useful tests include urine drug screening, serum thyroid-stimulating hormone, complete blood count, chemistry panel, a and a history of central neurologic illness, infection, or trauma. Many common medications may contribute to psychiatric symptoms. One of the main factors in diagnosis is the presence of chronic ADHD symptoms since childhood, without a major depressive episode. Several other scales have been developed for diagnosis.

Further Readings: Amen, Daniel. 2001. *Healing ADD: The breakthrough program that allows you to see and heal the 6 types of ADD.* New York: Berkley Books; American Academy of Pediatrics. "AAP Policy: Clinical Practice Guidelines." http://aappolicy.aappublications.org/practice_guidelines/index.dtl. Accessed 5/20/2009; American Psychiatric Association. 2004. *Diagnostic and Statistical Manual of the American Psychiatric Association.* 4th ed. Arlington, VA: American Psychiatric Association; Barkley, R. A. 2002. International Consensus Statement on ADHD. *Clinical Child and Family Psychology Review* 5(2):89-110; Boutros, Nash. 2005. A four-step approach for developing diagnostic tests in psychiatry: EEG in ADHD as a test case. *Journal of Neuropsychiatry Clinical Neuroscience* 17:455–464; Brown, Thomas E. 2005. *Attention deficit disorder: The unfocused mind in children and adults.* New Haven: Yale University Press; From the Heart Media. "Featured Shows: Our Shows with Daniel Amen." http://www.straightfromtheheart.com/author_amen.htm. Accessed 5/20/2009; Global ADHD Working Group. 2005. Global consensus on ADHD/HKD. *European Child Adolescent Psychiatry* 14:127–37; Gozal, David, and Dennis L. Molfese, eds. 2005. *Attention deficit hyperactive disorder: From genes to patients.* Totowa, NJ: Humana Press; Katusic, S. K. et al. 2005. Case definition in epidemiologic studies of ADHD. *Annals of Epidemiology* 15:430–37; World Health Organization. "F84 Pervasive Development Disorders." *International*

Table 9 Gathering Historical and Contextual Information about the
Person with ADHD

Medical history	Did the mother abuse drugs, have toxin exposure, or pregnancy complications? Were there complications during pregnancy or labor? Was there a traumatic brain injury or genetic disorder? What is the general health history of the child, including chronic illness, vision or hearing problems, and use of present medications? Does the child have sleep problems?
Developmental history and status	Was there a delay in the child's walking or talking? Has the child developed self-help skills? Has the child regressed in development? Are there persistent problems with language or motor skills? What is the current status in school?
Environment and social history	What is the nature of housing and the neighborhood? Is it public housing? Who are the members of the household? What is the stability of the household? Are there frequent moves? How would the parent describe the school environment now and over the past few years? What is the disciplinary style of the parent? Are there other sources of support, such as church or supportive relatives? Is there a history of abuse or neglect? Are there family stresses, such as loss of job, divorce, or death in the family? What is the cultural affiliation of family and relation to the local cultural mainstream?
History of the problem	Did the symptoms begin prior to age 7? When did the symptoms first draw the attention of parents, teachers, or others? How would the parent rate the symptoms in hindsight? Are there comorbidities? Has the person had prior psychological, psychiatric, and academic assessments? What are the prior attempts at intervention such as discipline at home and school interventions, such as Individualized Education Plans or 504 plans?
Family psychiatric history	What is the family's history of learning, scholastic, attention, or behavior problems? Is there a family history of neurological disorders? Is there a family history of psychiatric disorders, including personality disorders and chemical dependency?

Statistical Classification of Diseases and Related Health Problems. 10th ed. (ICD-10), Geneva, Switzerland, WHO, 2006; Zametkin, A. J. et al. 2009. Cerebral glucose metabolism in adults with hyperactivity of childhood onset. *New England Journal of Medicine* 323:1361–66.

Diagnostic and Statistical Manuals

The Diagnostic and Statistical Manuals are considered the "bible" of mental illnesses used for diagnosing psychiatric disorders. The books have been influential because they determine the status of a mental disorder and define what is and what is not a mental disorder. The manuals have also a great impact on society because as mental disorders are determined, public awareness, as well as industries' relating to mental health care, has grown. The manuals are responsible for the explosion of research and sales of pharmaceuticals relating to mental health.

DSM versions have a checkered history. The first versions were simple listing of common mental illnesses. In 1968, the second edition of the Diagnostic and Statistical Manual (DSM-II) added Hyperkinetic Reaction of Childhood disorder to its list of disorders. It used only one sentence to tell that the disorder is characterized by restlessness, distractibility, overactivity, and short attention span, especially in young children. The manual took its clue from the researcher Chess who believed this disorder was benign and usually diminished by adolescence; he considered this hyperkinetic action simply normal and really an insignificant problem.

In 1980, the publication of DSM-III showed a major change from DSM-II. This manual changed the concept from Hyperkinetic Reaction of Childhood to ADD with or without hyperactivity. The new diagnostic criteria emphasized inattention and impulsivity as defining features of the disorder and produced a more specific symptoms list.

In 1994 the Diagnostic and Statistical Manual of Mental Disorders, 4th ed., text revision (DSM-IV-TR), was published. According to the DSM-IV-TR, patterns of behavior indicate three types of ADHD: predominantly hyperactive-impulsive, predominantly inattentive, and combined, which may display both symptoms.

DSM-IV-TR turned a thin guidebook into an 886-page "bible" that expanded the meaning of mental illness. Some traits that were once associated with simple personality traits, such as shyness, became symptoms of social anxiety disorder. Drugs were developed for those mental disorders. Kent Garber in a January 7, 2008, article in *U.S. News and World Report* quoted a 2006 study that found that more than half of the researchers who worked on the manual had at least one financial tie to the drug industry.

Beginning in 2008, the American Psychiatric Association (APA) will develop a new edition of DSM. The target date for completion is 2013. APA pledges to avoid any appearance of conflict of interest by carefully screening the taskforce. The members will be asked for detailed financial information about stocks, honoraria, and consulting fees from drug interests. Although receiving fees does not necessarily indicate influence on decisions made for the manual, the APA desires to maintain transparency in erasing any appearance of conflict of interest.

The impact of the diagnosis of ADHD and related disorders will likely be changed in some ways. However, until the next version of the manual, DSM-IV-TR will hold for diagnosis. *See also* Diagnosis of ADHD.

Further Readings: American Psychiatric Association. 2004. *Diagnostic and Statistical Manual of the American Psychiatric Association.* 4th Ed. Arlington, VA.: American Psychiatric Association; Barkley, Russell. 2006. *Attention-deficit hyperactivity disorder: A handbook for diagnosis and treatment.* 3rd ed. New York: Guilford Press; Garber, Kent. 2008. Who's behind the bible of mental illness? *U.S. News &World Report* (December 31, 2007/January 7, 2008):25–26.

Diet. *See* Feingold Diet; Nutrition.

Discrimination in Employment

In 1990, Congress established the Americans with Disabilities Act (ADA). This Act was designed to end discrimination in the workplace and provide equal employment opportunities for people with disabilities. ADA provides for mental and physical conditions, such as cerebral palsy or visual impairment. However, for a person with ADHD to qualify, a simple diagnosis is not sufficient.

According to *ADDitude*'s "What You Need to Know about the Americans with Disabilities Act," to qualify for coverage, the following conditions must be met:

- The disability must cause a significant impact or limitation in a major life activity or function.
- The person must be regarded as having a disability.
- The individual must have a record of having been viewed as being disabled.
- The applicant must also be able to perform the essential job functions with or without accommodations to qualify as an individual with a disability under the meaning of the Act.

ADA applies to the following employers:

- Private employers
- State and local governments
- Employment agencies
- Labor organizations
- Labor-management committees

An employer or potential employer cannot ask questions about one's medical or psychiatric history. An exception exists if the applicant asks for accommodations during the hiring process and the disability is not obvious. The employer may ask for reasonable documentation. However, the employee may want to tell the employer about ADHD because not doing so could be a legitimate defense for the employer if a question arises leading to a lawsuit.

The person with ADHD may ask for reasonable accommodations, which may be required unless there would be an undue hardship on the employer, such as being too expensive or creating other problems within the workplace. Such accommodations could include the following:

- Job restructuring
- Part-time or modified work schedules
- Reassignment to a vacant position
- Adjusting or modifying examination, training materials, or policies

Some legal twists may come with the interpretation of this law. If medication controls ADHD, the person may not fit within the definition of disability. Liken this to a person who has a vision problem, but glasses correct the problem; if ADHD is successfully corrected by drugs, then it might be difficult to claim the condition as an impairment.

A person with ADHD who believes he or she has been discriminated against may contact the U.S. Equal Employment Opportunity Commission within 180 days of the alleged discrimination. Contact information is in Appendix B.

Further Reading: "What you need to know about the Americans with Disabilities Act." *ADDitude* http://www.additudemag.com/adhd-web/article/pront/674.html. Accessed 5/20/2008.

Dopamine

Dopamine is one of two neurotransmitters that are important in ADD and ADHD. The other neurotransmitter is norepinephrine. Dopamine is both a hormone and neurotransmitter, which occurs in a wide variety of vertebrates and invertebrates. In the brain dopamine activates five types of dopamine receptors: D1,D2, D3, D4, and D5. Arid Carlsson and Niels Ake-Hillarp, Swedish scientists, discovered dopamine in 1952. Carlsson won the 2000 Nobel Prize in Physiology or Medicine for showing that dopamine is a neurotransmitter, in addition to being a precursor or forerunner of norepinephrine (noradrenaline) and epinephrine (adrenaline).

Chemically dopamine is a member of the catecholamine family, a class of molecules that serve both as neurotransmitters and hormones. The chemical formula is $C_6H_3(OH)_2\text{-}CH_2\text{-}CH_2\text{-}NH_2$. It is a monoamine compound containing nitrogen formed from ammonia by replacement of one or more of the hydrogen atoms. As a neurotransmitter, dopamine is "packaged" after manufacture in the brain into chemicals that help transmit electrical impulses in the brain from one neuron to another. The chemical is stored in tiny bubbles called vesicles, located near the back end of each neuron. When a message comes through a neuron, the vesicles release small amounts of the neurotransmitter to help carry the electrical impulse across the synapse or gap between neurons. The action is very quick. Each molecule of a transmitter stays on the receptor for only about 50 milliseconds (one thousandth of a second). Twelve messages can be carried across the synapse in 1 millisecond. Any transmitter not used in the process is pumped back into the vesicle by specialized cells called transporters. This movement allows the system to reload for more action in a fraction of a second. At any one given time, vast numbers of messages are surging through millions of circuits in the brain all supported by neurotransmitters.

Dopamine has many functions in the brain, including important roles in behavior and cognition, motor activity, motivation and reward, inhibition, sleep, mood, inattention, and learning. The neurons whose primary neurotransmitter is dopamine are located in the ventral tegmental area of the midbrain, substantia nigra, and the arcuate nucleus of the hypothalamus. Dopamine is believed to provide a teaching signal to parts of the brain responsible for acquiring new behaviors and is also related to the reward system and acquiring of habits. In the frontal lobes, dopamine controls the flow of information from other areas of the brain. Disorders of dopamine in this area can cause a decline in neurocognitive functions, including memory, attention, and problem solving. Reduced dopamine concentrations in the prefrontal cortex are thought to contribute to ADHD. D1 receptors are responsible for the cognitive-enhancing effects of dopamine.

Both cocaine and amphetamines inhibit the reuptake of dopamine, but in different ways. Cocaine blocks the dopamine transporter and then inhibits dopamine uptake, creating an overabundance of dopamine within the neurotransmitters. Amphetamines are similar in structure to dopamine and can enter the terminal of the presynaptic neuron by way of its dopamine transporter and also by diffusing through the neural membrane. When the stimulants enter, they force dopamine molecules out of their storage vesicles and expel them into the synaptic gap.

Depletion of dopamine in the brain is associated with several pathological conditions. It is the hallmark of Parkinson's disease and has been studied for connections to schizophrenia, autism, ADHD, and drug abuse.

Further Readings: "Dopamine (definition)." http://www.mederms.com/script/main/art.asp?articlekey=14345. Accessed 7/1/2008; Heijtz, R. D. et al. 2007. Motor inhibitory role of dopamine D1 receptors: Implications for ADHD. *Physiological Behavior* 92(1-2):155–60; "Ventral Tegmental Area." http://www.ncbi.nlm.nih.gov/pubmed/16338078. Accessed 6/18/2009.

Dore Treatment

The Dore Program is a treatment that tailors eye, balance, and sensory exercise performed at home 5–10 minutes a day. The program requires one center visit every 6 weeks. Dore is designed as an alternative to medication for children and adults with ADHD. Practitioners are found in major areas such as Boston, Chicago, Dallas, Denver, Los Angeles, and Phoenix.

Created by Wynford Dore, a successful British businessman, the program supports the idea that the cerebellum is the root of the problem, and the exercises are designed to target cerebellar dysfunction. Some ADHD experts, such as Dr. Edward Hallowell, author of *Driven to Distraction*, believe that his is a ground-breaking new treatment for ADHD, which has benefited over 50,000 people. Hallowell believes this new procedure is the most exciting new treatment to appear since the advent of stimulants in 1937.

Douglas, Virginia I.

Virginia Douglas, Professor Emerita at Montreal's McGill University, has been a pioneer in the study of ADHD and was among the first to make this a field of respected scientific inquiry. She demonstrated that one could conduct both basic and meaningful research on a clinical population of children. She was among the first researchers to conduct controlled drug trials and to propose behavior modification to improve problems of attention and impulsivity. Her classic article in the 1970s, "Stop, Look, and Listen," was the primary stimulus for the change in the name of the characteristics of the diagnostic category from an emphasis on hyperactivity to an emphasis on attention.

She developed one of the two models of hyperactivity and influenced the research in the area during the 1970s. Douglas was one of the first to develop a battery of measures of various behavioral and cognitive domains. She found that hyperactive children did not necessarily and uniformly have more reading or learning disabilities than other children.

Her model found that four deficits accounted for the symptoms of ADHD:

1. Children had difficulty with the investment, organization, and maintenance of attention and effort.
2. Children had difficulty controlling impulses.
3. Children had difficulty in adapting to various situations.
4. Children have a desire to seek immediate reinforcement.

The research of Douglas and her team are credited with the reasons the disorder was renamed attention deficit disorder (ADD) in 1980 with the publication of Diagnosis and Statistical Manual III (DSM-III; American Psychiatric Association 1980). In the official revised taxonomy, deficits in sustained attention and impulse control were formally recognized as of greater significance in diagnosis than hyperactivity. She now studies the cognitive and neuropsychological deficits of children with ADHD and is interested in the effects of pharmacotherapy, cognitive training, and reinforcement on these children's deficits.

Further Readings: Berman, T., Douglas, V. I., and Barr, R. G. 1998. Effects of methylphenidate on complex cognitive process in attention-deficit hyperactive disorder. *Journal of Abnormal Psychology* 88:90–105; Douglas, V. I. 1998. Cognitive control processes in attention-deficit hyperactive disorder. In *Handbook of disruptive behavior disorders*, edited by H. C. Quay and A. E. Hogan, Chapter 5, 105–38. New York: Plenum Publishing; "Virginia I. Douglas." McGill University. http://www.psych.mcgill.ca/faculty/douglas.html. Accessed 5/20/2009.

Drug Interventions

Drug treatment of a person with ADHD always requires the services of a physician. Although nonmedical specialists, such as psychologists, educators, and social workers may provide useful information, they are not trained to use and cannot provide medications. Before initiating any treatment, the first concern for a parent of a child with ADHD or an adult who thinks he/she may have the problem is to be sure of a proper diagnosis. *See* Diagnosis.

Dr. Melvin Oatis, a New York University pediatric specialist in a discussion presented at the Attention Deficit Hyperactive Disorder (ADHD) AMA briefing stated that once the diagnosis is clear, it is important to tailor the treatment to their specific impairments. He emphasized that it is important to determine where (and when) children with ADHD are having the most difficulty. Is the problem at school, home, or both? Are they having trouble with their relationship with peers? Is this a problem that is specific to one area of their lives or is it more global. Dr. Oatis offers the following examples for doctors and parents to ask?

- What are the symptoms of impairment?
- What time of day is the person having the problem? Is he or she in trouble the first thing in the morning or is it at the end of the day? Is the first teacher in the morning or the last teacher in the afternoon the most frustrated?
- Does the person wake up with difficulties that last until they shut their eyes at night?

These types of questions can guide the doctor to the right medication.

S. K. Katusic et al. (2005) suggests a multistep procedure for case definition and identification, which includes the use of school and medical records, a computerized diagnostic index, private psychiatric records, and an combination of DSM-IV-TR questionnaire and clinical records. Because no gold standard for diagnosis of ADHD exists, data from multiple sources and procedures are usually collected in clinical practice.

Drugs used in ADHD are grouped in two major categories: stimulants and nonstimulants. Both work by affected specific neurotransmitters—dopamine and norepinephrine—within the brain. Low levels of dopamine appear to play a role in inattention and hyperactivity, whereas low levels of norepinephrine may contribute to inattention and the inability to control impulsive behavior.

- Stimulants block the reuptake of both dopamine and norepinephrine (dual reuptake inhibitors) and exert effects in the frontal cortex of the brain to help with organization. *See* Reuptake.
- Nonstimulants block the reuptake of norepinephrine more selectively than they do other neurotransmitters.

Stimulants

Stimulant medications or cerebral stimulants have been used in the treatment of ADHD for a very long time. Although the exact mechanism of action is not fully understood, several theories have been proposed. Stimulants are believed to inhibit the reuptake of dopamine and norepinephrine and thereby increase release of these transmitters from the neuron. Reuptake means that the neurotransmitters are taken back into the chemical system, and therefore they do not function properly. Stimulants allow these actions of reuptake to be stopped or slowed down to various degrees and channel the neurotransmitter to work. Individuals appear to react to stimulants in various ways. For this reason, failure of therapy with one agent does not mean the class is not effective and another agent within the class may work. If responses are ineffective, a stronger dose may be used, allowing for sufficient times between these doses. The word titration is used to refer to the different doses.

The most common stimulants are *d*-amphetamine and methyphenidate (MPH). *d*-Amphetamines have several trade names, the most common being Dexedrine; Ritalin is the trade name for MPH. Amphetamine was first used for the treatment of ADHD children in 1937; MPH has been used since the 1960s. A common drug pemoline (Cylert) was introduced in Europe a number of years before being approved in the United States. Pemoline was removed from the Canadian market in 1999 because of safety consideration; the U.S. FDA removed it from the market in 2005 because of liver toxicity.

Extensive experience with these medications is one of the advantages of using them; long-term information of their safety and efficacy is available. Currently there are 10 commonly used stimulant medications that are distinguished by their mode of delivery to the body. Medications can either be short- or long-acting; short-acting formulations are effective for 2 to 4 hours; long-acting formulations can last 8 to 12 hours. Also, long-acting formulations differ in how much drug is released into the body immediately compared to what is released over time. For example, one formulation may release 50 percent of the medication immediately, with the remaining 50 percent slowly entering the blood stream. Another formulation releases only 30 percent immediately with a slow release of the remaining 70 percent. The value of answering the questions about the time of difficulty can be seen here. Choosing the right medication often means finding the delivery system that works best for the individual.

Longer-acting formulations of both MPH and amphetamine have entered the market. One new delivery system is based on a "bead" technology, in which long- and short-acting beads release the drug, mimicking twice-daily dosing and allowing for extended duration of effect. Another long-acting formulation uses an osmotic release oral system (OROS), in which an immediate release of part of MPH is contained in the capsule's overcoat, with the remainder of the drug osmotically released over the course of several hours. A formulation of mixed amphetamine salts (MAS) contains both *d*- and *l*-amphetamine isomers (forms of the drug) and is designed to give a double-pulsated delivery of amphetamines that prolongs its release. A new transdermal system delivers the drug in a discreet, clear patch that is applied once daily and releases a consistent amount of drug while the patch is worn and for about 3 hours after the patch is removed. Extended release formulations provide longer durations of action of 8 to 10 hours, resulting in the need for fewer daily administrations and eliminating the need to take medication while at school.

Adderall, approved in 1996 as a treatment of ADD/ADHD, is a cocktail or mixture of four drugs from the amphetamine family, which includes dextroamphetamine saccharate, amphetamine aspartate USP, and dextroamphetamine sulfate USP. Adderall is classified as a respiratory and cerebral stimulant. As a result, it has a broad spectrum of symptom coverage. It tends to last for about 6 hours per dose and can cover the entire school day. Some physicians say that it appears to be less harsh than Ritalin. However, concerns of the possibility of cardiovascular problems caused sales of Adderall XR to be suspended for 6 months in 2005. Similar concerns with Concerta related to psychiatric problems evoked further investigations by the FDA in July 2005, but the agency was not convinced there was enough evidence to declare a cause-effect relationship and decided more investigation was needed.

Researchers at the University of California, San Diego, researched a patch containing MPH, the ingredient found in Ritalin. The patch provides a steady level of drug through the skin to the blood stream and offers an alternative to twice-daily pills. The patch may reduce some of Ritalin's side effects, such as jitteriness and stomachaches because the effects are often due to fluctuations of MPH blood levels associated with taking the short-acting oral form of the drug several times a day.

Stimulants enhance the availability of dopamine, the neurotransmitter, to allow greater control over sustained attention. Table 10 lists the major stimulants used for ADHD.

Table 10   Major Stimulants for ADHD

Brand Name and Manufacturer	Generic Name	Duration of Effect (hours) and Available Dosage (mg)	FDA Approval
Ritalin, Novartis; Methylin, Alliant	MPH	8; 5, 10, and 20	An older medication
Ritalin-LA, Novartis	MPH	6-10; 20, 30, and 40	2002
Dexedrine, Glaxo-Smith-Kline; Dextrostat, Shire	Dextroamphetamine	6; 5	Older formulation
Metadate-CD, Celltech Group PLC	MPH-HCl	6-10; 10 and 20	2001
Concerta, McNeil Consumer & Specialty Pharmaceuticals	OROS MPH	9-12; 18, 27, 36, and 54	2000
AdderallXR, Shire	MAS	10-12; 5, 10, 15, 20, 25, and 30	2001
Focalin, Novartis	*d*-MPH	6-19; 10, and 20	2001
FocalinXR, Novartis	*d*-MPH HCl—extended release	9-12; 5, 10, and 20	2004
Daytrana, Shire	MPH transdermal patch system	Up to 12; 10,15, 20, and 30	2006
Vyvanse, Shire	Lisdexamfetamine dimesylate	Up to 12; 30, 50, and 70	2007

MPH, methylphenidate; MAS, mixed amphetamine salts.

Table 11   Nonstimulant Medications for ADHD

Name	Registered Name	Comments
Atomoxetine	Strattera; Eli Lilly and Company	Approved 2002
Pemoline	Cylert	Effective with ADHD but questions about the effect on liver; withdrawn from the United States in 2005
Bupropion HCl	Wellbutrin	Antidepressant
Imiprine HCl	Tofranil	Antidepressant
Nortriptyline HCl	Pamelor	Antidepressant
Clonidine HCl	Catapres	Used to treat high blood pressure; effective in managing ADHD, conduct disorders, and sleep disorders
Guanfacine	Tenex; INTUNIV	Decreases fidgeting and restlessness; increases ability to tolerate frustration

Nonstimulant Medications

When the popular medications are not effective, physicians will try other drugs. The first nonstimulant medication approved by the Federal Drug Administration (FDA) for use with ADHD was atomoxetine (Strattera), a long-acting medication taken once every 24 hours. Atomoxetine blocks the presynaptic norepinephrine transporter in the prefrontal cortex. This drug needs to build up a therapeutic level in the bloodstream, and it is important that the person does not miss a dose. The once-a-day dosing allows patients to be more easily controlled. Atomoxetine has been shown in clinical studies to be superior to placebo in reducing impulsivity, hyperactivity, and inattention. Gibson et al. (2006) did a metaanalysis comparing atomoxetine with psychostimulants in five head-to-head trials for the treatment of ADHD. Generally, few significant differences were found on the ADHD Rating Scale. Tolerability was similar; however, more long-term safety data are needed to establish its place in the treatment of ADHD.

Pemoline (Cylert) was used at one time but because of reported cases of liver infection was taken from the market in 2005. Some children are receiving guanfacine HCl (Tenex), which decreases fidgeting and restlessness, increases ability to tolerate frustration, and increases attention. Some antidepressants include bupropion HCl (Wellbutrin), imiprine HCl (Tofranil), and nortriptyline HCL (Pamelor). Clonidine HCl (Catapres) is used to treat high blood pressure but has been found an effective manager for ADHD core symptoms, conduct disorders, and sleep disorders. Table 11 lists the nonstimulant medications used for ADHD.

Deciding on a Stimulant or Nonstimulant

When deciding on a stimulant or nonstimulant, the doctor must assess and compare the profiles of different side effects. Table 12 compares the side effects of stimulants and nonstimulants. Another consideration is the onset of action; stimulants work more quickly than nonstimulants.

Table 12 Comparative Side Effects

Stimulants	Nonstimulant (Atomoxetine)
Headache	Stomachache
Stomachache	Decreased appetite
Decreased appetite	Nausea or vomiting
Sleep disturbance	Dizziness
Potential effect upon growth, especially height	Tiredness/sedation
Moodiness	Mood swings
An association with tics	In adults, side effects may differ

There has long been the hypothesis that children with ADHD are delayed in maturation. Swanson et al.(2007) studied the Multimodal Treatment Study of ADHD (MTA) at 3 years' follow-up. When the team compared a nonmedicated subgroup with a sample of patients who took stimulants, they found unexpected results. This study found the opposite; their data showed that children who took drugs experienced an accelerated growth rate in preadolescence and adolescence that than a maturation delay.

Emerging Treatments

An emerging treatment is lisdexamfetamine dimesylate (Vyvanse), a stimulant. In November 2007 Shire Pharmaceuticals announced that that *Biological Psychiatry* had published the results of a study showing that Vyvanse provided efficacy in children with ADHD for up to 12 hours. This Phase II randomized, double-blind, placebo-controlled, and active-controlled crossover classroom study in children aged 6 to 12 examined the efficacy and safety of Vyvanse (30, 20, or 30 mg and Adderall XR (mixed amphetamine salts extended-release 10, 20, or 30 mg) or placebo. Vyvanse provided a consistent time to maximum plasma concentration from patient to patient and demonstrated efficacy up to 12 hours after administration, which is something that parents are interested in because it may help improve their family and homework time in the evening. Patients in the study also developed significant improvement in math problems attempted compared to placebo. Vyvanse is currently approved in the United States for treatment in children aged 6 to 12 years. The U.S. FDA approved the additional dosage strengths: 20, 40, and 60 mg in January 2008. A supplemental New Drug Application (sNDA) for Vyvanse treatment of ADHD in adults is currently under review for adults.

Lisdexamfetamine dimesylate is a prodrug, which means it is an active drug that is covalently bonded to the amino acid L-lysine. In February 2007, the FDA approved lisdexamfetamine for treatment of ADHD in the United States. The following is the mode of action of the drug: after oral ingestion, lisdexamfetamine is converted to L-lysine, a naturally occurring amino acid and to active *d*-amphetamine; the effect is consistent throughout the day; the normal gastrointestinal pH does not affect the process. There is reduced potential for abuse, overdose toxicity, and drug tampering.

The drug remains biologically inactive until it is metabolized in the body. This delayed metabolism results in lower potential for abuse and diversion because it does not produce the same euphoric effects as its active drug counterpart. The possibility of substance abuse is reduced because this multistep drug is something that one can mimic or create only in a sophisticated laboratory, not in a kitchen. The yield is very low, and it is difficult to convert this drug to agents of abuse. Lisdexamfetamine dimesylate also provides overdose protection; the enzyme system appears to limit the amount of active drug that is available by restricting release. The ability of lisdexamfetamine dimesylate to produce euphoria was much lower than that of the active parent drug dextroamphetamine. Rapid uptake in the brain is not seen with this particular medication. This prodrug is not affected by gastrointestinal pH and is unlikely to be affected by alteration in normal GI transit systems.

Drug Holidays

Some patients may initiate taking a "holiday" from their medication regimes. Faraone et al. (2004) surveyed patients in a psychiatric environment and in a primary care setting. They found that 24 percent of patients in the psychiatric environs and 17 percent in primary care took drug holidays. Patients initiated it 57 percent of the time. Some evidence supports the idea that drug holidays may reduce insomnia and appetite suppression without a significant increase in symptoms. However, other studies show no benefit. There are no clear guidelines on whether to use drug holidays, and the decision to implement them is determined by the degree of the problems related to the symptoms.

FDA Approval of Drugs

The path to FDA approval is not always smooth and may take years. All pharmaceuticals in the United States must go through an approval process by the FDA through its Center for Biologics Evaluation and Research (CBER). Drugs for ADHD and related comorbid conditions are no exceptions. To have a drug approved, it must go through a long, rigorous period of development, testing, and then close scrutiny once it gets on the market. It may take 10 to 15 years for a new formulation to come to the market. *See also* Clinical Trials and Medical Approval.

Even after years of scrutiny and tests, problems may arise after approval. For example, the FDA has issued a public health advisory regrinding the development of suicidal tendencies in patients treated with atomoxetine, and a "black box" warning was added to the labeling of that drug. The FDA has further mandated that all drugs approved for the treatment of ADHD carry guides to inform patients about the potential for cardiovascular risks and adverse psychiatric symptoms. Some adverse events such as sudden death in patients with underlying serious heart problems and a slight increased risk for drug-related psychiatric adverse events, such as hearing voices, was also found. Guides for patients, families, and caregivers will now be included in the package inserts with all ADHD prescriptions. With the significant abuse of some medications, regulatory actions from the FDA and Drug Enforcement Agency will be coming. Expect in the future ways to

Tips for Taking ADHD Medications

Medications can help children with ADHD, but it is absolutely essential that the medications be taken carefully and according to the doctor's orders. The following are some ideas for safety in taking medications:

- Children and teenagers should never be in charge of their own medications.
- To avoid side effects, give medications with food, encourage healthy snacking, and plan for a dinner later at night.
- At home, keep medication locked in a childproof container. Psychostimulant drugs such as methylphenidate and amphetamines are nervous system stimulants. An overdose can cause severe confusion, agitation, and accelerated heart rate and is potentially fatal. Children age 5 and younger are especially sensitive to drug overdoses.
- If sleeping is a problem, try to give medication earlier in the day. Avoid sleep aids, such as sleeping pills.
- Never send medication to school with your child. Deliver the medication to the school nurse or health office yourself. School districts may have varying policies for taking medications at school. Check with your school district about the policy for taking medications at school; some districts require the prescription from the doctor to be on file in the school office.
- Talk to the child about medications. Make sure he or she understands that it is not permitted to give or sell medication to others. Request that he tell you immediately if classmates pressure or threaten.

Source: Adapted from Lerche Davis, Jeanie. "Tips for reducing side effects." WebMD. http://www.webmd.com/add-adhd/guide/reduce-side-effects-adhd-medications. Accessed 5/20/2009.

prevent potential problems as an added assurance for safety for patients, caregivers, and prescribers.

Some new formulations of drugs in novel classes are being studied. ABT-089 is a partial nicotinic receptor agonist for possible treatment for ADHD in adults. Also, the extended-release alpha-2-adrenoreceptor agonist guanfacine has passed the Phase I safety trials for treatment in adults.

Despite some advantages of drug therapy, not all people are comfortable with the use of long-term medications for children with ADHD. When first confronted with the prospective use, some parents may be hesitant. However, ADHD is a quite serious and disabling disorder, and if medications can help, parents should consider all options when making a decision. The important item for parents is to be patient and seek out a correct diagnosis.

A 2007 study has shown global use of ADHD medications has risen dramatically from 1993 to 2003. Published in the National Institute of Mental Health publication *Health Affairs*, researchers examined data from 70 countries in North America, Europe, and Northeast Asia and found among 5 to

19 year olds, use of medications to treat ADHD has increased by 274 percent. The United States prescribes the most ADHD medications, but its share of the worldwide market declined from 87 percent in 1993 to 83 percent in 2003. According to lead author of the study, Dr. R. M. Scheffler, ADHD is poised to become the world's leading disorder treated with medication; however, he emphasized the importance of clearly identifying the benefits and risks of these treatments and promoting careful prescribing and monitoring practices.

Further Readings: Faraone, S. V. et al. 2004. Attention-deficit/hyperactivity disorder in adults: A survey of current practice in psychiatry and primary care. *Archives of Internal Medicine* 164:1221–26; Gibson, Aaron P. et al. 2006. Atmoxetine versus stimulants for treatment of attention deficit/hyperactivity disorder. *Annals of Pharmacotherapy* 40:1134–42. DOI 10.1345/aph.1G. Published Online, May 30, 2006. http://www.theannals.com/content/vol40/issue6/. Accessed 5/20/2009; Katusic, S. K. et al. 2005. Case definition in epidemiologic studies of ADHD. *Annals of Epidemiology* 15:430–37; Oatis, M. D. "Treatment-pharmacology." Discussion presented at the Attention Deficit Hyperactive Disorder (ADHD) AMA Media Briefing; September 9; New York, NY, 2004; Scheffler, R. M. et al. 2007. The global market for ADHD medication. *Health Affairs* 26(2, March/April):450-57; Swanson et al. 2007. Effects of stimulant medication on growth rates across 3 years in the MTA follow-up. *Journal of American Academy of Child and Adolescent Psychiatry* 46:1014–26; Wender, Paul. 1987. *The hyperactive child, adolescent, and adult: Attention deficit disorder through the lifespan.* New York: Oxford University Press; "Vyvanse." http://www.vyvanse.com. Accessed 5/20/2009.

DSM-IV. *See* Diagnosis of ADHD; Diagnostic and Statistical Manuals.

Due Process Hearing for Students with ADHD. *See* Individuals with Disabilities Education Act (IDEA).

Dyslexia

Dyslexia is one of many comorbid or coexisting conditions with ADHD. The general public is still confused about what truly defines a child with dyslexia, and educators are also frustrated about the best way to teach these students. The word "dyslexia" comes from two Greek words, *dys* meaning "difficult with" and *lex* meaning "word." Dyslexia is an inherited condition that makes it extremely difficult to read, write, or spell in the native language, although the person may have average or above intelligence. A person with dyslexia has difficulty processing words or reading.

Several studies correlate ADHD with reading difficulties. It is commonly believed that the person with dyslexia sees letters or words that are reversed or scrambled visually. British and Scottish physicians first described dyslexia in the late 1800s and called it "congenital word blindness." A Pittsburgh physician, E. Bosworth McCready, in1909 reported 41 cases of "word blindness" worldwide, but the American who left an indelible stamp on dyslexia was Samuel Orton, who studied Iowa farm boys whose vision was excellent but could barely read. He noted how they reversed and mixed up letters.

From studies researchers have found that dyslexia is a neurological disorder that interferes in processing language. The condition varies in degrees

Famous People with Both ADHD and Dyslexia

Some of the world's most accomplished people have had ADHD and dyslexia. See how many your can recognize. Here is a partial list: Alexander Graham Bell, Cher, Winston Churchill, Tom Cruise, Walt Disney, Thomas Edison, Albert Einstein, Benjamin Franklin, Judge J. H. Gallet, Danny Glover, Whoopi Goldberg, Bruce Jenner, Magic Johnson, John Kennedy, John Lennon, Carl Lewis, Greg Louganis, Wolfgang Mozart, General George Patton, Pablo Picasso, Charles Schwab, and Woodrow Wilson.

Source: LD Research Foundation. http://www.ldrfa.org/?pID=34. Accessed 6/18/2009.

of severity. The condition may manifest itself in sound processing, reading, writing, spelling, handwriting, and sometimes in arithmetic. The cause of dyslexia is elusive, just like the cause of ADHD, although suspected genetic links appear to exist for both conditions.

Some physicians, using functional magnetic imaging (fMRI) studies, have questioned old ideas about the cause of dyslexia and have found that blood flow in a different part of the brain shows a weakness in the area that decodes the sounds of written language. Dr. Marcel Just, a brain researcher at Carnegie Mellon University, Pittsburgh, found that a region that is just above the left ear at the junction of the brains temporal and parietal lobes is the area that lights up brightly on brain scans of normal readers who can sound out words. As readers become more skilled, an area further back in the brain next to the visual processing area starts to show greater activity. When one first learns to read, it takes a lot of effort, but after you have read a word a certain number of times, these nerve endings come together, and then the word is stored in the word-form area in the occipito-temporal area of the brain.

Other researchers suspect that both dyslexia and ADHD are connected to the corpus callosum, the large structure that connects the two hemisphere of the brain. The role of the corpus callosum is to pass information from the left hemisphere to the right and vice versa; the two hemispheres must work efficiently for information to be passed between the two halves of the brain. Scientists suspect that the front part of the corpus callosum is smaller in children with dyslexia. The fact that the corpus callosum is larger in professional musicians than in nonmusicians has led some researchers to suggest that playing instruments involves a lot of crossing to keep hands moving together. Regular practice can strengthen the corpus callosum. Such programs as the Dore Program, Interactive Metronome, and primitive reflex–based treatment such as INPP may train the brain.

Because reading is the basis for all learning, parents should not let children lag in their instructions. Children need a multisensory approach; if they do not pick up phonics by the third grade, they will be stuck at a second grade reading level. Although parents cannot insist that children receive a particular kind of methodology, such as Orton Gillingham, or Lindamood, they do have the right under Individuals with Disabilities Education Act (IDEA) to provide special teaching.

Researchers believe that the "whole language" approach to reading does not work well for those with dyslexia. The best interventions are the letter-to-sound decoding techniques that are even more detailed and concrete than regular phonics classes. A study called Power4Kids is an example of letter-to-sound program. Also computer games, such as Wii Drums and Wii Fit may help. *See also* Specific Learning Disability (SLD).

Further Readings: "ADHD and Dyslexia," http://www.healthyplace.com/communities/add/judy/dyslexia_1 htm. Accessed 7/13/2008; "Famous People with ADHD and Dyslexia." http://www.ldrfa.org/?pID=34. Accessed 7/13/2008; Myomancy, ADHD, Dyslexia, and Autism. "The Corpus Callosum, Dyslexia, and ADHD." January 2008. http://www.myomancy.com/2008/01/the-corpus-callosum-dyslexia-and-adhd. Accessed 5/20/2009.

E

Economic Impact of ADHD. *See* Costs of ADHD.

Education

The educational needs of a child with ADHD are considerable. Because of dwindling resources in many school districts, many children are not able to receive the full support they require. Demands for the classroom appear contradictory: the student needs both flexibility and structure. The classroom must be a consistent and predictable setting that provides much structure and limited distractions, but flexibility in addressing each child's learning style.

Few educators are familiar with major findings from recent scientific studies of ADHD. For years most educators, physicians, psychologists, and parents have considered ADHD as a cluster of behaviors and as a label for students who are disruptive in class and who won't stop talking. Increasingly, scientists are realizing that it is a complex syndrome of impairments that affect the executive or management function of the brain. *See also* Teaching Children with ADHD.

Emotional Disturbance (ED)

A child with ADHD may have an emotional disturbance. Although the term may be thrown around loosely, the Americans with Disabilities Act (1990) has a specific definition, especially when it comes to children in school. The term "emotional disturbance" means a condition exhibiting one or more of the following characteristics over a long period of time and to a degree that adversely affects a child's educational performance. The following characteristics must apply:

- The child has an inability to learn that cannot be explained by intellectual, sensory, or health factors.
- The child has an inability to build or maintain satisfactory interpersonal relationships with peers and teachers.

- The child displays inappropriate types of behavior or feelings under normal circumstances.
- The child has a general pervasive mood of unhappiness or depression.
- The child has a tendency to develop physical symptoms or fears associated with personal or school problems.

The term includes schizophrenia and other mental illnesses but does not apply to children who are socially maladjusted, unless it has be determined that they have an emotional disturbance.

Some children with ADHD will develop maladaptive behaviors and will need an emotionally supportive environment with firm expectations for behavior. If the child with ADHD is determined eligible under ED criteria, parents will want to be sure they receive concrete instruction in behavior-change strategies to meet behavioral goals.

Further Reading: "Texas Partners Resource Network." http://www.PartnersTX.org. Accessed 5/18/2009.

Enuresis. *See* Bedwetting.

Environment

Although ADHD is suspected to be a highly inherited psychiatric condition, environment also plays a role. Studies have consistently associated the following environmental factors with the development of ADHD:

- Prenatal exposure to drugs such as nicotine and cocaine
- Maternal depression
- Negative parenting styles
- Exposure to lead and other kinds of environmental toxins

Some scientists theorize that the pregnancy and birth experiences of the mother are substantial factors relating to brain injuries and ADHD. Inattention to proper prenatal care may lead to low birth weight and hypoxia or diminished oxygen at birth. Hypoxia can cause serious brain damage or may result in conditions that show up later as learning disabilities.

Many toxins can cause damage to the developing fetus. If the mother uses cocaine during pregnancy, it can lead to birth insults that may affect the developing brain. Fetal exposure to alcohol has been linked to ADHD. Others argue that stress and poor nutrition during pregnancy can cause babies to have more allergic reactions that may cause developmental problems.

Barkley (2006) discussed environmental factors, including pre- and peri-natal abnormalities, central nervous system infections, and reactions to sugar and food additives, as proposed correlations of ADHD. For example, a 2002 study indicated that smoking and eating a high-carbohydrate, high-sugar diet during pregnancy appeared to be related to behavior problems in toddlers. Smoking lowers blood oxygen levels that are critical in fetal development, especially fetal brain cells. These two factors combined may evoke ADHD in children.

Some nutritional studies in children have found the following correlations with ADHD:

- Calcium deficiency.
- High serum copper.
- Iron deficiency can cause irritability and attention deficits.
- Magnesium deficiency may lead to fidgeting, anxiety, restlessness, psycho-motor problems, and learning difficulties.
- Malnutrition in general is related to learning disabilities; the child does not have to look malnourished, a forgotten fact in affluent countries.
- Dyslexic children appear to have abnormally low zinc metabolism and high copper metabolism.
- Iodine deficiencies have been linked to learning difficulties.

ADHD also occurs in certain biological conditions. Children born with Fragile X syndrome, a genetic condition carried on the X chromosome, are often hyperactive and have attention deficit. Children also born with fetal alcohol syndrome are known also to have attention problems.

However, these factors collectively explain only a small proportion of the variance in ADHD. Many of the same genetic factors have been related to substance abuse, making scientists suspect that exposure in the environment may release the genetic propensity for the condition. Some have related heredity and environment to the metaphor: genetics loads the gun but the environment pulls the trigger.

Further Reading: Barkley, Russell. 2006. *Attention-deficit hyperactivity disorder: A handbook for diagnosis and treatment.* 3rd ed. New York: Guilford Press.

Evolutionary Aspects of ADHD

Thom Hartman in his book *Attention Deficit Disorder: A Different Perception* hypothesizes that people with ADD are the leftover hunters, those whose ancestors evolved and matured thousand of years in the past in hunting society. Although some may disagree with Hartman's hypothesis regarding ADHD, it is an interesting one to note. According to Hartman, many instances exist of genetic diseases that represent evolutionary survival strategies. For example, sickle cell disease evolved to make victims less susceptible to malaria. When living in the jungles of Africa, those with the sickle cells had a powerful evolutionary tool against death; in malaria-free countries, the condition has become a liability. Children who inherited Tay-Sachs, a genetic disease of the Jews of Eastern Europe, have relative immunity to tuberculosis, a condition that was rampant in Jewish ghettos of the past. Cystic fibrosis, a condition carried by one in 25 Americans, is thought to have developed as a protection against the cholera epidemics that periodically swept Europe.

Thus, Hartman argues that if these diseases could evolve according to Darwin's theory of natural selection, the traits for surviving in a society of hunters and gatherers also could enhance survival. He describes a number of attributes that are beneficial to those in the hunter societies and prevalent in people with ADHD. Whether the person was chasing buffalo in North America, deer in Europe, or wildebeest in Africa or spearing fish in a stream, these hunters developed a set of mental and physical skills to survive. They needed to constantly monitor the environment and notice everything.

Survival was based on those who were brave and impulsive, with a thirst for excitement that sent them better equipped to pursue the game for survival. They could also hyperfocus on details to track animals and to notice differences in their environment. Hunters think visually, describing their actions in terms of pictures, rather than words or feelings. When farming was introduced, the people had to be patient, methodical, and more passive. However, human survival depends on both the farmers and hunters.

Schools are not designed for hunters but for the more patient farmers. According to Hartman, ADHD children would not be considered deficient if they were allowed to follow their nature. The modern classroom that is overcrowded and based on visual learning forces children to comply or fail. Hartman sides with parents who do not want their children labeled and who believe that children should be children. They want to explore the world, run, play, and fidget. Being distracted, impatient, and impulsive are hallmarks of childhood.

Further Reading: Hartmann, Thom. 1997. *Attention deficit disorder: A different perception.* Grass Valley, CA: Mythical Intelligence Press.

Executive Function

Executive function (EF) in ADHD refers to management of the cognitive functions of the brain. ADD is not merely a deficit of attention as well as excessive movement but a deficit in the brain circuits that prioritize, integrate, and regulate other cognitive functions. EF provides the mechanism for self-regulation.

Thomas E. Brown, Ph.D. (2005) uses the metaphor of the symphony orchestra to show EF. All the members of the orchestra can play their instruments beautifully, but if no conductor organizes the players of individual instruments to begin or to convey the overall interpretation of music as a whole, the orchestra will not produce good music. Everyone will be doing his or her own thing. Symptoms of ADD can be compared to impairments, not in the work of the individual musicians, but in the orchestra's conductor. On occasion persons with ADD may be able to do well an individual task that they are interested in, but the problem lies in their chronic inability to activate and manage these functions in the right way at the right time. Therein lies the similarity to the orchestra: The problem lies not with the individual musicians who can play instruments perfectly but with the conductor, who must start and guide all the individual players.

Brown uses another illustration given by Martha Bridge Denckla, Johns Hopkins, describing patients with high intelligence and no specific learning disabilities but who have problems dealing with tasks. She compares these people to a disorganized cook trying to get a meal on the table. A person, who has a well-equipped kitchen and shelves stocked with all the essentials, is preparing lasagna. She can even read the recipe. However, she forgets to thaw the meat, searches through the shelves to find the spices, and forgets to turn on the heat in the oven. This cook is motivated but disheveled and is unlikely to get her dish on the table in time. This metaphor again describes the executive function of a person who wants to accomplish a task but is unable to get it all together.

Brown relates three concepts to EF: intelligence, awareness, and the brain's signaling system:

1. EF and intelligence. As seen in the example of the disorganized cook, disorganization can be independent of general intelligence. Persons can be extremely bright on standard measurements of IQ, but this has little to do with whether they meet the diagnostic criteria for ADD.
2. EF and awareness. The metaphor of a person getting ready to fix a screen on his window shows how awareness plays into the picture. He went to the basement to get some nails and found the garage was a mess, so he started cleaning it. He decided to put up some pegboard to hang tools, so he jumped in the car to go to the store to buy it. At the store, he found paint on sale and realized the porch needed painting; he forgot the pegboard. The original focus and awareness of his intent of fixing the screen was lost.
3. EF and the brain's signaling system. Considerable evidence exists that those with ADD have significant impairments in the executive functions of the brain. EF is not concentrated in one area of the brain but is decentralized and supported by many complex networks within the prefrontal cortex. Some essential EF functions are related to the amygdala and subcortical structures, whereas others depend of the reticular portions of the cerebellum. *See also* Brain and ADHD. Complex neuronal networks and signals move signals along with two important neurotransmitters: dopamine and norepinephrine.

Brown describes six executive functions that are impaired in ADD syndrome:

1. Activation. Organizing, prioritizing, and getting ready to work
2. Focus. Keeping on task
3. Effort. Keeping alert, maintaining effort, and regulating speed
4. Emotion. Managing frustration
5. Memory. Using working memory and accessing recall
6. Action. Keeping self-control

Further Readings: Barkley, Russell. 2006. *Attention-deficit hyperactivity disorder: A handbook for diagnosis and treatment.* 3rd ed. New York: Guilford Press; Barkley, R. 1997. *ADHD and the nature of self-control.* New York: Guilford Press; Brown, T. E. et al. 2006. ADHD gender differences in a clinic-referred sample. In *Attention-deficit hyperactivity disorder: A handbook for diagnosis and treatment.* 3rd ed., edited by Russell Barkley. 108. New York: Guilford Press. Also presented at the annual meeting of the American Academy of Child and Adolescent Psychiatry, New York, October 1989.

F

Feingold, Benjamin F.

Dr. Benjamin Feingold was a pediatric allergist who made a correlation between certain foods and additives and children's behavior and ability to learn. He read the research of Dr. Richard Lockey from Mayo Clinic who had designed a diet for allergies that focused on exclusion of specific foods and had helped some patients with allergies. Building on that diet, he presented a paper in June 1973 to the American Medical Association that stated that salicylates, artificial colors, and artificial flavors cause hyperactivity in children. The presentation of that paper began his quest for answers to the problems of attention and hyperactivity.

Born in Pittsburgh, Pennsylvania on June 15, 1899, Feingold graduated from the University of Pittsburgh with an M.D. in 1924. He studied extensively in the United States and in Germany, and after several distinguished positions, joined the Kaiser Foundation Hospital and Permanente Medical Group in 1951 to establish a Department of Allergy. His research led him to conclude that the items people take into their mouths affect behavior.

When he presented his report to the AMA in 1973, the science of nutrition was in its infancy. The idea that biochemicals in food might affect behavior was not accepted. However, Feingold was convinced of the connection and developed the Feingold Diet (also known as the Feingold Program), which he claimed could help both children and adults and had no side effects (Feingold 1974). He spent his professional life traveling throughout the world to encourage his diet and the formation of support groups for people with attention and behavior disorders. From these support groups, the Feingold Association of the United States was formed.

The Feingold Diet remains controversial. He wrote several books about the diet, along with a cookbook. Many mainstream physicians deny the claims as unproven; others consider his recommendations as scientifically solid. However, Feingold decorated his office with notes and pictures from those that he helped and referred to them as "my kids."

Further Readings: Feingold, B. F. 1973. *Introduction to clinical allergy.* New York: Charles C. Thomas; Feingold, B. F. 1974. *Why your child is hyperactive.* New York:

Random House; Feingold, B. F. 1979. *The Feingold cookbook for hyperactive children.* New York: Random House.

Feingold Diet

Although most people think of diet plans as ways to lose weight, some diets, such as the Feingold Diet, are based on the concept that certain foods can affect behavior. In 1974 Dr. Benjamin Feingold wrote the book *Why Your Child Is Hyperactive,* espousing what he called the "KP" or "Kaiser-Permanente" diet, named after the medical center where he practiced and taught (softcover published in 1985). In 1979 he and his wife wrote *The Feingold Cookbook*, and the name Feingold Diet began to stick.

To treat and prevent hyperactivity, Feingold and his followers recommend a diet that eliminates foods with salicylates, artificial flavors, and artificial colors. The diet has been the subject of many studies with diverse findings. In 1989 the National Institutes of Health held a consensus conference; the panel concluded that the evidence presented at the time warranted further research.

The Feingold Program is build on elimination of the following items from the diet:

- Artificial or synthetic food colorings
- Artificial flavoring such as aspartame, saccharin, and cyclamates
- Three antioxidant preservatives: BHA, BHT, TBHQ

Feingold pointed out that food dyes and preservatives came from petroleum. Other additives that are of concern are: monosodium glutamate (MSG), fluoride, corn syrup, sulfites, sodium benzoate, and calcium propionate.

The Feingold Diet is set up in stages or weeks. During the first week of the program all foods that have natural salicylates are temporarily removed from the diet and nonsalicylates take their place. The foods that have natural salicylates are almonds, apples, apricots, all berries, cherries, cloves, coffee, cucumber and pickles, currants, grapes and raisins, nectarines, oranges, oil of wintergreen, peppers, plums and prunes, tangerines, tea, and tomatoes. Of course, all aspirin and medicines containing aspirin are removed. The following nonsalicylates that are tolerated by most people are substituted: avocado, artichokes, asparagus, alfalfa sprouts, banana, bamboo shoots, bean sprouts, beans, eggplant, figs, grapefruit, guava, kiwi, lemons, lettuce, lentils, pears, peas, persimmons, pineapple, pomegranate, potatoes, pumpkin, beets, broccoli, brussels sprouts, cabbage, cantaloupe, carrots, cauliflower, celery, coconut, dates, limes, mushrooms, mangoes, melons, okra, olives, onions, papaya, parsley, parsnips, radishes, rhubarb, rutabaga, spinach, squash, turnips, water chestnuts, watercress, watermelon, yams.

According to Feingold, salicylate sensitivity is a very big problem and doctors often do not recognize it. They may realize that the child is sensitive to aspirin but are unaware that grapes or tomatoes can have a serious effect on one who is sensitive to them. Another area of sensitivity may be the use of additives in nonfood products such as toothpaste, vitamins, medicine, lotions, and even colored play dough.

People usually find it takes about 2 weeks to become accustomed to the new diet, which eliminates many old favorites. The time for the program to take effect varies from 3 days to about 3 weeks, according to Feingold. Since Feingold first described the elimination diet, several other physicians have added other items such as flour, milk, chocolate, corn, nuts, and all processed foods.

The Feingold program offers people a food list and shopping guide with acceptable name brands on its Feingold Association Web site. The site emphasizes that one cannot determine the level of salicylates in food by just looking at the nutrition facts label or product contents. For example, Eggo Homestyle Waffles are not acceptable but Eggo Buttermilk Waffles are, according to the site. Sugar is not restricted but anything that has corn syrup is because it is processed and chemical-laden. Although the Web site does offer lots of information, for participants to have access to starting the program, they must pay about $77 for a food list and shopping guide, regular updates, and a companion book.

The Feingold site is filled with testimonials from parents who describe changes in their children's behavior while using the diet. On the pro-Feingold side, the Center for Science in the Public Interest issued a 32-page report in 1999 that cites 17 controlled studies that found diet affects behavior. It also cites six studies that did not detect changes in behavior with changes in diet. However, the Center does believe that if there is a chance that diet will help some children, it is worth trying before treating the child with stimulants or other drugs.

However, critics of the Feingold Diet point to the studies that show no behavioral improvement on the diet. Several critics express the idea that the potential benefit should be weighed against the potential harm of teaching children that their behaviors and school performance are related to what they eat rather than what they feel and depriving the child of receive proper professional help. A fact sheet from the Web site of Children and Adults with Attention/Deficit Hyperactivity Disorder lists the Feingold diet as a controversial treatment for ADHD. Research into the issue is continuing.

Further Readings: "CHADD: Children and Adults with Attention Deficit/Hyperactivity Disorder." http://www.chadd.org. Accessed 5/20/2009; Feingold, B. F. 1973. *Introduction to clinical allergy.* New York: Charles C. Thomas; Feingold, B. F. 1974. *Why your child is hyperactive.* New York: Random House; Feingold, B. F. 1979. *The Feingold cookbook for hyperactive children.* New York: Random House; Hersey, Jane. 1996. Why can't my child behave? A comprehensive guide to the Feingold program. Riverhead, NY: Feingold Association of the United States. http://www.feingold.org/pg-book.html. Accessed 5/20/2009.

Feingold Foundation

The Feingold foundation is a support group for those people who are involved in following the Feingold Diet. It was founded by a group of parents in May 1976 and was named in honor of Dr. Feingold. The association publishes the Feingold newsletter *Pure Facts* ten times a year. They also publish lists of acceptable foods such as ice creams, potato chips, mixes, candy, beverages.

Further Reading: Feingold Association of the United States. http://www.feingold. org. Accessed 5/20/2009.

Fetal Alcohol Syndrome (FAS)

Children with fetal alcohol syndrome (FAS) and those with ADHD have many similar problems. Fetal alcohol syndrome is caused when the mother drinks alcohol while pregnant. Alcohol is recognized as a potent neurotoxin when delivered to a developing fetus through the placenta. Jones and Smith (1973) first described FAS as a complex pattern of minor malformations that identifies a group of children who have been exposed to prenatal alcohol. These children have distinct facial and other features and are at risk for a number of physical and neurological problems. Also, some children with prenatal exposure to alcohol may develop a less severe form called alcohol-related neurodevelopmental disorder (ARND). The exact amount of alcohol that affects the children is unknown. A study by the National Institute of Drug Abuse reported that 18.8 percent of mothers had used alcohol during pregnancy.

Children with FAS have multiple cognitive and behavioral issues, including learning disabilities, language disabilities, memory problems, and mathematical difficulties. The children may also display problems with paying attention; poor impulse control, a lack of self-control; temper outbursts, little control of temper; learning difficulties, problems in school; learning difficulties, problems in school; and social and behavior problems.

Bhatara et al. (2006) in a review of charts from a large referral center found that 41 percent of FAS children had ADHD, and 17 percent had a learning disorder. Sixteen percent met the criteria for oppositional defiant disorder. These comorbidities are also found with ADHD.

Treatment of comorbid FAS and ADHD are limited. A study with four participants found stimulants to improve symptoms of hyperactivity as measured on the Connor Parent Rating Scale (CPRS) but not inattention. Research with animal models has led some to believe that stimulants may help. Some physicians have noted improvement in behavior with stimulant therapy but also difficult and unusual side effects.

In a 1997 study from Emory University, researcher Claire Coles examined how children with FAS learn compared to children with ADHD The study compared 122 teens ages 14 and 15 with FAS to a group of 27 teens of he same age with ADHD. According to Coles, children with FAS could focus on tasks, but had trouble using the newly learned information and switching attention to a new task. They had trouble learning new material, but once they did they were as good as anyone else. Children with ADHD could not focus well and keep their attention on things. They could not focus on computer tasks, but the children with FAS were happy with doing the same thing over and over. These differences may explain why drugs such as Ritalin, which help focus attention, do not help children with FAS, who can focus but need help changing focus, according to Coles.

Many children are misdiagnosed. The problem may be FAS, but the children are diagnosed as having ADHD. The difference is that the genetically based ADHD is quite different from the structural brain injuries acquired when the mother drank alcohol during pregnancy. Misdiagnosis leads to treatments that are not correct for either disorder.

Further Readings: Bhatara V. et al. 2006. Association of attention deficit hyperactivity disorder and gestational alcohol exposure: An exploratory study. *Journal of Attention Disorders* 9:515–22; "Drug Exposed Babies or Fetal Alcohol Syndrome vs. ADHD." http://newideas.net/adhd/about-attention-deficit/fas-drug-exposed-adhd. Accessed 7/13/2008; Jones, K. L., and D. W. Smith. 1973. Recognition of the fetal alcohol syndrome in early infancy. *Lancet* 2:1267–71; "Treatment for Fetal Alcohol Syndrome May Be Inappropriate." 1997. http://emory.edu/EMORY_REPORT/erarchive/1997/April/erapril.14/4_14_97 Fetal Accessed 7/13/2008 Wehrspann, Bill. 2006. ADHD related to fetal alcohol syndrome. *Medscape Psychiatry & Mental Health* 11(2).

Focalin and FocalinXR

Focalin and FocalinXR are methylphenidate hydrochloride (MPH) compounds and are registered trade marks of Novartis Pharmaceuticals. Focalin is different from the other compounds in that it is made of just one part MPH and leaves out another part that is inactive and may contribute to side effects. In substances like Ritalin medicines are made of two isomers or forms of the compound; Focalin uses only one of these isomers, allowing the person to use a lower dose of the medicine. However, a 2004 study in the *Journal of the American Academy of Child Psychiatry* concluded that Focalin is as effective and safe as Ritalin but did not show it had superiority in efficacy or safety.

FocalinXR is a once-a-day treatment for ADHD in children, adolescents, and adults. Taken in the morning, it is an effective treatment that starts working quickly and lasts throughout the day. It is available in four strengths: 5-, 10-, 15-, and 20-mg capsules.

Like other MPH preparations, Focalin should not be used if the person has significant anxiety, tension, or agitation, allergies to MPH, glaucoma, tics, Tourette's syndrome, or a family history of Tourette's syndrome. The person should not take a monoamine oxidase inhibitor (MAOI) for 14 days before or 14 days after using Focalin.

The doctor should be informed if there are past or current heart abnormalities or if there is a family history of such conditions. If the person has depression or bipolar disorder or if a family member has a history of psychotic illnesses including suicide, that individual should not take a stimulant drug. Patients with a history of seizures should not take stimulants. Just like other stimulants, abuse of FocalinXR can lead to dependence. *See also* Methylphenidate (MPH).

Further Readings: Wigal, S. 2004. A double-blind, placebo-controlled trial of dexmethyphenicate HCl and d, l-ThreoMPH HCl in children with ADHD. *Journal of the American Academy of Child Adolescent Psychiatry* 43(11):1406–14; Novartis Pharmaceuticals Corporation. "FocalinXR Prescribing Information Sheet." May 2005. http://www.pharma.us.novartis.com/products/name/focalin.jsp. Accessed 5/20/2009.

Food Additives

According to the Food and Drug Administration (FDA), a food additive is a substance or its byproducts that are used to affect the characteristics of a food. They are usually chemicals but do not include spices, seasonings, and flavorings. The additive may become part of the food product directly or indirectly during preparation, storage, or packing. Direct additives are added to a product to preserve or replace a specific feature. Indirect additives are found in tiny amounts and get into foods during growing, storing, and packaging.

About 3,000 additives are used in small amounts to prevent spoilage and extend shelf-life. In America over 10,000 chemical additives are legally approved. Highly processed and packaged foods usually contain the most additives.

Monitoring additives in the food supply is one of the jobs of the FDA. In 1906 the Pure Food and Drug Act was passed, which gave the government control over the safety of the food supply chain. Before this time, food processors used many harmful substances to preserve products. For example, formaldehyde was added to milk; sulfurous acid preserved meat; borax was added to butter. The following is the history of government efforts at regulation of additives:

- 1938. The Food, Drug, and Cosmetic Act gave FDA additional control of ingredients in food and labeling of food.
- 1958. A Food Additives Amendment required manufacturers to prove and additive's safety. Part of this amendment was the Delaney Clause that prohibits additives that cause cancer in humans or animals, even in the tiniest amount.
- 1960. The Color Additive Amendment required prior approval of all dyes used in foods, cosmetics, and drugs. Of 200 of the original additives, only nine were approved.

The FDA has an Adverse Reaction Monitoring System (ARMS) where complaints arising from a particular food additive are investigated. To report an adverse reaction to an additive, FDA in Appendix B, Organizations.

Some studies have shown that additives can cause reactions. Dr. Michael Lyon is a proponent of the new science of functional medicine. He says that because ADHD may be inherited, sensitivities to certain chemicals may fit into this picture. These are not true allergies but are sensitivities that may affect the ability of the liver or other systems to detoxify these chemicals. Therefore, the toxic buildup may affect the behavior adversely. Eliminating these additives may pay great dividends in improved behavior, according to Dr. Lyon.

The following are some of the food additives that some individuals may be sensitive to:

- Sulfites. Sulfites are compounds of sulfur and are used as a preservative in canned vegetables, dehydrated vegetables, dried fruits, peeled and processed potatoes, shrimp, wine, beer, and other processed products. These additives are known to cause adverse reactions in people who are sensitive to them. In 1986 the FDA banned their use on fruits and vegetables to be eaten raw. The Center for Science in the Public Interest (CSPI) is a consumer advocacy group that monitors food safety and questions the safety of additives.

- Artificial sweeteners. Sweeteners such as aspartame, saccharin, and acesulfame K are controversial, and studies are inconclusive. Stevia is a less controversial artificial sweetener that is 200 to 300 times sweeter than sugar and is used in Japan.
- Antioxidants. Antioxidants prevent fats in foods from becoming rancid. Butylated hydroxytoluene (BHT) and butylated hydroxyanisole (BHA) are commonly used antioxidants. The FDA has determined that small amounts are not harmful; however, some people who are sensitive to the substances may develop rashes. Propyl gallate, an antioxidant commonly used with BHA and BHT, may have cancer-causing properties; CSPI recommends avoiding propyl gallate because testing has been inadequate.
- Color enhancers. Food dyes were originally derived from coal-tar oil, but today are made from petroleum. One of the underlying principles of the Feingold Diet is that food dye or coloring could be a source of ADHD. The top six food coloring offenders are Blue No. 1, found in baked goods and candies, Citrus Red 2 used to color the skins of oranges, Green No. 3 used in baked goods; Red No. 3, used in baked goods; Yellow No. 5 (tartrazine), used in cereals and other foods; and Yellow No. 6, found in many processed foods.
- Flavor enhancers. One of the most common flavor enhancers monosodium glutamate (MSG) can cause reactions such as nausea, headaches, sweating, and burning sensations in people who are sensitive. MSG is found in bouillon cubes, hot dogs, frozen foods, instant soup, poultry, restaurant foods, salad dressings, sauce mixes, seafood, stews, and other processed foods.
- Antimicrobial preservatives. Nitrates and nitrites are used a preservatives in processed meats such as bacon, bologna, hot dogs, and corned beef. Nitrites and nitrates contain small amounts of nitrosamines, which are known as cancer-causing agents.
- Fat substitutes. These substances may cause mild to severe cramps and also inhibit the absorption of certain fat-soluble vitamins. These may be found in chips, crackers, and other processed foods.
- Hydrogenated fats. Trans-fatty acids have been recognized as a source of health problems. The substances are found in baked goods, chips, margarine, vegetable shortening, and many processed foods.
- Other additives. Phosphates and potassium bromate are additives that are used in the bread-making process. Sugars, including dextrose and corn syrup, are highly suspected of contributing to ADHD. Other substances that may contribute to ADHD include carrageenan, a derivative of sea weed, and xanthan gum, derived from the fermentation of corn sugar using *Xanthomonas campestris*, a bacterium.

The following is a list of suggestions for avoiding food additives in the diet:

- Eat only fresh, wholesome food such as fresh vegetables, fruits, and whole grains.

- Shop around the edge of the supermarket where the fresh foods, dairy, and meats are found. The aisles with canned goods also have additives and preservatives.
- Learn to read labels to avoid the substances that are questionable.
- Eat fewer foods with labels.
- Eat organically grown fruits and vegetables, organically raised livestock and eggs, and kosher meats.
- When eating out at restaurants, know the additives that may be in foods and ask about them.
- Carry a list of the additives that you want to avoid and refer to it often.

Further Readings: Center for Science in the Public Interest (CSPI). http//www. cspinet.org. Accessed 5/20/2009; Lyon, M. 2000. *Healing the hyperactive brain: Through the new science of functional medicine.* Calgary, AB, Canada: Focused Publishing; Rhodes, Richard. 1998. *Deadly feasts.* New York: Simon & Schuster; Schwartz, George R. 1988. *In bad taste: The MSG syndrome.* Abingdon, UK: Health Press.

Fragile X Syndrome

Fragile X Syndrome (FXS) and ADHD are associated in that many children with FXS also have ADHD. FXS is the most common form of mental retardation and is so called because of the mutation or defect on the X chromosome. Children with FXS usually look much more like each other than their families. They may have a characteristic long face pattern, tooth and jaw misalignment, certain muscle and skeletal abnormalities, and autism. The children often appear normal in infancy but develop typical physical characteristics during their lifetime. They also may have puffy eyes, flat feet, and a hollow chest and be double-jointed. The symptoms do not appear as pronounced in females as males. Because of advances in science and genetic testing, the number of children diagnosed with Fragile X has increased over the last decade. A simple test is available to see if the woman is a carrier of the mutated gene.

The most prevalent behavior of children with Fragile X are attention problems and hyperactivity, similar to those of ADHD. The attention deficit and hyperactivity is frequently treated with medication, generally central nervous system stimulants such as Ritalin or Dexedrine. However, children with FXS appear to have more specific side effects, which include irritability and poor appetite. Amantidine has been especially successful in treating hyperactivity and attention difficulties in children with low IQs. Also children with FXR and ADHD may benefit from a tricyclic antidepressant or major tranquilizer. Some times they experience mood swings and temper tantrums and may need lithium or fluoxetine (Prozac).

A 2008 study showed that L-acetyl carnitine (LAC), a variety of amino acid, may have promise in reducing hyperactive behavior in FXS boys with ADHD. M. Guulia Torrioli and a team in Rome, Italy studied 51 boys between the ages of 6 and 12 with both FXS and ADHD. Subjects had reduced hyperactive behavior and better attention, including no side effects. Patients receiving LAC also increased their sociability.

Children with FXS and ADHD often react strongly to changes in environment, which may increase behavioral difficulties. Because of the hypersensitivity to the environment, they have difficulty screening out light, noise, colors, and odors. FXS is similar to autism in that children may flap their arms, bite their hands, and respond negatively to being touched. However, one difference is that they may be friendly and sociable.

Early intervention is essential in helping children with FXS become integrated into society. Treatment should be tailored to meet each child's specific needs.

Further Readings: "Facts about Fragile X Syndrome." http://www.childdevelopmen tinfo.com/disorders/facts_about_fragile_x_syndrome.htm. Accessed 7/13/2008; "For Boys with Fragile X Syndrome and ADHD, New Hope Found in Non-Stimulant Medication." http://www.medicalnewstoday.com/articles/98191.php. Accessed 7/13/2008; "Fragile X Syndrome." http://www.med.umich.edu/1libr/yourchild/fragileex.htm. Accessed 7/13/2008.

Functional Magnetic Resonance Imaging (fMRI)

Functional magnetic resonance imaging (fMRI) is a new neuroimaging technique that measures tiny metabolic changes in the brain. It is becoming an important tool of choice for learning how normal, diseased, or injured brains are working. fMRI has been used to study the functioning brain of people with ADHD.

Physicians use fMRI to examine the anatomy of the brain and to determine which part of the brain is handling functions such as thought, speech, movement, and sensations. fMRI permits investigators to simultaneously produce high-resolution anatomical images as well as information regarding changes in blood flow between an active and resting brain. The advantage of fMRI compared to PET or SPECT is that it is noninvasive and the subject is not exposed to ionizing radiation.

The technical explanation of the fMRI reveals that images of blood flow are based on the varying magnetic properties between oxyhemoglobin, blood cells that have oxygen, and deoxyhemoglobin, the blood cells that have carbon dioxide and no oxygen. When brain activity is increased beyond a certain threshold, the amount of oxygen in the blood support to that brain region surpasses the amount of oxygen being used. The ratio of oxyhemoglobin to deoxyhemoglobin increases and is detected by the scanner. The method has commonly been referred to as the blood oxygen level–dependent or BOLD technique. A variation of fMRI, T2 relaxometry, has been utilized to evaluate steady-state perfusion of various brain regions over time.

The traditional MRI unit is a large cylindrical tube surrounded by a circular magnet. The person lies on a moveable examination table that slides into the center of the magnet. In an fMRI examination, the person is asked to perform a particular task during the imaging process that causes increased metabolic activity in the area of the brain responsible for the task. The activity, which includes expanding blood vessels, chemical changes, and the delivery of extra oxygen can then be recorded on the MRI images. The person may be asked to perform a variety of small tasks, such as tapping the thumb against each of the fingers on the same hand, rubbing a block of sandpaper, or answering simple questions. The individual must be perfectly still while the images are being recorded in the circular-shaped tube surrounded by a circular magnet.

Further Readings: Gozal, David, and Dennis L. Molfese, eds. 2005. *Attention deficit hyperactive disorder: From genes to patients.* Totowa, NJ: Humana Press; Radiological Society of North America. 2008. "Functional MR Imaging (fMRI)—Brain." http://www. radiologyinfo.org/en/info.cfm?pg=fmribrain&bhcp=1. Accessed 7/13/2008.

G

Gender

Gender comparisons of ADHD suggest that girls and boys with ADHD are quite similar in their symptoms, but girls may manifest somewhat lower levels and are considerably less likely to manifest aggressive behavior. Girls with ADHD have a lower risk of ODD, CD, and acting-out behaviors than boys, although they may show more depression than boys and a somewhat lower levels of intelligence.

According to Barkley (2006), boys are three times more likely to have ADHD than girls and five to nine times more likely than girls to be seen by physicians. Brown et al. (2006) found that girls were more socially withdrawn and had the internalizing symptoms of anxiety and depression than did boys but had similar evaluations on clinical measures of their symptoms.

Individual studies can vary depending on whether the source of the samples is from the clinic or the community, whether the information is from parent, teacher, or tests, and certain characteristics as socioeconomic group and age. Gaub and Carlson (1997) conducted a metaanalysis (a study of all the studies) on gender differences in samples of children with ADHD and concluded there were no gender differences in impulsiveness, academic performance, social functioning, fine motor control, and family factors. Girls were found to be more impaired in their intelligence, less hyperactive, and less likely to demonstrate aggression, defiance, and conduct problems. Evaluations from the community showed that girls were less aggressive. One problem with the studies of gender to date is that they have used only small samples of girls. *See also* Women.

Further Readings: Barkley, Russell. 2006. *Attention-deficit hyperactivity disorder: A handbook for diagnosis and treatment*. 3rd ed. New York: Guilford Press; Brown, T. E. et al. 2006. ADHD gender differences in a clinic-referred sample. In *Attention-deficit hyperactivity disorder: A handbook for diagnosis and treatment*. 3rd ed., edited by Russell Barkley. 108. New York: Guilford Press. Also presented at the annual meeting of the American Academy of Child and Adolescent Psychiatry, New York, October 1989; Gaub, M., and Carlson, C. L. 1997. Gender differences in ADHD: A meta-analysis and critical review. *Journal of the American Academy of Child and Adolescent Psychiatry* 36: 1036–45.

Genetics

In the past decade, several exciting developments in the understanding of the genetic basis of susceptibility to ADHD have emerged. Studying the genetics of ADHD is similar to studying behavior traits, such as alcohol abuse or other addictions. In a given population behaviors vary from those who have opposite tendency to those who exhibit the behavior in the extreme. ADHD is viewed as the extreme of certain behavioral traits that vary genetically throughout the entire population. Some scientists agree that genes predispose one to hyperactive and attention behaviors. However, little research exists into the genetics of people with the disorder.

Researchers now believe that a gene variation associated with ADHD first appeared between 10,000 and 40,000 years ago and was probably a significant advantage to the early humans who had it. Possessors of these traits would have more likely survived the times. Thom Hartman in his book *Attention Deficit Disorder: A Different Perception* writes that people with ADD are the leftover hunters whose ancestors evolved and matured thousands of years in the past in hunting societies. *See* Evolutionary Aspects of ADHD. However, the exact etiology of ADHD is unknown, but a substantial genetic element is implicated in family, twin, and animal studies.

How does one go about finding the genes that are responsible for behaviors? Three ways of looking for genes exist: twin studies, quantitative trait loci (QTL) or family studies, and animal models. Finding a gene for a disease that cannot be traced to a single gene is a challenge. For example, the gene that causes cystic fibrosis has been traced to a single gene. However, many traits, including behaviors, are quite complex, and the necessary studies are difficult to do. Interaction between multiple genes are involved.

Twin Studies

The genome for individual humans is about 99.9 percent identical, in contrast to the great variety among dogs. For example, a Great Dane is very different from a miniature poodle, not only in size but also in basic body functioning. With humans, a relatively less narrow range exists. For behaviors and traits, there is a normal range in which humans fall and just how much is genetic and how much is environment is always debated. Obviously, environment does account for some of the differences in the range of variation in traits.

Studies of identical twins who were raised apart have contributed to the understanding of the effect of genetics and environment. Identical twins, also called monozygotic (MZ) twins, share identical heredity because one sperm from the father fertilizes one egg from the mother. After fertilization the egg splits into two cell masses to from two zygotes that develop into two identical individuals. In contrast, fraternal or dizygotic twins (DZ) are the result of two eggs fertilized by two sperm and are no more alike than other brothers and sisters. Scientists have found in comparing MZ and DZ twins that there is greater similarity between the MZ twins, indicating a genetic effect. The strength of the effect is called heritability.

Several studies of family and twins have shown that parents with ADHD are more likely to have children with ADHD than parents without this diagnosis. In 1995 Levy and Hay studied twins in Australia and found a 91 percent concordance of ADHD in monozygotic or identical twins. Concordance is a term used in genetics to describe a likeness or a match. Several studies worldwide in the early 1990s, including one by Biederman et al., reflected this same 91 percent ratio; dizygotic twins or fraternal twins have a concordance of 30 to 40 percent. A specific study in 2000 showed that children with an identical twin having ADHD are more likely to have it too. The heritability of ADHD is about 80 percent (70–95 percent of trait variation in the population), which is close to the heritability of human height.

Also, a two-way connection between ADHD and depressive disorders in many generations has shown a possible genetic link. Several studies suggest that the incidence of ADHD in offspring of adults with recurrent depression is higher than in the general population and that first-degree relatives of juveniles with ADHD show higher rates of major depressive disorders. Scientists also know mood disorders are highly heritable. In a 2004 twin study, M. J. Rietveld and colleagues found that ADHD is one of the most heritable psychiatric disorders, estimated at 80 percent. Thus the connection between ADHD and mood disorders indicates a genetic component.

Genes involved in the transmission of dopamine, a neurotransmitter, have been reported in people with ADHD. Genes that encode the D2 and D4 dopamine receptors and the dopamine transporter genes appear to show mutations in ADHD. A problem with this approach in studying ADHD is that identical twins discordant for ADHD are rare. Most research suggests that ADHD arises from a combination of various genes, many of which affect dopamine transporters. Suspect genes include the 10-repeat allele of the DAT-1 gene, the 7-repeat allele of the DRD4 gene, and the dopamine beta hydrozylase gene DBH TaqI.

QTL

QTL uses maps of generations to trace and locate various genes. Using the genome of the mouse, researchers have made maps of genes that are common for certain traits. QTL discovery is the first step in identifying genes that influence complex traits. The approach is tedious and is limited by the low precision of the DNA region. Behavioral traits pose special and difficult problems.

To date there have been few QTL association studies in ADHD. Several family studies have investigated the effect of comorbid disorders in ADHD. These studies suggest that relatives of probands with ADHD and comorbid conduct disorder are at greater risk for ADHD than relatives of probands with ADHD alone. The proband is the family member though whom a family's medical history comes to light. For example, a proband might be a baby with Down syndrome; the proband may also be called the index case. Given the difficulty of defining the diagnostic phenotype, more objective measures of behavior are essential. However, advances in gene mapping technology may identify new genes and new neurological targets.

Research to pinpoint the abnormal genes is honing in one two genes: a dopamine-receptor (DRD) gene on chromosome 11 and the dopamine-transported gene (DAT1) on chromosome 5. Several studies have found evidence that children with ADHD have genetic variations in one of the dopamine-receptor genes (DRD4). Several other studies have found abnormalities of the dopamine-transporter gene (DAT1) in children with severe forms of ADHD.

Animal Models

Animal models have become an important tool for understanding the predisposing biological factors for attention deficit and hyperactivity. In animals, attention deficits and hyperactivity have been produced mainly through deprivation models, lesion models, and genetic models.

In deprivation models, rats are reared in social isolation or undergo prolonged parental separation as infants. The social manipulations during the maturation period lead to attention deficits and hyperactivity.

In the lesion approach, the brain is damaged through surgical or toxicological interventions. A number of areas in the brain that are considered to be critical for attention are rendered inoperative, and then the group with lesions is then compared to a normal control group without lesions. X-rays targeted at the hippocampal area are sometimes used to produce the granular cell degeneration and deficits linked to ADHD. However, one problem with these models is that the specific area of the brain that controls certain behaviors is necessary to select the proper target.

Genetic models have also been developed in mice and rats. The system of neurotransmitters, which include dopamine, serotonin, and norepinephrine, has come under scrutiny because studies in neuroimaging have consistently points to chemical pathways in the frontal lobe. Each of these neurotransmitters has candidate genes for genetic analysis.

Molecular biology has provided powerful tools to study genes: transgenic animals. The term transgenic refers to the process of transferring genetic information from one organism to another. By introducing new genetic material into a cell or individual, a transgenic organism is created that has new characteristics that it did not have before. Scientists are able to "knock out" normal genes and "knock in" a gene they may be interested in.

One pair of animal models, the Naples high- and low-excitability rat models, has been used to investigate the neural basis for ADHD. The Naples rats are two genetic strains of the Sprague-Dawley rats developed in Naples, Italy. Scientists studied the rats as they ran mazes, such as the Lat maze, hexagonal tunnel maze, and asymmetric radial arm maze, to determine their low or high activity rate. Rats that were vulnerable to high activity were bred together; those with low activity levels were bred together. When compared to randomly bred rats, the Naples high- and low-excitability rat strains are hyperactive and hypoactive, respectively. The Naples strains did not differ in learning abilities but rather in motor reactivity, frequency of crossings and rearing in mazes, and attention. The Naples high excitability rats model the ADHD plus variant, and the Naples low-excitability rats model ADHD minus variant.

Hyperactive knockout mice can be viewed using the link at the following Web site: http://www.med.yale.edu/chldstdy/plomdevelop/genetics/01febgen.htm. You will need Realplayer software.

Molecular genetic studies have produced evidence for the involvement of dopamine in ADD. The gene encoding the dopamine transporter DAT1 was the initial candidate gene studies. This gene is of particular interest as the principal target for methylphenidate (Ritalin) and other psychostimulant medications. The area of interest is a 40-base pair sequence in an untranslated region of the DAT1 gene found on chromosome 5. Several studies have replicated the location of this gene, but others have not. So despite compelling evidence for a genetic basis for ADHD, the findings to date are not definitive. There are many susceptibility genes, and evidence is emerging that there are many subtypes of ADHD.

Cytochrome oxidase, a mitochondrial enzyme, is a marker of metabolic activity. This chemical is the oxygen-activation enzyme for the function of all plant and animal cells and is the site of the process where energy is conserved for synthesis of ATP, the substance the neurons use for energy. Noted differences in this chemical in specific regions of the cerebral cortex and limbic are noted between the high-excitability and low-excitability strains and the randomly bred rats. Observed prefrontal cortex difference may underlie the differences in goal-directed attention.

Little research has been done on the genetic brain differences in brain differences that predispose certain individuals to ADHD subtypes. Human studies with neuroimaging techniques have reported that certain regions in the prefrontal cortex, basal ganglia, and cerebellum are smaller or show abnormal metabolism in children diagnosed with ADHD. However, it is not possible to tell which of the brain differences may be related to genetic factors, which are the consequences of living with ADHD, and which neural connections correlate with various behavioral responses.

The hunt is on for specific genes for ADHD. The problem is that ADHD is not a single entity, but rather different subtypes that vary dramatically in clinical presentation. These subtypes are related to neuropsychological processes called endophenotypes, which are more closely linked to genes associated with ADHD. Faraone and colleagues (2005) did a metaanalysis of all molecular genetic studies on the heritability of ADHD. A metaanalysis is a study of all the written literature available on a subject; the results are then tabulated statistically as to findings. The researchers found seven genes that are consistently associated as risk factors for ADHD. All seven genes are involved in neurotransmission. A large number of people with ADHD do not have these risk alleles and many people with without ADHD may have the alleles. . However, people with one of these alleles are highly likely to develop ADHD. According to Kollins, genetic factors are clearly most strongly associated with the development of ADHD, but it is not a foregone conclusion that if parents have ADHD, the children will have it but the odds are increased dramatically. Unfortunately, scientists do not know who is going to have the disorder and who is not.

New research into the role of the serotonin system is emerging. *See also* Serotonin. The research into the molecular genetics involved in the transmission of ADHD across generations will continue as more sophisticated techniques in the area develop. Such research offers promise for eventual diagnostics such as genetic tests for ADHD, for subtyping ADHD, and for research into pharmacological agents for treating ADHD.

Further Readings: Faraone, S. V. et al. 2005. Advances in Genetic and Neurobiology Update. *Biological Psychiatry* 57:1313–23; Gonzalez-Lima, F. 2005. Cortical and limbic systems mediating the predisposition to attention deficit and hyperactivity. In: *Attention deficit hyperactivity disorder research,* edited by Michelle P. Larimer, 1–18. New York: Nova Science Publishers; Hartmann, Thom. 1997. *Attention deficit disorder: A different perception.* Grass Valley, CA: Mythical Intelligence Press; Kirley, Aiveen. 2005. Scanning the genome for attention deficit hyperactive disorder. In *Attention deficit hyperactive disorder: From Gene to patients,* edited by David Gozal and Dennis Molfese. Totawa, NJ: Humana Press, 2005; Kollins, S. H. et al. 2005. ADHD and Smoking. *Archives of General Psychiatry* 62:1142–47; Rietveld, M. J. et al. 2004. Heritability of attention problems in children: Longitudinal results from a study of twins, age 3 to 12. *Journal of Child Psychology and Psychiatry* 45:577–88.

Giftedness

Many intellectually gifted children exhibit behaviors similar to ADHD. It may be possible for children to be gifted with ADHD, and the dangers of misdiagnosis are possible when the evaluation is not thorough. According to the research by Cramond (1995), the most important distinctions between the child with ADHD and the gifted child are the situation and variability of task performance. Activities of children with ADHD tend to be both continual and random; gifted children actions are more episodic and directed to specific goals. Children with ADHD are inconsistent in almost all tasks in all settings, except television or computer games. Gifted children may do well in classes that are enjoyable and challenging.

The gifted child may be deemed as inattentive or bored. Described as hyperactive, the child may have high energy. When considered difficult, the gifted child may question authority. Researchers have found several differences exist between gifted children and nongifted children with ADHD. For example, Kaufman et al. (2000) found that gifted children with ADHD are more impaired than other ADHD children. Obviously, educators and parents may miss gifted children with milder forms of ADHD. High ability can mask ADHD because attention deficits and restlessness tend to make test scores lower. When targeting children for a gifted program, schools rely on certain tests; the gifted child with ADHD may be distracted and not perform well on these test. Likewise, teachers may focus on the disruptive behaviors or gifted ADHD students and fail to see their ability. Moon (2002) believes that gifted children who are not recognized and who do not receive appropriate services are later at risk for developing learned helplessness and chronic underachievement.

Barkley (2006) states that as a group ADHD children tend to lag two to three years behind their age peers in social and emotional maturity, and gifted children are no exception. However, Niehart et al. (2002) found that as a group, gifted children without ADHD tend to be more similar in their cognitive, social, and emotional development to children two to four years

Gifted with ADHD

Michael Kearney, who graduated from college at the age of 10, was diagnosed as a toddler with ADHD and prescribed Ritalin. His parents declined medication and decided to nurture Michael's genius with education. He started school at the age of 3, entered junior college at 6, and graduated from the University of South Alabama at the age of 10. His father Kevin refused the notion that his inattention is due to lack of attention and believed that actually he has an attention surplus. The fact that Michael was so much faster than the average and has usually figured out what you are going to say in 2 seconds makes him look like he is not paying attention, and it drives teachers crazy.

Source: LD Research Foundation. http://www.ldrfa.org/?pID=34. Accessed 6/18/2009.

older than children their own age. According to Niehart, the research shows that lack of intellectual challenge and little access to others with similar interests, ability, and drive are often risk factors for gifted children and contributes to social and emotional problems.

The gifted student with ADHD exists between two worlds. A bright individual is more self-aware and is likely to perceive himself as inadequate. If the task is repetitive or below the student's achievement level, he will tune out and miss vital information. When engaged, the same student can perform brilliantly. Teachers may interpret this as laziness. Depending on the state, gifted students who are identified with ADHD may qualify for a 504 plan and an IEP for special services and accommodations.

Further Readings: Barkley, Russell. 2006. *Attention-deficit hyperactivity disorder: A handbook for diagnosis and treatment.* 3rd ed. New York: Guilford Press; Cramond, Bonnie. 1995. "The Coincidence of Attention Deficit Hyperactive Disorder and Creativity." http://www.borntoexplore.org/adhd.htm. Accessed 6/29/2008; He@lth Consumer. "Gifted Children with ADHD." http://www.athealth.com/consumer/disorders/adhdgifted.html. Accessed 5/20/2009; Kaufman, F. et al. 2000. *Attention deficit disorder and gifted students: What do we know?* Storrs, CT: National Research Center on Gifted and Talented, University of Connecticut; Moon, S. 2002. Gifted children with attention deficit/hyperactivity disorder. In *The social and emotional development of gifted children: What do we know?* edited by M. Niehart et al., 193–204. Waco, TX: Prufrock Press; Niehart, M. et al. 2002. *The social and emotional development of gifted children: What do we know?* Waco, TX: Prufrock; Watkins, Carol. 2006. "The Gifted Student with ADD: Between Two Worlds." http://www.ncpamd.com/Gifted_ADD.htm. Accessed 5/20/2009.

Guanfacine

Unlike other ADHD medications that work indirectly in the prefrontal cortex, guanfacine works directly as it binds specifically to the alpha-2A adrenergic cell receptors in the prefrontal cortex. The prefrontal cortex is the area of the brain associated with executive function, behavioral inhibition, regulation of attention, distractibility, impulsivity, and frustration tolerance.

The selective alpha-2A agonist strengthens working memory and assists firing of the neurons in the prefrontal cortex. Guanfacine is not a controlled substance and does not appear to have a known mechanism for potential abuse of dependence.

Tenex, a formulation of guanfacine, is an orally administered centrally acting antihypertensive agent that may confer less of a risk of sedation and hypotensive effects than clonidine. Clinicians have been increasing their use of guanfacine in treating ADHD. It may be considered for children older that 7 years or adolescents with ADHD or other comorbid conditions after treatment with established medications such as stimulants or antidepressants.

In May 2008, Shire Pharmaceuticals announced findings from analyses of pivotal trials of INTUNIV, a once-daily formulation of guanfacine that provides a steady delivery of drug throughout the day and is designed to minimize the fluctuations between peak and trough concentrations as seen with immediate release guanfacine. In Phase III clinical trials all patients treated with INTUNIV showed significantly greater improvement on rating scales than the group receiving placebo. Safety data showed that adverse events reported were generally mild and moderate, with the most common complaint being the feeling of sedation.

Further Reading: "Shire Investigational Nonstimulant INTUNIV Showed Significant Efficacy in Reducing ADHD Symptoms. http://www.medicalnewstoday.com/articles/106801.php. Accessed 5/28/2008.

H

Hearing Loss and ADHD

Many children who are diagnosed with ADHD may have a common hearing disorder. According to Dr. Fred Bess, Vanderbilt Medical Center, five million school-aged children or 11.3 percent of all school children in the United States show some degree of hearing impairment. Dr. Bess found that 5.4 percent of children in schools have "minimal sensorineural hearing loss" (MSHL) that may go unrecognized. At the same time ADHD is the most commonly diagnosed behavioral disorder in childhood. Dr. Bess believes the two problems—ADHD and MSHL—overlap and are easily confused when children are observed.

Children who are deaf or hard of hearing may have ADHD, just like other children, but hearing difficulties may cause the child to appear inattentive, bored, and unable to focus. A recent study by an audiologist compared children with ADHD and MSHL. Both groups have academic difficulty and give inappropriate responses to questions. Neither group completed assignments and had trouble listening to oral presentations. Following directions was a problem. Both groups exhibited low self-esteem and tended to repeat grades.

In young children a common type of hearing loss called conductive hearing loss is generally correctable through medical and surgical options. Conductive hearing losses include broken eardrums, middle ear infections, ear fungus, or other hearing problems that may block the path of sound. Researchers have determined that 50 percent of children between birth and 5 years of age will experience a conductive hearing loss. Another study from the American Academy of Audiology noted that about 80 percent of elementary students suffer temporary hearing loss at sometime during the school year. These losses were generally undetected by parents and teachers.

A test called the Screening Instrument for Targeting Educational Risk (SIFTER) can diagnose the problem. Unfortunately, comprehensive audiologic evaluations are often not part of ADHD/ADD protocols.

Further Reading: Ulrich, Margie. "ADHD/ADD or Hearing Loss?" http://www.health articles.org/adhd_add_hearing_loss_071304.html. Accessed 8/9/2008.

Heart Disease and Cardiovascular Problems

ADHD may relate to the cardiovascular system in several instances. Heart disease and cardiovascular problems affect the blood and oxygen flow to the brain, causing defective blood vessels that can affect behavior. Some heart and cardiovascular problems can cause behaviors that mimic ADHD. Psychostimulants commonly prescribed to children with ADHD have been effective in controlling the symptoms in many children. However, these stimulants do have known and well-described cardiovascular effects on blood pressure and pulse in particular. In August 2006, amphetamine-based drugs such as Adderall and Dexedrine had a new, expanded black box warning for increased risk of sudden death in patients with heart problems. The FDA panel had considered putting the warning on all stimulant drugs that treat ADHD but stopped short because the members did not agree on the warnings.

Robert Findling (2008), Director of Child and Adolescent Psychiatry at Case Western Research University in Cleveland, has expressed concern that a group of youngsters who may have undetected cardiovascular disease and for whom stimulants may put a greater risk for heart disease. Findling suggests several aspects of patient history to observe:

- Does the child have a history of dizziness or fainting or shortness of breath with exertion?
- Does the child have irregularities in pulse and blood pressure?
- Is there a family history of sudden cardiac death, dysrhythmias, Wolff-Parkinson-White syndrome, or long QT syndrome?
- Is the child taking other medications that might interact to cause problems?

Some doctors propose that youngsters undergo an electrocardiogram (ECG) before the initiation of stimulant treatment. This proposal is controversial. In April 2008, the American Heart Association recommended that physicians order an ECG after diagnosing the ADHD and before administering stimulants. The main position for this assertion is that it is better to be safe than sorry. Proponents quote the 2003 statistics that an estimated 2.5 million children in the United States took medication for ADHD. Surveys show that about 33 to 42 percent of cardiac patient have ADHD; up to 2 percent of healthy school-aged children have potentially serious undiagnosed conditions identified by ECG.

Others argue that the procedure is not really necessary for all children and it will frighten people away from therapy. Also they are concerned with the effects of the EKG on those that have no cardiovascular symptoms.

Further Readings: Findling, Robert. 2008. "AHA Recommendations on Cardiovascular Monitoring in Patients with ADHD and Heart Disease." Medscape Psychiatry and Health. http://www.medscape.com/viewarticle/574540_print. Accessed 8/11/2000, Hitti, Miranda. 2006. "New Heart Alert for Some ADHD Drugs." http://www.webmd.com/add-adhd/news/2006822/geart-alert-adhd-drugs. Accessed 8/11/2008; Hughes, Sue. 2008. "Children with ADHD Should Have ECG before Taking Stimulant Drugs." http://www.theheart.org/article/858823.do. Accessed 8/11/2008.

Herbal Medicine

One of the most popular alternative therapies for ADHD is use of herbal medicines or phytotherapy. Since the beginning of time, herbal medicine has been used in healing. Not only have plants provided food, but they have also been used in treatment for different kinds of disorders. A person who treats individuals with plants is called an herbalist. Herbalists, like other complementary therapists, seek to treat people rather than just diseases. As a complementary or alternative therapy, herbal therapy includes a host of treatments that are not part of Western medicine or scientific or evidence-based medicine.

According to herbalists, the following plants are helpful:

- Ginkgo (*Ginkgo biloba*) helps increase cerebral blood flow and is reputed to restore memory and increase concentration and focus. Ginkgo brings greater oxygenation to the brain and improves brain flow metabolism.
- Brahmi (*Bacopa monniera*) is an Ayurvedic herb with a long history as a brain enhancer. It supposedly protects the brain from free radical damage while stimulating improved learning and cognitive function.
- Siberian ginseng (*Eleutherococcus senticosis*) helps modulate stress reactions by stimulating brain activity and causing a release of body energy.
- Goto kola (*Centella asiatica, Hydrocotyle asiatica*) are herbs that reduce corticosterone blood levels during stress and are helpful for nervous disorders and vascular problems of the brain. This herb should not be confused with the caffeine containing Kola nut.
- Green oats (*Avena sativa*) are fresh green seeds that are a mild antispasmodic and nourishing nerve tonic.
- St. John's Wort (*Hypericum perforatum*) is an anti-inflammatory sedative used for depression, fear, insomnia, anxiety or feelings of worthlessness.
- Kava kava (*Piper methisticum*) is a sedative, hypnotic, and antispasmodic used to relieve tension headaches, insomnia, and ADHD. Unlike most sedatives, users claim they can still perform cognitive functions.
- Skullcap (*Scutellaria lateriflora*) is a sedative and cerebral vasodilator used for insomnia, restless sleep, agitation, nervous exhaustion, and nervous system weakness after prolonged illness.
- Cat's claw aids the immune system and decreases gut permeability to certain peptides that can trigger allergic responses in the brain.
- Valerian root calms and relaxes nervous tension.
- Chamomile (*Matricaria recutita*) has a calming effect especially on babies and small children.
- Echinacea stimulates properties that protect against illnesses that could disrupt intestinal function.
- Aloe vera reduces toxins that affect the intestines and the brain.

People must never self-medicate with herbs; combining them requires a certain degree of knowledge and skill. The advice of a trained and experienced herbalist is essential for those who seek complementary strategies.

Further Readings: Cooper, Paul, and Katherine Bilton. 1999. *ADHD: Research, practice and opinion.* London: Whurr Publishers; Dye, John M., N. D. "ADHD Treatments: Herbal Medicine." 2000. http://www.healing-arts.org/children/ADHD/herbal.htm. Accessed 7/20/2008.

History of ADHD

Early History

ADHD is not just a fad that has been created in the latter half of the 20th century. It is documented in history. In 493 B.C. Hippocrates, the great physician on the Greek island of Cos, described a condition in patients who had quick sensory experience and whose souls moved quickly on to the next impression. Believing that an imbalance of the four humors—water, fire, earth, and air—cause all diseases, Hippocrates attributed this condition to an over-balance of fire over water. He recommended a diet of barley rather than wheat bread and fish rather than meat; adding water, drinks, and natural and diverse physical activities were also recommended.

William Shakespeare, the famous British writer and poet, was a keen observer of behavior. He described how King Henry VIII had a serious malady of attention.

Thom Hartmann in his book *Attention Deficit Disorder: A Different Perception* proposes that ADD is a genetic disease that represents evolutionary survival strategies. Sickle cell disease, Tay-Sachs disease, and cystic fibrosis developed to protect people against certain diseases that were prevalent at the time. Hartmann argues that the attention deficit gene enabled those people in a hunting society to survive. The hunters have certain attributes, such as constantly monitoring the environment, thinking visually, and loving action, but hating mundane work; those characteristics made them successful. A failure to have the characteristics might have meant death in the forest.

History is full of references to people fitting the pattern of symptoms of inattention, restlessness, hyperactivity, and impulsivity. Hartmann said that in medieval Europe they possibly would be burned at the stake for being touched by demons. Native Americans might have elevated the person to greatness as a medicine man or shaman. He also questions what would have happened in history if Thomas Edison, Benjamin Franklin, Nostradamus, George Fredrick Handel, Salvatore Dali, Wolfgang Mozart, Ernest Hemingway, or Van Gogh had been medicated back to "normal."

As early as the 17th century, the philosopher John Locke described a perplexing group of young students who, try as hard as they could, would not keep their minds from straying. Abraham Lincoln's third son Tad was a holy terror in the White House, often chasing his brother through the Oval Office. Tad was reported to have major learning problems.

The German physician Heinrich Hoffman wrote one of the first references to a child with hyperactivity. In 1845 he penned a group of poems about the childhood problems that he saw in his practice; he called his character Fidgety Phil. Fidgety Phil did all the annoying things that one sees in a hyperactive individual, including leaning back in his chair and eventually pulling the table cloth off the table, causing all the food to land on the floor. *See also* Hoffman, Heinrich, and Sidebar 14.

History of ADHD Timeline

Concepts of ADHD have changed throughout the years. Even the name has changed from attention deficit disorder in the first DSM-III-R Manual to attention-deficit hyperactivity disorder in DSM-IV-R. The following timeline shows some of the major events in the history of ADHD.

495 B.C.	Hippocrates describes a conditions in which people move quickly from one thing to another
1845	Dr. Heinrich Hoffman writes about Fidgety Phil.
1902	Dr. George Still describes the first clinical ADHD-like behaviors; ADHD is considered a defect of moral control.
1908	Dr. Arthur Tredgold builds on Still's ideas and stresses the need for special education.
1918	The great influenza epidemic leaves survivors who had encephalitis with ADHD-like behaviors.
1937	Dr. Bradley found amphetamines helped hyperactive children.
1956	Ritalin (methyphenidate) is introduced for narcolepsy
End 1950s	It was generally accepted that hyperactivity was the result of brain damage called minimal brain disorder (MBD).
1960	Stella Chess proposed the "hyperactive child syndrome" and separated this from the idea of MBD.
1968	Hyperkinetic reaction of childhood is mentioned in DSM-II.
1969	Conners developed the first rating scale.
1970s	Research took a great leap with more than 2,000 studies, texts, and journal articles on the subject.
1970s	Two diverse models developed. Wender continued the idea of MBD; Douglas believed that sustained attention was the main problem and designed the first battery of tests.
1970	B. F. Skinner develops behavioral modification.
1975	Dr. Feingold proposes that ADHD is the result of eating food and dyes that cause allergies and develops a diet.
1975	Passage of PL-94-142 for special education for students with disabilities.
End 1970s	Interest in adult ADHD develops.
1980	Attention deficit disorder with or without hyperactivity is in DSM-III.
1990s	Decade of the brain ushers in neuroimaging, genetics, and other studies.
1994	Attention-deficit hyperactivity disorder is in DSM-IV.
1996	FDA approves Adderall for treatment of ADHD.
2002	Strattera is approved.
2007	Vyvanse (methyphenidate) patch is approved.

Two Early Pioneers: George Still and Alfred Tredgold

The first serious scientific studies of the phenomenon of inattention and hyperactivity are generally credited to George Still and Alfred Tredgold. In a series of three published lectures to the Royal College in 1902, Still described 43 children in his practice who had serious sustained attention problems. He referred to the philosopher/educator William James who said that paying attention is an important element in the classroom for the "moral control of behavior." The children that Still described were often aggressive, defiant, resistant to discipline, and excessively emotional or passionate. According to Still, they showed little inhibitory control over their behavior and were also lawless, spiteful, cruel, and dishonest. They were insensitive to punishment and might continue a behavior, even though they were physically disciplined for it.

Still was convinced that these children displayed a major "defect in moral control" in their behavior and that they had perhaps acquired the condition as a secondary effect of an acute brain disease. He found the condition in 23 of his cases of children who were mentally retarded, but it also appeared in 20 children of near-normal intelligence. Some chronic cases developed into criminals, although not all. He concluded that a defect in moral control arose from three district impairments:

- A defect of cognitive relation to the environment
- A defect of moral consciousness
- A defect in inhibitory volition

Still observed that a greater proportion exist in males compared to females (3:1), and most cases appear before the age of 8. He observed that many of his patients had abnormal physical appearances, such as an abnormally large heads, malformed palates, or increased epicanthic folds over the eyelids. He called these deformities the "stigmata of degeneration." These children had more accidents and were a threat to the safety of other children because of their aggressive or violent behavior. A study of their biological family trees showed the relatives displayed more alcoholism, criminality, and affective disorders such as depression.

According to Still's observations, some of the children displayed a history of brain damage or convulsions. A few had associate tic disorders or "microkinesia"; this was the first time ADHD was possibly connected to comorbid conditions.

The family life of the children with hyperactivity played an important part in the development of Still's theories. Many of the children came from chaotic families, but others came from parents who seemingly tried to give the children a good upbringing. Still believed that when poor child rearing was involved, the children should be exempt from the category of lack of moral control; that belief was reserved for those who were raised in good families but still displayed morbid failure. For the children with good raising, he proposed possibly a hereditary condition or possibly pre- or postnatal brain injuries. He hypothesized that deficits in inhibition, moral control, and attention were all related to each other and to the same underlying neurological deficit. He also speculated about a syndrome where intellect was dissociated from the will and that condition might be a result of nerve cell modification. He also believed that temporary improvements might be found with changes in the environment or by using medications.

Alfred Tredgold in 1908 built on Still's idea that undetected damage accounted for the late-arising behavioral and learning deficiencies. Both of the physicians believed that the defect was permanent but could be helped by changes in the environment and possibly by medications. They strongly stressed the need for special educational environments. However, it would be 70 years before their ideas would take hold; the psychoanalytic and behavioral views overemphasized poor child rearing as largely causing such behavior disorders in children. Today, the children that Still and Tredgold described probably would be not only classified with ADHD but also with oppositional defiant disorder and most likely a learning disability.

History From 1920 to 1950

The Great Influenza Pandemic of 1918 resulted in 650,000 deaths in North America. There were many complications of the flu that resulted in pneumonia and a brain disease called encephalitis. It was noted that many of the children who survived encephalitis had serious behavioral and cognitive deficits. Three papers by Ebaugh, Strecker, and Stryker appeared in the mid-1920s, which described children with symptoms that are currently ascribed to ADHD. The children were described as inattentive, impulsive, disorganized, memory deficient, and often socially disruptive. The condition was called "postencephalitic behavior disorder" and was clearly he result of brain damage. Many of the children were recommended for care outside of the home, and in spite of the view that these children were hopeless, some improved with simple behavior modification and increased supervision.

Origins of Brain-Damage Syndrome

When the encephalitis epidemic appeared to cause changes in behavior manifestations, investigators explored the possibility of other causes of brain injury. In 1936, a study associated head trauma to attention deficit. This investigation led to later studies such as a 1938 study relating inattention and hyperactivity to epilepsy, a 1943 study relating the condition to lead toxicity, and a 1953 study correlating with measles. Terms describing the conditions during this era were "organic driveness" and "restlessness" syndrome. Many of the children in these studies had mental retardation, obvious brain damage, and more serious behavior problems than those associated today with ADHD, and decades elapsed before investigators began to separate the ideas of intellectual delay, learning disabilities, or other neurological deficits from those of the maladjustment in these children in earlier studies.

During this era researchers began to notice the striking similarity between hyperactivity in children and the behavior of primates with frontal lobe lesions. Some investigators had studied the frontal lobes of monkeys for more than 60 years, beginning when Ferrier published his study in 1876. He noted that the lesions in the frontal lobe resulted in excessive restlessness, poor ability to sustain interest in activities, aimless wandering, and excessive appetite. Levin in 1938 postulated that severe restlessness in children could be the result of defects in the forebrain structures, although he had little evidence to back up this conjecture. During this era, mild forms of ADHD were thought to be the result of poor parenting, which caused spoiled children, or of poor environment. This idea of poor parenting was resurrected in the 1970s and remains today among many lay people and critics of ADHD.

In the decade of the 1940s children who were hospitalized in facilities and who demonstrated attention deficit symptoms were assumed to have brain damage whether there was any evidence to support this idea. Strauss and Lehninen published a study using the term "brain-injured child" and applied it to those with problem behaviors. They even argued that the behavior was evidence of brain damage. In their classic text, these researchers recommended placing these children in smaller, more carefully regulated classrooms and reducing the amount of stimulation in the environment. For example, in this sterile and austere classroom, teachers could wear no jewelry or brightly colored clothing, and no pictures could be on the wall to distract students. This text was used as a guide to special education services adopted later in U.S. public schools. Many of the guidelines recommended in this text were incorporated into the initial Education for All Handicapped Children Act of 1975 (PL 94-142) mandating special education for children with learning disabilities and behavioral disorders and later in the Americans with Disabilities Education Act of 1990.

The Rise of Drugs for ADHD

In the 1930s some researchers used pneumoencephalograms to study the brains of disruptive youths. This procedure involved injecting air into the brain and then using electrodes to trace brain patterns. To counteract headaches as a result of the experiments, the researchers gave the children drugs, especially amphetamines. They noted that both behavior and academic performance improved. In 1937 Dr. Bradley of Providence, Rhode Island, reported that a group of children with behavioral problems improved after being treated with stimulant medications. Later studies in the 1950s confirmed a positive response in half or more of hyperactive children when given amphetamines. Ritalin was first produced in 1950 and was initially used to treat narcolepsy, chronic fatigue, and depression and to counter the effects of other medications. By the 1970s stimulant medications were becoming the treatment of choice for behavioral symptoms now associated with ADHD. In 1996, the FDA approved a second medication, Adderall, for the treatment of ADHD.

The 1950s and The Emerging Hyperkinetic Syndrome

In the 1950s standards for human experimentation were not the same as they are in the 21st century. Many of the experiments today would be considered unusual and definitely not acceptable medical procedures. In the early 1950s Laufer and colleagues performed a study of the effects of the "photo-Metrozol" method, in which a drug metronidazole (Metrozole) were administered to a child and then lights were flashed before the eyes. The researcher compared the amount of drug required to induce a muscle jerk of the forearms, as the spike wave brain pattern was measured on an electroencephalogram. The study found that children with hyperactivity required less Metrazole to evoke a response than those without hyperactivity. The finding suggested that hyperactive children had a lower threshold for stimulation, possibly in the thalamic area. This study has never been replicated, and it would probably never pass an institutional review board for human experimentation. However, the study was a milestone in the history of the disorder because it indicated that a specific mechanism such as low cortical thresholds or over stimulation might give rise to the disorder. By the end of the 1950s it was generally accepted that hyperactivity was a brain-damage syndrome, even when there was no evidence of actual damage.

The Period 1960 to 1969

In the late 1950s and 1960s critical reviews appeared questioning the concept of brain damage in those who displayed only the symptoms of hyperactivity. The idea of minimal brain disorder (MBD) was scrutinized. In 1966, a task force from the National Institute of Neurological Diseases and Blindness questioned applying the idea of brain damage and found at least 99 symptoms for the disorder. They proclaimed the idea as vague, over-inclusive, or of little or no prescriptive value. The term "minimal brain disorder" would die a slow death and be replaced by more specific and observable terms, such as dyslexia, language disorders, learning disabilities, and hyperactivity, designated "minimal brain dysfunction."

In 1960 Stella Chess urged researchers to focus on hyperactivity and defined the hyperactive child as one who carries out activities at a rate of speed that is higher than the normal rate of the average child or as one who is constantly in motion or both. Chess described the characteristics of 36 children from her practice that included 881 children and found that males outnumbered females in a ratio of 4 to 1. The children were referred before age 6, and educational difficulties were common. She also noted impulsive, aggressive behavior, and poor attention span. However, she maintained that the condition was relatively benign and that most children would outgrow it, but the ideas were important for the following four reasons:

1. Activity became the defining feature.
2. Objective evidence was considered beyond just the subjective reports of parents and teachers.
3. Blame was taken away from the parents.
4. The idea of hyperactivity was separated from the concept of brain damage.

In 1968, an important development in treatment occurred that seemed insignificant at the time. The second edition of the Diagnostic and Statistical Manual (DSM-II; American Psychiatric Association) added Chess's designation "hyperkinetic reaction of childhood" to its list of disorders. It used only one sentence to state that the disorder is characterized by restlessness, distractibility, overactivity, and short attention span, especially in young children. Taking the clue from Chess, writers of the manual stated that hyperkinetic disorder is a benign disorder that usually diminishes by adolescence.

By the end of this decade the prevailing idea was that hyperkinetic disorder was no longer ascribed to brain damage but instead, the focus was on brain mechanisms. The symptoms included a higher activity level than those displayed by a normal child. The condition was considered benign, with interventions to include short-term treatment with stimulant medications until it was outgrown in puberty. Classrooms were to provide little stimulation.

The Decade of the 1970s

During the 1970s research into hyperactivity took a great leap. More than 2,000 studies, clinical and scientific textbooks, and special journal issues were published. The topic was becoming an important subject in the scientific, educational, and lay communities. The defining features of hyperactivity were broadened to include attention span, low frustration tolerance, and aggressiveness. However, some researchers persisted with the concept of MDB, which included motor clumsiness, cognitive impairments, and parent-child conflict.

Two diverse models of ADHD emerged: the model supported by of Paul Wender and the one of Virginia I. Douglas. Paul Wender insisted that the essential psychological characteristics of children with MBD consisted of six clusters of symptoms:

1. Motor behavior
2. Attention and perceptual-cognitive functioning
3. Learning
4. Impulse control
5. Interpersonal relations
6. Emotion

Many of the ideas that Still first developed were echoed by Wender.

The second was the model of Douglas, which included attention and impulse control in hyperactive children. At the Canadian Psychological Association in 1972, Virginia Douglas presented the presidential keynote address, which has become of historical importance in ADHD studies. She argued that deficits in sustained attention and impulse control were more likely than just hyperactivity to cause difficulty for students. She presented a thorough battery of objective measures of various behavioral and cognitive domains that had never been used before in research on ADHD. She did not believe that students with ADHD necessarily had more reading or other difficulties than other children, did not manifest right-left discrimination patterns, and had no difficulties with short-term memory. Douglas and the McGill University team found that hyperactive children had their greatest difficulties on sustained attention, such as continuous-performance tests, which lasted for several hours. One of her colleagues Gabrielle Weiss later found that although some of the problem may disappear as the children go through adolescence, many of the problems persist through life. *See also* Wender, Paul; Douglas, Virginia I.

Other Historical Developments in the 1970s

Several other important historical developments arose in the 1970s including the rise of medication therapy, the environment as a cause, development in assessments, passage of Public Law 94-142, the rise of behavior modification, the focus on psychophysiology, and an emerging interest in adult ADHD.

Use of medication therapy in this decade developed rapidly. Numerous studies showed that hyperactive children could benefit from the use of stimulants. The development of rigorous methodology in scientific research was also seen. More than 120 studies were published through 1976; use of medications in ADHD was quickly becoming the best-studied therapy in child psychiatry. With the use of stimulants came criticism both from within and without the profession that drugs were being overused. These reports prompted a Congressional review the use of psychotropic drugs for school children.

As a backlash against the use of drugs for behavior problems, the belief that hyperactivity was the result of environmental causes arose. This idea coincided with the popular interest in health goods, extending life expectancy, psychoanalytic theory, and behaviorism. Benjamin Feingold (1974) saw hyperactivity as a result of allergic or toxic reactions to food additive, dyes, and preservatives. These views became widespread. A National Advisory Committee on Hyperkinesis and Food Additives (1980) convened to review the evidence of Feingold's claims and did not support his claims. The idea remains popular among certain groups; however, the main thrust now is to focus on sugar as a cause of hyperactivity. *See also* Feingold, Benjamin F.; Food Additives.

Another side of the environmental view was that of poor child rearing and poor child behavior management. Both the psychoanalysts and behaviorists supported this view for different reasons. Psychoanalysts said that parents who tolerated negative behavior in their infants would react with an outlook that encouraged hyperactivity in their developing children. Behaviorists stressed that poor conditioning of children to stimulus control and instruction could give rise to noncompliant behavior. Both groups singled out mothers as the causal connection.

A second trend that developed in the 1970s was that of the use of behavior modification. Educational interventions that were originally developed for children with mental disabilities were adapted to other areas, including management of the regular classroom. Behavior modification is based on the work of B. F. Skinner and uses rewards and consequences to manage children. Although the method is somewhat effective, it has not been shown to be as effective as stimulant control. However, most of current thinking is that training parents and teachers in behavior modification, along with stimulant medication gives a comprehensive management approach for the disorder. *See also* B. F. Skinner in Behavior Modification.

A third hallmark of this era was the development of parent and teacher rating scales. In 1969 C. Keith Conners developed the Conners Rating Scale for the assessment of symptoms of hyperactivity. These scales became the gold standard for rating children for clinical and research use, but would later be criticized for pairing hyperactivity with aggression. However, the creation of the scales was a historic milestone in the analysis and treatment of ADHD.

Passage of Public Law 94-142

An important development was the passage of PL 94-142 in 1975 mandating special educational services for physical, learning, and behavioral disabilities of children, in addition for those services available for children with mental retardation. This law gave financial incentives for states that adopted the law and encouraged immediate implementation by all of them.

The decade also saw advances in a number of studies that sought to correlate physical and mental responses. Studies measuring electrical skin responses, heart rate acceleration and deceleration, brain waves, pupil responses, and other physical responses were correlated with over- or under-arousal of the central nervous system. Many of these studies were flawed in methodology and had contradictory findings but possibly served to put to rest the idea of the over stimulated cerebral cortex as the cause of the symptoms in hyperactivity.

A last area of importance was the emerging interest in adult hyperactivity. Initial interest is traced back to the latter part of the 1960s with the publication of several studies demonstrating the persistence of hyperactivity/MBD into adulthood. Such observations would be quite prophetic as research in the next 20 years would show.

The 1970s closed with several views on the table: hyperactivity was not the only behavioral deficit, but poor attention and impulsivity were also important. Brain damage was seen as playing a very minor role. Environmental causes, especially related to diet, pollutants, and child rearing were presented as alternative treatments for pharmaceutical treatment. Special education programs grew as a result of consciousness and law. American professionals tended to view the disorder a common, in need of medication; Europeans continued to believe that the disorder was uncommon and defined by several over activity and associated with brain damage.

The Period 1980 to 1989

This period began with the publication of DSM-III (American Psychiatric Association, 1980) with a major change from DSM-II. This manual changed the concept from Hyperkinetic Reaction of Childhood to ADD with or without hyperactivity. The new diagnostic criteria emphasized inattention and impulsivity as defining features of the disorder and produced a more specific symptoms list.

This decade is characterized by an increase in research on hyperactivity that began in the 1970s. More books, conferences, and scientific papers appeared during this decade than in any other previous historical period. The period would end with serious challenges to the idea that attention deficit is the core behavioral problems with ADHD.

The following important advances developed during this decade:

- Development of research diagnostic criteria. With the development of DSM-III, others were assessing development of specific diagnostic criteria. Discussion of ADD+H and ADD-H (with and without hyperactivity) became prevalent. There was a drive to determine more specific descriptions of the condition. Efforts led to an international symposium in 1988 to develop a general consensus that research on ADHD should have the following criteria:

  1. Reports on behavior from adults should be from at least two settings, such as home, school, or clinic
  2. Endorsement of at least three of four difficulties with activity and three of four with attention
  3. Onset behavior before age of 7
  4. Duration of at least 2 years
  5. Significantly elevated scores on parent/teacher ratings of ADHD symptoms
  6. Exclusion of autism and psychosis

- Subtyping of ADD. Also important in this era was the development of useful subtypes.
- ADD becomes ADHD. Late in the 1980s the DSM was revised, resulting in the renaming of the disorder to ADHD. The single symptom list was replaced by three separate symptoms of inattention, impulsivity, and hyperactivity.
- ADHD as a motivation disorder. A large discussion loomed over the role of motivation during this decade, but by the end of the decade researches began to agree this was also a factor.
- Increasing role of social ecology. Greater research into the social-ecological impact of ADHD symptoms on children, their parents, siblings, and peers was conducted. These studies included the effects of stimulant medications on children with ADHD within the social setting.
- More sophisticated research. Designs in research were improving.
- Developments in assessment and therapy. Comparisons of single and combined treatments were more common, and specific training manuals for families of children with ADHD and oppositional behavior were published. A similar increase in more rational approached to classroom management of children with ADHD developed during this time. A fourth area of development was that of social skills training for children with ADHD.
- Public awareness of ADHD. National networks began to develop and political action organizations such as CHADD and the Attention Deficit Disorder Association developed.

The decade closed with a professional view that ADHD is a developmentally disabling condition with a strong biological and hereditary predisposition and can have a negative impact on lives of children. Effective treatment involves multimodal interventions.

The Period From 1990 to 1999

The decade of the 1990s was the decade of the brain and great advances were made in understanding brain function because of neuroimaging. Also, research in genetics led to the possibilities of an inherited condition. This decade also saw an emphasis on adult ADHD:

- Neuroimaging. In 1990 Alan Zametkin and colleagues of the National Institute of Mental Health published a landmark study that evaluated brain metabolic activity in 25 adults with ADHD who had a history of the disorder in childhood and who also had children with the disorder. Using a PET scan, the researchers found reduced activity in the frontal and striatal areas of the brain. Although there were some difficulties in replicating the study, the report does stand out as an important beginning in the field of neuroimaging. By the end of the decade researchers were using MRI and functional MRIs (fMRIs).
- Genetics. Although some genetic studies had been done previously, researchers in the 1990s ushered in new studies. Biederman and colleagues clarified and strengthened the evidence of the familial nature of ADHD. Large scale twin studies also were carried on to support the idea. Advancing techniques in molecular biology to analyze DNA also supported the ideas that the genetic component was strong.
- A best selling book by Hallowell and Ratey, *Driven to Distraction*, was published in 1994. This broadened the emphasis on ADHD as an adult condition and made an impact on adult psychiatry and treatment.
- In 1994 new diagnostic criteria were written and brought forth in DSM-IV.
- A new multisite study called the MTA was begun. This study focused on combinations of treatments that were effective for subgroups of ADHD.

By the end of the 1990s there was a shift to the idea that physiology and genetics influenced ADHD more than environment and society. This expansion led to greater acceptance of ADHD as a disability. Political activity resulted in increased eligibility for those with ADHD entitlements, under the IDEA, and legal protection, under the Americans with Disabilities Act.

The 21st Century

The study of heredity, molecular genetics, and brain imaging continues with more advanced technology. ADHD is now recognized as a universal disorder with every growing international acceptance as a chronic and disabling disorder, for which a combination of medications and psychosocial treatments and accommodations may offer the most effective approach to management.

Further Readings: Barkley, Russell. 2006. *Attention-deficit hyperactivity disorder: A handbook for diagnosis and treatment.* 3rd ed. New York: Guilford Press; Conners, C. Keith. (2008). "CRS-R (Conner's Rating Scales-Revised)." http://www.pearsonassessments.com/test/crs-r.htm. Accessed 7/4/2008; Douglas, V. I. 1998. Cognitive control processes in attention-deficit hyperactive disorder. In *Handbook of disruptive behavior disorders*, edited by H. C. Quay and A. E. Hogan, Chapter 5, 105–38. New York: Plenum Publishing; Hallowell, Edward M., and John J. Ratey. 1994. *Driven to distraction: Recognizing and coping with attention deficit disorder from childhood through adulthood.* New York: Touchstone Press; Wender, Paul. 1987. *The hyperactive child, adolescent, and adult. Attention deficit disorder through the lifespan.* New York: Oxford University Press.

Hoffman, Heinrich

Dr. Heinrich Hoffman, a physician and writer, was first credited with describing children with ADHD. A psychiatrist and writer of books on medicine and psychiatry, he later established an asylum in Frankfurt, Germany. At the time of the mid-19th century, few children's books were in existence. He could find none that were suitable for reading to his 4-year-old son, Carl Philipp, so he decided to write and illustrate a book of poems for him.

The book *Der Struwwelpeter* is a series of ten stories or poems that describe children who are not behaving; each one has a moral and an unhappy ending as a result of the behavior. Two of the stories, *Zappelphilip* or "Fidgety Phillip" and *Hans-Guck-in-die-Luft* or "John-Look-in-the Air" are strongly believed to describe persons with ADD. The drawings impressively depict the behavior of a child that today would be diagnosed as ADHD. Medical historians point to the fact that ADHD has been around for a long time and is not a creation of modern times. In fact, ADD in Germany is often called the "Zappelphilip-Syndrom."

These stories written in 1845 are somewhat notorious for perceived brutal treatment of erring children. In *Zappelphilip*, in spite of his parents' pleas to be a little gentleman, Fidgety Phillip simply would not sit still at dinner table. He wiggled and giggled and tilted his chair back like a rocking horse. He became wilder by the minute, when suddenly his chair slipped out from under him. He grabbed the tablecloth, pulling the dishes and food all over on top of him. At the end of the poem, poor Mama and Papa wonder what they will do for dinner.

John-Look-in-the Air is the story of a boy who is so inattentive and not paying attention that he walks into the river. He is soon rescued but loses all his belongings. Hoffman's *Der Struwwelpeter* has become a popular German children's book and is a classic of children's literature. The tales have been dramatized and have been sellouts at various literary festivals. A museum is dedicated to *Der Struwwelpeter* in Frankfurt.

Further Readings: Thome, Johannes, and Kerrin Jacobs. 2004. Attention deficit hyperactive disorder (ADHD) in a 19th century children's book. *European Psychiatry* 19(5 August):303–6; ADHD Strategies. "The Story of Fidgety Phillip: The First Known Written Description of ADHD." http://www.adhdstrategies.com/FigetyPhillip.asp. Accessed 5/20/2009.

Homeopathy

Some practitioners of homeopathic medicine have suggested that the techniques and strategies of homeopathy can be useful in treating ADHD. Homeopathy is classified as alternative medicine.

The German physician Samuel Hahnemann (1753–1843) founded the practice of homeopathy near the beginning of the 19th century. He joined the Greek terms *homoios* meaning "similar" and *pathos* "suffering." Positing these two ideas against each other is the basis of homeopathy, which treats disease by introducing remedies that create symptoms that are similar to

"The Story of *Zappelphilip* or Fidgety Phillip"

"Let me see if Philip can
Be a little gentleman;
Let me see if he is able
To sit still for once at table:"
Thus Papa bade Phil behave; And Mamma looked very grave.
But fidgety Phil,
He won't sit still;
He wiggles, And giggles,
And then, I declare,
Swings backwards and forwards,
And tilts up his chair,
Just like any rocking-horse—
"Philip! I am getting cross!"
See the naughty, restless child
Growing still more rude and wild, Till his chair falls over quite.
Philip screams with all his might,
Catches at the cloth, but then
That makes matters worse again.
Down upon the ground they fall,
Glasses, plates, knives, forks, and all.
How Mamma did fret and frown,
When she saw them tumbling down!
And Papa made such a face!
Philip is in sad disgrace.
Where is Philip, where is he?
Fairly covered up you see!
Cloth and all are lying on him; he has pulled down all upon him.
What a terrible to-do! Dishes, glasses, snapped in two!
Here a knife, and there a fork!
Philip, this is a cruel work.
Table also bare, and ah!
Poor Papa and poor Mamma look quite cross, and wonder how
They shall have their dinner now.

Source: *Struwwelpeter*, a series of poems for children written in 1845 by German psychiatrist Dr. Heinrich Hoffman. http://www.adhdstrategies. com/FigetyPhillip.asp. Accessed 5/20/2009.

those caused by the disease itself. There are three basic principles of the treatment:

- A medicine that in large doses produces symptoms of the disease will cure that disease if used in small doses.
- When diluted, the medicine's curative powers are enhanced, and all the poisonous side effects are lost.
- Homeopathic medicines are prescribed individually, and the whole person is studied according to his or her temperament and response.

Homeopathy is a process in which remedies are given to help the person regain health by stimulating the body's natural healing potential. Almost since its creation, homeopathy has been controversial.

Homeopathic physicians generally take a holistic perspective and examine each child with hyperactive behaviors as an individual. They believe that each child manifests an individual set of symptoms. The homeopathic practitioner examines the symptoms of each part of the person and the condition around those symptoms and tries to find a correlation or meaning in the interrelationship of those symptoms. Their complex medical chest includes more than 4,000 remedies.

Homeopathy may be used in ADHD to avert drastic intervention or the use of drug therapy such as Ritalin. Homeopathy considers use of drugs simply as a treatment and not a cure. The substances for homeopathic treatment may be a plant, mineral, metal, or animal substance or may be such things as moonlight, sunlight, or magnetism. Some of the remedies recommended by homeopaths for ADHD are the following:

- Sulphur for children who are always fidgeting or fingering things
- Tuberculinum, a miasmic remedy, meaning it comes from noninfective tuberculosis cells, for inner restlessness
- Medorrhinum, another miasmic condition made from gonorrhea cells, used in ADHD
- Lycopodium for those who have severe attention deficit
- Argentum nitrium for those who are anxious and lack confidence.

Few objective studies have been performed on homeopathic treatments. One study was published in the *British Homeopathic Journal*, October 1997, in which 43 children with ADHD were given a homeopathic treatment or a placebo for 10 days, and then the parents ranked them for behavior. Two months after the study ended, 57 percent showed improvement with homeopathy and had continued to improve, even though they discontinued the homeopathic remedies; 19 percent experienced positive results, but only while taking the homeopathic medicines. This study found that three homeopathic medicines were most helpful for ADHD:

- Stramonium for children who suffered fears or symptoms of posttraumatic stress disorder
- Cina for children who were physically aggressive
- Hyoscyasmus niger for children with manic or sexualized symptoms

Homeopathic doctors realize the pros and cons of their treatment. One of the pros is that it treats the whole person at the root of the problem and is considered safe without the side effects of stimulants and other medications. The treatments use natural, nontoxic medicines to heal physical, mental, and emotional symptoms. The treatment, which is inexpensive and cost effective, seeks to heal physical, mental, and emotional ailments.

The physicians recognize that their treatment does not suit everyone. The patient and parents must be good observers and be able to relate the history of the experiences of the person with all their conditions. Some children, especially teenagers, may resent close scrutiny of their behavior and fight the process. Another downside is that homeopathy sets off a process of self-healing and does not always work instantly to relieve symptoms. It requires patience and a willingness to put lots of effort into the treatment process.

Homeopathic remedies must never be self-administered. Only a practitioner can give advice on use of these remedies.

Further Readings: "ADHD: Treatments Homeopathic Therapies" http://www.healing-arts.org/children/ADHD/homeopathy.htm. Accessed 8/3/2008; Cooper, Paul, and Katherine Bilton. 1999. *ADHD: Research, practice and opinion.* London: Whurr Publishers; "How to Treat ADHD with Homeopathy." 2006. http://www.ehow.com/how_2052053_ treat-adhd-homeopathy.html. Accessed 8/3/2008; "The Homeopathic Treatment of Children with ADHD and Similar Behavioural Learning Disorders." http://www.holos-homeo pathy.com/ADHD_information_1.htm. Accessed 8/3/2008.

Hyperactivity

According to DSM-IV-TR, hyperactive children always seem to be in constant motion. It does not take long to recognize children with hyperactivity. At school, they may climb under the table, get constantly out of their seats, and run around the room. They may talk constantly and bother things that belong to other children, who consistently complain about them. When playing games, they prefer not to listen to rules and get in trouble for not following rules or staying in line. Sitting still at dinner or during a school lesson or story can be a difficult task. They may swing their legs, move their feet, or drum their pencils. Hyperactive teenagers and adults may always appear restless. They become easily bored and have the need to roam or wander. Certain jobs that require long periods of quiet or concentration are difficult. However, they may try to do too may things at one time but not accomplish any of them.

Overexcitablity and Giftedness

In the 1960s Kazimerz Dabrowski proposed his Theory of Positive Disintegration, which stated that people born with over excitabilities had a higher level of development potential than others. Several researchers have over the past decades tried to map out the correlation between children who are over excitable, ADHD, and giftedness. It appears that over excitabilities can be used to predict giftedness.

Dr. Samuel Johnson: Gifted and ADHD

Dr. Samuel Johnson was a brilliant literary character of the 18th century. He created one of the first dictionaries of the English language and was so influential that his era in literature is known as the age of Johnson. However, Fanny Burney, a fine English lady and novelist, meeting him at the home of Sir Isaac Newton was totally disturbed by his appearance. She described that his mouth was almost continually opening and shutting as if he were chewing. He had an annoying and really strange method of frequently twirling his fingers and twisting his hands. His body was in perpetual motion as he see-sawed up and down. His feet were never quiet for one moment.

As the group met in the library, he was fixed on his books. He stood away from the group and read to himself, but when he was taken from his books, he participated in clever conversation. Although he could talk about any subject, his dress looked like he just came in from the road, according to Ms. Burney.

Source: Burney, Fanny. "Diary of Fanny Burney." http://www.edprint. demon.co.uk/johnson/sam-fanny.html.

Dabrowski described five types of over excitabilities:

1. Psychomotor. This type of excitability expresses an excess of energy that is defined as constantly moving, rapid speech, impulsiveness, and restlessness.
2. Sensual. This person has great sensory awareness in the form of touch, taste, or smell. It may be expressed as a sharp sense of esthetics.
3. Imagination. The individual uses vivid imagery, metaphor, visualization, and inventiveness. The imaginations may include vivid dreams, fear of the unknown, poetic talent, or just enjoying fantasy.
4. Intellectual. This person persists in asking probing question, pursuing knowledge, discovery, theoretical analysis and synthesis, and independence of thought. This type is not the same as IQ, which is the ability to solve a problem; it is the pleasure and excitability of tackling the problem.
5. Emotional. This type of over excitability concerns deep relationships, concerns with death, feeling of compassion and responsibility, depression, need for security, self-evaluation, shyness, and concern for others.

People can have all five over excitabilities or just a few. The correlation of these excitabilities with the symptoms of ADHD can be readily made. Someone with psychomotor over excitability has a high likelihood of meeting the DSM-IV criteria for ADD with hyperactivity. On the other hand, someone without the psychomotor movement but with imagination might be described as inattentive. Many gifted children are underachievers in school. One study shows that as many as 45 percent of children with IQs above 130 are underachievers.

Another reason a gifted child may be labeled ADHD is negative behavior in the classroom. When gifted children respond in a perceived negative fashion, they display traits similar to ADD. Teachers like to think gifted students are compliant and obedient and are not inclined to think that a child who is gifted could be acting out. Researchers considering gifted children argue that behavior problems are developed in response to inappropriate curricula and instructional methods or the climate created by teacher and classroom peers. *See also* Giftedness.

Further Readings: Ackerman, Cheryl. 1997. Identifying gifted adolescents using personality characteristics: Dabrowski's overexcitabilties. *Roeper Review—A Journal on Gifted Education* 19(June, 3):229–36; Johnson, C. 1981. Smart kids have problems, too. *Today's Education* 70:27–29; DeLisle, J. R. 1992. *Guiding the social and emotional development of gifted youth: A practical guide for educators and counselors.* New York: Longman; Reid, Brian et al. 1995. Square pegs in round holes—These kids don't fit: High ability students with behavior problems. The National Research Center on the Gifted and Talented. http://www.gifted.uconn.edu/NRCGT.html.

Hypoglycemia

The first time one suspects that a person has ADHD is when the person is inattentive and overactive. ADHD is not diagnosed using brain scans, blood tests, or other tests, but rather by observing how the person behaves. The problem of using behavior for diagnosis is that many other conditions also may show these same behaviors. One of the most common conditions that is overlooked in diagnosis is hypoglycemia or low blood sugar.

The following are the common complaints of people with hypoglycemia:

- Forgetful, especially of people's names
- Difficulty in school although intelligence is normal
- Tendency to insult people without meaning to
- Itching and crawling sensation in the skin
- Cannot get organized
- Difficulty handling stress
- Cries easily
- Gets angry easily
- When depressed, eating ice cream or candy picks them up
- Needs coffee or caffeine in soft drink to keep going
- Bothered by light
- Night sweats
- Sensitive to color, sound, and odor
- Dizziness when getting up quickly from a reclining position
- Frequent colds
- Dry mouth
- Drowsiness after a sweet or starchy meal
- Has nightmares often
- Have difficulty keeping a job

People with hypoglycemia have many of the same behavior problems as those with ADHD. Certain drugs, hormone deficiency, organ failure, liver problems, or alcohol may cause hypoglycemia, but the most common cause is a poor diet heavy in refined sugars and flours. Poor nutrition may also be one of the mitigating factors in ADHD.

Serotonin, one of the neurotransmitters involved in ADHD, is also related to hypoglycemia. A person low in serotonin will be inclined to consume greater amounts of sugar in an attempt to increase serotonin production, which may lead to sugar addiction. Insulin is produced to process the sugar in the body, and such addiction can lead to insulin resistance. At first it starts at a mild level but over time unstable concentration of blood sugar causes diabetes. Also, erratic sugar levels in the blood and brain explain some of the variable psychological symptoms of hypoglycemia.

According to the ADHD Help Center, changing the diet to natural whole foods such as fresh fruits and vegetables can alleviate and even reverse the symptoms of ADHD and hypoglycemia. The Center recommends the following:

- Eliminate all sugar, aspartame or NutraSweet from the diet; stevia is the only sugar substitute that should be used.
- Eliminate fast food and school lunches from the diet.
- Eliminate processed foods that might have monosodium glutamate (MSG), preservatives, food dyes, or other chemicals.
- Drink filtered water and fresh vegetable juice.
- Eliminate soft drinks, caffeinated beverages, and cow's milk from the diet.
- Eliminate white bread and white rice from the diet; instead use whole grain breads, brown rice, and other grains.

Many of these recommendations are similar to those of other diets. However, most nutritionists recommend similar changes in the diet for healthy living.

Further Readings: "Attention Deficit Disorder or Hypoglycemia?" http://www.add-adhd-help-center.com/newsletter/newsletter_15nov03.htm. Accessed 8/6/2008; "The Serotonin Connection." http://www.hypoglycemia.asn.au/articles/serotonin_connection.html. Accessed 8/6/2008.

Impulsivity

According to DSM-IV-TR, impulsive children seem unable to curb their immediate reactions or think before they act. Among the characteristics of ADHD, impulsivity is one of the most common. Although every child wants what he wants when he wants it, the child with ADHD acts without reflection or consideration of the consequences. The child with ADHD behaves like a child several years younger than his chronological age.

The impulsive child becomes upset when things do not go his way. He may kick, break toys, or hit children who stand in his way. He may act on the spur of the moment, rushing into the street or climbing on things without thinking the object could be dangerous. He received more cuts, bruises, and trips to the doctor than most children.

Impulsivity also manifests itself in poor planning and judgment. Although it may be difficult to tell exactly how much planning is expected of young children, those with ADHD appear to have less than other children their age. They are disorderly and disorganized. Impulsivity combines with their distractibility to produce messy rooms, sloppy dress, unfinished assignments, and careless reading and writing.

A related problem is bladder and bowel control. When children with ADHD are younger, they may soil or wet themselves slightly during the day. They appear to pay no attention to their pressing needs. Although bedwetting occurs in about 10 percent of 6-year-old boys, it appears to be more common in children with ADHD. Bedwetting itself has been related to unusually deep sleep and sometimes to symptoms of anatomical abnormalities or psychological problems. However, bedwetting may be the result of ADHD and respond to the general treatment prescribed for it.

Children with ADHD may display social impulsivity or antisocial behavior. Although other children may lie or play with matches, the child with ADHD does not learn to control these impulses. ADHD does not explain why children do these things; it may be that the child wants something that another has. However, whatever the situation, a twofold approach is required: Deal with the specific motivation and increase the ability for self-control.

Impulsivity in the Lincoln White House

A child with impulsivity lived in the Lincoln White House. Abraham Lincoln's third son Tad fit the picture of impulsivity, inattention, hyperactivity, and restlessness. He would burst into the Oval Office while chasing his brother. He had learning problems too. His mother hired tutor after tutor to come into the White House to help him, but they all quit, saying that he was not teachable. In fact, Mary Todd Lincoln might have had ADHD herself. She was always overspending the White House budget and caused embarrassment and ridicule to the president. One time President Lincoln was reviewing the troops, and Mrs. Lincoln saw him speak to a young captain's wife. She immediately started screaming at her husband and the woman in front of the entire crowd.

Further Readings: Barkley, Russell. 2006. *Attention-deficit hyperactivity disorder: A handbook for diagnosis and treatment.* 3rd ed. New York: Guilford Press; Barkley, Russell. 2002. ADHD and accident proneness. *ADHD Report* May:2–5; Barkley, R. A. 2001. *Taking charge of ADHD.* New York: Guilford Press; Wender, Paul. 1995. *Attention deficit hyperactive disorder in adults.* New York: Oxford University Press.

Inattention

According to DSM-IV-TR, children who are inattentive have a hard time keeping their minds on any one thing and may get bored with a task after only a few minutes. If they are doing something they really enjoy, they have no trouble paying attention, but focusing deliberate, conscious attention to organizing and completing a task or learning something new is difficult. DSM-IV-TR describes the following signs of inattention:

- Often becoming easily distracted by irrelevant sights and sounds
- Often failing to pay attention to detains and making careless mistakes
- Rarely following instructions carefully and completely losing or forgetting things like toys, pencils, books, and tools needed for a task
- Often skipping from one uncompleted activity to another

Children displaying the predominately inattentive type of ADHD are seldom impulsive or hyperactive, but they are not paying attention, appear to be daydreaming, may be easily confused, slow moving, and lethargic.

Further Reading: American Psychiatric Association. 2004. *Diagnostic and statistical manual of the American Psychiatric Association.* 4th ed. Arlington, VA: American Psychiatric Association.

Incidence of ADHD

ADHD and ADD are present in all populations with varying prevalence. Because of differing criteria used for diagnosis and methods of evaluations, comparisons between countries are difficult.

Thomas Edison: Inattentive and Different

Young Thomas Edison, known as Al, angered his schoolmaster with his dreamy, distracted behavior. He often floated off during recitations and preferred to draw in his notebook. One day Edison heard the teacher say that he was addled and it was useless keeping this boy in school any longer. When he told his mother that he had heard what the teacher said, she ran down to the school and told the teacher that Al had more brains than the teacher. She began home schooling him and was determined that the school or teacher would not hobble the full sweep of her boy's imagination.

Al was always investigating happenings. An angry ram attacked him while he studied a bumblebees' nest in a pasture. While exploring new ways to shorten a skate strap, he cut off the tip of his middle finger with an ax. When he hypothesized that birds could fly because they ate worms, he mashed up a concoction of worms and convinced a girl to drink it to see if she could fly. She got sick, and he got the switch.

Al started working for the railroad at age 13. He was working on a chemistry experiment when he set fire to a train. Naturally, he lost his job on the railroad. Later, he was fired or quit various jobs in several fields.

Source: Baldwin, Neill. *1995. Edison: Inventing the century.* New York: Hyperion.

Most researchers suggest that ADD affects 10–20 percent of the school age population. The ratio of males to females in the general population is 3:1; however, in clinical populations the ADD ratio varies from 6:1 to 9:1. For girls, the condition may be recognized later in life. ADHD referrals contribute to up to 30–40 percent of all clinic referrals.

Individualized Education Plan (IEP)

Children with ADHD may or may not qualify for an Individualized Education Plan (IEP). If children are diagnosed with ADHD, it does not mean that they will qualify for special services. A study team is convened to determine if the child should be placed for these services. If it is determined that the child's condition may interfere with his educational progress, then the child may be considered. However, because most children respond to medication or other behavioral interventions, most children with ADHD do not qualify. However, if learning disability, physical disability, conduct disorder, or oppositional defiance are present, the person may qualify under specific provisions of the Individuals with Disabilities Education Act (IDEA). Another option for children with ADHD who do not qualify under the IDEA is to request a 504 plan. *See also* Section 504.

The IEP is a formal document, developed by parents, teachers, and related services personnel, that sets forth how a child with disabilities is to receive a free appropriate public education in the least restrictive environment. PL-94-142 called the Education for All Handicapped Children Act was enacted in 1975 as a response to increased awareness of the need to properly educate children who had disabilities, and judicial ruling required states to provide an education for students with disabilities if the states was providing education for those without disabilities. Thus all 50 states were impacted by this legislation. Not only did the law require a "free and appropriate education" in the "least restrictive environment" but required an IEP for students. The IEP lays out a per-child plan of annual goals for the child, how the student's attainment of those goals will be determined, and the specific services the child may require and prescribes any adjustments or substitutions in the assessments to be used with the child.

In 1997 PL 94-142 was reauthorized and labeled the IDEA and called for states and districts to identify curricular expectations for special education students that were as equal as possible, given the curricular expectations established for all other students, and to report those results to the public. There were no penalties for those that did not comply, and therefore many states did not do so. Unlike IDEA, No Child Left Behind enacted on January 6, 2002 put in place serious penalties for noncompliance. Its aim was that all children would demonstrate improvement on state-chosen tests linked to each state's curricular aims. The law sets forth 12-year goals of having 100 percent of all students score at a "proficient" or higher level on No Child Left Behind Act (NCLB) tests by the 2013–2014 school year.

Accountability is straightforward. Students' test scores must improve on a regular basis over a dozen years in order to reflect substantially improved student learning. States are allowed some flexibility in deciding how many more students must have a higher score each year on that state's test. If a school fails to make adequate yearly progress (AYP), the school is first publicly proclaimed to be deficient and then is placed on a sanction-laden improvement track that can, in a very few years, cause the school to be taken off the list by the state. Not making the AYP goal is quite serious and has district and state consequences.

An IEP must spell out accommodations or adaptations that must be provided for students with disabilities during instruction and assessment. The adaptations will give the student a fair opportunity to succeed and be assessed accurately. The purpose of the accommodation is to eliminate or at least reduce the effects of the student's disability. They do not lower expectations or alter what is being measured.

In 2005 the Council of Chief State School Officers (CCSSO) broke down these accommodations into four categories as follows:

1. Presentation. Allow the students to access information in ways that do not require them to visually read standard print. These alternate modes of access are auditory, multisensory, tactile, and visual.
2. Response. Allow students to complete activities assignments and assessments in different ways or to solve or organize problems using some type of assistive device or organizer.
3. Setting. Change the location in which a test or assignment is given or the conditions of the assessment setting.

4. Timing and scheduling. Increase the allowable length of time to complete an assessment or assignment and change the way the time is organized.

The IEP is a legal document that is intended to have parents work with teachers to improve their children's education. Parents can challenge a district is an IEP is not followed properly.

Further Readings: Popham, W. James. 2006. *Assessing students with disabilities.* New York: Routledge; Thompson, Sandra J. et al. 2005 *Accommodations manual: How to Select, administer, and evaluate use of accommodations for instruction and assessment of students with disabilities.* 2nd ed. Washington, D.C.: The Council of Chief State School Officers, August, 2005.

Individuals with Disabilities Education Act (IDEA)

Children with ADHD may or may not qualify under Individuals with Disabilities Act (IDEA). In order to receive services, the condition must have an effect on that individual's education to the extent that it requires delivery of special education programs and related services. Education for All Handicapped Children's Act (EAHCA) was renamed IDEA in 1990, and a few new provisions were added. The original act included three major provisions:

- A free appropriate public education (FAPE)
- An individualized education program (IEP)
- Due process procedures

In 1997 IDEA was changed to affect eligibility, programming, private school placements, discipline, funding, attorney's fees, discipline resolutions, and procedural safeguards.

However, the general definition of a child with disabilities did not change, but the policy was clarified. During this reauthorization of IDEA, the Department of Education (DOE) took the position that it was not necessary to include ADHD as a separate category of disability. Their position was that children with ADHD were potentially eligible for special education and related services under the existing disability categories in Part B of IDEA. Part B requires that State and local education agencies provide a free and appropriate public education to all eligible children with disabilities. The agencies still have an affirmative obligation called "child find" to locate, identify, and evaluate all children who have a disability or who are suspected of having a disability and are in need of special education and related services. A local school district may not refuse to evaluate a child for special education and related services solely because he or she has been identified as ADHD. However, parents need to know that the diagnosis alone is not sufficient reason for schools to provide special education. The following are some additional points relating to IDEA:

- Before a child with ADHD can receive special education and related services, the district must conduct an evaluation.

- A multidisciplinary team must conduct the evaluation, including at least one person who is knowledgeable about the child's diagnosis.
- Under Part B, eligible children will be provided special education and related services through an IEP.
- To be eligible for special education under Part B, a child must be evaluated as having one or more specific physical or mental impairments and must need special education and related services as a result of the impairment.
- For all children with ADHD, the manifestation of their disabilities may be different from one another, that is, some children will have difficult paying attention, others may have problems with hyperactivity or acting out behaviors, and still others will have impulsive behaviors that need attention.
- Children with ADHD may need services under one or more of the existing categories, such as other health impairment (OHI), emotional disturbance (ED), or specific learning disability (SLD). OHI is considered when ADHD is a chronic or acute health conditions, a child has limited alertness to school work because of the ADHD, and ADHD adversely affects educational performance.
- When a child is found not to be eligible under Part B, he may meet the requirements of Section 504 of the Rehabilitation Act of 1973. This Civil Rights Act prohibits discrimination on the basis of disability by any program receiving federal funding.

On December 3, 2004, the president signed the IDEA 2004, the bill reauthorizing IDEA 1997. This act changes how many service are provided to student but does not change the districts' basic obligation to provide FAPE. Most provisions became effective July 1, 2005. The following is a summary of the changes:

- District's disciplinary authority. Lots of confusion existed over the meaning of disciplining for students with disabilities, especially those with ADHD. Many children with ADHD are seen in discipline offices. If the diagnosis is simply ADHD, then they are disciplined as other students. However, if they have comorbid conditions, such as conduct disorder (CD) or oppositional defiant disorder (ODD), it must be determined if the act was related to the disability. A provision of IEDA is that if misbehavior was caused as a manifestation of the disability, then that should be considered when looking at his consequences. This led to situations where students who were in special education would not be disciplined, and regular students who had done the same thing might be suspended or expelled from school. Under the old rule, there were four questions. IDEA 2004 clarified the relationship with two questions:

1. Did the disability cause the conduct?
2. Did the district's failure to implement the IEP cause the misconduct?

- If either of the answers is "yes," then the conduct was a disability manifestation. Also under the new rule, the district will be able to use a 45-day interim alternative placement for students who cause serious bodily injury to another. Previously, this option was available only for drug and weapons offenses. Also, time was extended from 45 days to 45 school days. The district may remove the students from the classroom and place him or her in an alternative setting during the appeals process. Previously, the stay-put provision barred alternative placement during the appeal.

- Writing and changing IEPs. Districts will no longer have to include benchmarks and short-term objective in IEPs, but they do have to describe how the student's progress toward annual goals will be measured. The IEP states when those progress reports will be made, such as quarterly or with report cards. The Education Department publishes models for IEPs that have individualized family service plans, procedural safeguards. A parent may agree to modify the IEP in writing without another formal meeting. An IEP team member may be excuses if the district and parents agree the member's services are not needed or the team member may submit written input before the meeting. The staff may use alternative meetings, such as videoconferencing and conference calls. Also the DOE gave 15 states the privilege of developing multiple-year IEPs that would last as long as 3 years.

- Evaluating students. The staff has more options even if parents refuse consent. For example, if Johnny manifests behaviors that staff is convinced needs attention, it may request an evaluation even if the parent does not want it. Although parent involvement is still an important part of the process, IDEA 2004 allows districts to initiate evaluations, under certain circumstances. Unless state law demands parental consent, the district may do an evaluation, but still must follow all procedural safeguards. In addition, if the parent does not consent, the district will not be liable for failing to convene an IEP meeting and not providing special education and related services.

- Identifying specific learning disabilities. Under IDEA 1997, the district was required to ask the question: Is there a severe discrepancy between the student's achievement and his or her intellectual ability? IDEA 2004 allows districts to use a process that determines whether the student response to scientific, research-based intervention. Thus educators have more flexibility in categorizing a student with a learning disability, even if he does not meet the former criteria for learning disabilities.

- Student transfers. Because a lot of confusion existed in the districts, the new IDEA language follows existing case law and says that students who transfer during one year from one district to another when the same state must receive comparable services until the old IEP is adopted or a new one is developed. If students transfer from out of the state, the district must conduct a new evaluation and then develop a new IEP; however, until the district conducts this evaluation, it must provide services comparable to what the children received before transferring.

- Due Process Hearings. To discourage litigation, new provisions limit the time within which due process hearings may be requested. Parents have 2 years from the date they know about the issues for due process. In the past, state law established the time limit. In hopes of resolving complaints before they go to a formal hearing, an alternative dispute resolution (ADR) must be heard within 15 days to try to settle the matter. Under IDEA 1997, parents who prevailed in due process cases were allowed to seek attorney's fees from the district; but if the district won, it could not pursue these fees. Under current law, the following three circumstances determine if the district may be awarded attorney's fees:

1. The due process request or lawsuit is frivolous, unreasonable, or without foundation.
2. The attorney continued to litigate after the litigation and truly became frivolous.

3. The due process request or lawsuit was filed for the wrong purpose, such as harassment, unnecessary delays, or needlessly increasing the cost of litigation.

If the parents filed suit for an improper purpose, then a district may be awarded the attorney's fees against that parent.

IDEA 2004 sets standards for highly qualified teachers that coincide with standards in the No Child Left Behind Act (NCLB). *See also* No Child Left Behind Act. All teachers must be certified or licensed in special education, and anyone hired after July 2005 must meet the requirement.

Many court cases have arisen as disputes between districts and parents. The district loses when it skirts due process or claims that it cannot perform a service because of cost. For the courts, the cost of services is not an issue. Parents lose when they bring frivolous and unreasonable cases.

Another issue causing a lot of litigation is the idea of inclusion. IDEA requires the states "to maximum extent appropriate ... educate children with disabilities ... with children who do not have disabilities." This preference for mainstreaming is the basis of inclusion. The same section also provides that "special classes, separate schooling, or other removal of children with disabilities from the regular educational environment occurs only when the nature or severity of the disability is such that education in regular classes with the use of supplementary aids and services cannot be achieved satisfactorily."

The 1983 *Roncker v. Walter* (700 F.2d 1058 6th Cir. 1983) cited three factors to be considered in inclusion:

- The comparative benefits of the two placements
- Any disruption by the student in nonsegregated setting
- The cost of mainstreaming the students

Because the student with ADHD may disrupt the regular classroom, many are placed in special classes and should not be there. The student with just attention or hyperactivity problems without learning disabilities or CD or ODD does not qualify under IDEA. However, many children with ADHD also have these comorbid conditions and will have an IEP or may qualify under a 504 plan. *See also* Americans with Disabilities Act; Individualized Education Plan (IEP); No Child Left Behind Act; Section 504.

Further Readings: Kelly, Evelyn B. 2006. *Legal basics: A handbook for educators.* 2nd ed. Bloomington, IN: Phi Delta Kappa International; Texas Partners Resource Network. http://www.PartnersTX.org. Accessed 5/20/2009; Zirkle, Perry A. 2005. *Section 504: Students issues, legal requirements, and practical recommendations.* Bloomington, IN: Phi Delta Kappa Educational Foundation.

Industrial and Environmental Toxins

ADHD has been correlated with exposure to numerous industrial and environmental chemicals. The long list includes cigarette smoke, lead, pesticides, gasoline fumes, herbicides, disinfectants, furniture polishes, air fresheners, mercury, manganese, fluoride, dry cleaning fluid, arsenic, PCBs, and all kinds of solvents. About 80,000 chemicals are registered in the United States, and about 1,000 are know to cause neurotoxicity in animals, and 200 are toxic to human brains. Five chemicals have been documented to affect human brain development.

Researchers Phillippe Grandjean, professor of environmental health at Harvard University, and colleagues have suggested that a number of chemicals may be causing a silent pandemic of brain disorders during fetal and childhood development. An important point is that although only moderate amounts of mercury, lead, or other chemicals may damage neurological function in adults, only small amounts are needed to affect the developing brains of babies, infants, and young children.

Researchers from Johns Hopkins examined the experimental effect of lead toxicity on the developing structure of the neocortex region in the brain. Stacked with layers of nerve cells, the neocortex has a critical role in processing information. Because of its plasticity during early childhood, it is highly vulnerable to damage.

Braun et al. (2006) cites numerous studies of a significant association between prenatal environmental tobacco smoke and ADHD behaviors. In case-controlled studies, investigators found a two- to fourfold increased risk.

Many poisons come from unexpected sources. Eating vegetables and fruits that are not thoroughly washed is a source. Beds and carpets are dangerous places in a house because they are full of different types of dust and other toxins that can cause hyperactivity, attention deficits, irritability, and learning problems. High levels of mercury can be found in dental fillings. Children whose mothers have mercury amalgam fillings and grind their teeth are a risk for exposure to high mercury levels. Many European countries have discontinued the use of mercury fillings because of possible side effects.

Further Readings: Braun, Joe et al. 2006. Exposures to environmental toxicants and attention deficit hyperactivity disorder in U.S. children. *Environmental Health Perspectives* 114(12):1904–09; ADD Information Library. "Mercury Poisoning, Heavy Metal or Chemical Toxicity, and Brain Development." ADHD Mental Health. http://www.newi deas.net/adhd/differential-diagnosis/mercury-chemical-toxicity. Accessed 8/08/2008.

Intelligence

When it comes to intelligence, many parents, educators, and scientists cannot figure out what is happening in the mind of people with ADHD. They do not perform well in school, may appear disinterested, and may completely disrupt a classroom or social situation. They may have moments of brilliance but other times are complete failures. People may consider them to be like the absent-minded professor and ask how can one who is so smart can be so dumb. They appear to have an odd type of intelligence that is difficult for those in the mainstream to understand.

The idea of multiple intelligences may shed some light on how people, including those with ADHD, think. Howard Gardner, Harvard psychologist, in his classic book *Frames of Mind: The Theory of Multiple Intelligences* proposes that intelligence is not based on just verbal or logical responses but actually is composed of seven different types:

- Linguistic intelligence. This type of IQ uses words to express ideas and is valued in school on achievement and intelligence or IQ tests.
- Logical-mathematical intelligence. People with this type of IQ display ability to use numbers and solve logical problems. These first two types are valued on IQ tests and in school.
- Musical intelligence. These children display music ability from very early years; they may have vocal perfect pitch or instrumental leanings.
- Bodily-kinesthetic intelligence. These children have great physical coordination that may lead to athletic excellence.
- Spatial intelligence. People with this ability can visualize objects in different dimensions; acclaimed artists, architects, and engineers have spatial intelligence.
- Interpersonal intelligence. People with this intelligence know how to understand and deal with people; they understand and relate to them; this group include teachers, sales people, ministers, and others who are interested in others.
- Intrapersonal intelligence. These people can look inside themselves and appears to understand intuitively where they are in life and how they fit into the scheme of things; they understand their abilities and limitations.

Some people add an eighth intelligence called naturalistic intelligence, the ability to understand and appreciate nature and the environment.

Howard Gardner also has written *Creating Minds: An Anatomy of Creativity Seen Through the Lives of Freud, Einstein, Picasso, Stravinsky, Eliot, Graham, and Gandhi* in which he illustrates the theory of multiple intelligences as he describes how great innovators for various fields used their intelligence and assesses the relative strength of the different types of intelligences.

Probably no one exemplifies Gardner's multiple intelligence theory better than Albert Einstein. Einstein has become known for his remarkable logical and spatial abilities. His theory of relativity in physics is so complex that few people understand it. However, he was very poor in relating to people or interpersonal intelligence. Mahatma Gandhi, the great leader of India's passive resistance movement against British rule, was articulate and personable. He had great linguistic and personal skills, but through his own admission could not draw a tree and had poor artistic abilities. Pablo Picasso, the famous abstract artist, could visualize space in art and painting but had great difficulties handling logical issues. He admitted that he did very poorly in school. Sigmund Freud, the founder of the psychoanalytic school of psychiatry, was quite adept in languages and communicating with people. However, when it came to musical talent, he was lacking. In fact, many of the geniuses of our age were real misfits in school.

Using Gardner's theory of multiple intelligences, Jeffrey Freed in his book *Right-brained Children in a Left-brained World* presents the idea that children with ADHD have the ability to think abstractly and visually. They may be powerful visual/spatial thinkers. Many of these children are dyslexic and do not do well in schools that have only traditional rote-type instruction.

According to right brain/left brain theory, people with ADHD may possibly be right brained. However, most instruction in school values left-brained skills. It is the right hemisphere of the brain that is associated with visual thinking as well as other traits. Freed cites how some of our most famous scientists and artists were very visual thinkers. Among these successful people with possible ADHD were Albert Einstein, Michael Faraday, English chemist and physicist, Thomas Edison, famous inventor, and Leonardo Da Vinci, the famous painter and early genius of science.

Further Readings: Freed, Jeffrey, and Laura Parsons. 1997. *Right-brained children in a left-brained world: Unlocking the potential of your ADD child.* New York: Fireside; Hartmann, Thom. 1996. *Beyond ADD: Hunting for reasons in the past and the present.* Grass Valley, CA: Mythical Intelligence Press; Gardner, Howard. 1993. *Frames of mind: The theory of multiple intelligences.* 10th ed. New York: Basic Books. http://www.born toexplore.org/addmult.htm. Accessed 5/20/2009; Gardner, Howard. 1994. *Creating minds: An anatomy of creativity seen through the lives of Freud, Einstein, Picasso, Stravinsky, Eliot, Graham, and Gandhi.* New York: Basic Books. http://www.bornto explore.org/addmult.htm. Accessed 5/20/2009; West, Thomas. *In the mind's eye: Visual thinkers, gifted people with dyslexia and other learning difficulties, computer images and the ironies of creativity.* New York: Prometheus Books, 1997.

International Consensus Statement on ADHD

In 2002 a consortium of distinguished scientists, researchers, and physicians gathered to issue a statement of their agreement about ADHD. Concerned about some of the portrayal of ADHD in media reports, the group expressed the fear that inaccurate stories about ADHD were spreading myths or were reporting that ADHD was either a fraud or a benign condition. Misperceptions may cause many individuals not to seek help of treatment. Such stories lead people to trivialize the condition and not consider it a valid condition. The group sought to help people understand that the views of a handful of nonexpert doctors who claim that ADHD does not exist are not substantiated by mainstream scientific views and studies.

Because of overwhelming scientific evidence, the U.S. Surgeon General, the American Medical Association, the American Psychiatric Association, the American Academy of Child and Adolescent Psychiatry, the American Psychological Association, the American Academy of Pediatrics, and others recognize ADHD as a valid disorder. The groups recognize that individuals who suffer from the disorder have a serious deficiency or failure that is universal to humans and that deficiency leads to harm for that person. The deficiency affects the life functioning of that individual.

The consortium emphasized the following points in this statement:

- Through numerous studies, specific brain regions, including the frontal lobe, its connections to the basal ganglia, and certain parts of the cerebellum link to ADHD.
- Most people with ADHD have less electrical activity in some areas of the brain and show less stimulation in one or more of these regions.

- Numerous studies of twins in the United States, Norway, Australia, and other countries have shown the condition to be inherited.
- Studies of twins have shown that family environment does not make a significant difference, although the consortium does recognize that the home environment does have an effect on individuals.
- Hundreds of studies show that education combined with family, education, and social accommodations can make a difference in the lives of individuals.
- ADHD is not a benign condition and can cause devastating problems for an individual.

The group laments that less than half of those with the disorder are receiving treatment. They implore the media to portray ADHD and the science about it as accurately as possible. Eighty-six scientists, researchers, and physicians signed the document.

Further Reading: Barkley, R. A. 2002. International consensus statement on ADHD. *Clinical Child and Family Psychology Review* 5(2):89–111.

Intestinal Parasites

In addition to parasite infestations that are indigenous in poverty pockets in the United States, many children and adults are immigrating and bringing parasites that practitioners in the medical community have not seen. However, parasites are increasing in the general population as a result of years of poor eating habits, overuse of medications, and increased exposure to these organisms. Presence of the parasites may cause inattentiveness, hyperactivity, and many of the symptoms found in ADHD.

All parasites live by feeding off the cells and tissues of the infected host. The effects of some parasites may mimic other conditions, including allergies, asthma, irritable bowel syndrome, heart disease, and ADHD. The following are the common intestinal parasites that may cause problems:

- *Giardia lamblia,* a common protozoan, causes giardiasis, which is transmitted through contaminated food or water. Infestation can lead to the malabsorption of nutrients and problems with listlessness and attention.
- Cryptosporidia are tiny protozoans that are also spread from contaminated food and water and person-to-person contact.
- Entamoebas are protozoans that can cause serious chronic problems even in healthy people; sometimes people contract these organisms in foreign travel.
- Worms such as hookworms or ascaris (stomach worms) cause weight loss and malnutrition; pinworms, which are common in children, may cause them to be listless and inattentive.

The fact that these parasites cause some of the same symptoms as many other diseases makes getting an accurate diagnosis difficult. Many doctors do not think these parasites can cause a health problem until many other possibilities have been exhausted, and time has allowed the parasites to do damage, including irreparable harm.

Further Reading: "Parasites." http://www.symmetry4u.com/Info/parasites.htm. Accessed 8/7/2008.

INTUNIV

Unlike other ADHD medications that work indirectly in the prefrontal cortex, INTUNIV a form of guanfacine works directly binding specifically to the alpha-2A adrenergic cell receptors in the prefrontal cortex. The prefrontal cortex is the area of the brain associated with executive function, behavioral inhibition, regulation of attention, distractibility, impulsivity, and frustration tolerance. The selective alpha-2A agonist strengthens working memory and assists firing of the neurons in the prefrontal cortex. Guanfacine is not a controlled substance and does not appear to have a known mechanism for potential abuse of dependence.

In May 2008, Shire Pharmaceuticals announced findings from analyses of pivotal trials of INTUNIV, a once-daily formulation of guanfacine, which provides a steady delivery of drug throughout the day and is designed to minimize the fluctuations between peak and trough concentrations as seen with immediate release guanfacine. In Phase III clinical trials all patients treated with INTUNIV showed significantly greater improvement on rating scales than the group with placebo. Safety data showed that adverse events reported were generally mild and moderate with the most common complaint side effects as the feeling of sedation.

Further Readings: "Shire Investigational Nonstimulant INTUNIV Showed Significant Efficacy in Reducing ADHD Symptoms." http://www.medicalnews today.com/articles/106801.php. Accessed 5/28/2008.

Iron Deficiency

Some researchers have found that iron deficiency is correlated with ADHD. Iron, an essential component of hemoglobin, the oxygen-carrying pigment, is an important mineral in the functioning of red blood cells. The lack of iron causes anemia and other problems.

Konofal et al. (2004) found that iron deficiency causes abnormal dopaminergic neurotransmission. Dopamine is one of the neurotransmitters that does not function properly in ADHD. He surmises that the lack of iron contributes to the physiopathology of ADHD. To evaluate the relationship of iron deficiency, Konofal studied 53 children with ADHD and 27 controls. The results suggested that low iron scores contribute to ADHD and that ADD children can benefit from iron supplementation.

Further Reading: Konofal, E. et al. 2004. Iron deficiency in children. *Archives of Pediatric Adolescent Medicine* 158(12):1113–15.

K

Klinefelter Syndrome

Klinefelter syndrome is a rare genetic disorder that is associated with an increased risk for ADHD. Humans normally have 46 chromosomes; females have two X chromosomes, and males have an X chromosome and a Y chromosome. Klinefelter syndrome results when males have at least one extra X chromosome (XXY). The syndrome occurs in about 1 in 1,000 males. The presence of the extra chromosome may cause some males to have some usual attributes: sparse body hair, enlarged breasts, and wide hips. The testicles may be small, and the voice may not be deep. They usually cannot father children. A degree of subnormal intelligence appears in some individuals; however, others appear normal and have no obvious symptoms. In this rare genetic disorder, some individuals may experience learning, behavior, and social problems.

The condition can be detected through a genetic test and treated with testosterone, the male hormone. Speech therapy and educational support can help those boys who have language, learning, or behavioral problems.

Further Readings: "Klinefelter's Syndrome." http://www.2.healthtalk.com/go/adhd/encyclopedia?p1/000382.htm. Accessed 8/11/2008; "What is Klinefelter's Syndrome?" http://men.webmd.com/tc/klinefelter-syndrome-topic-overview. Accessed 8/11/2008.

L

Laterality

Children with ADHD are often thought to prefer use of one side over the other. "Laterality" is the term that refers to the use of one side of the brain and body over the other. It often refers to the left-brain/right-brain dominance, as well as to use of the hand, foot, or eye on a particular side of the body. According to left-brain/right brain theorists, the left brain is the rational logical side of the brain where individuals process verbal, numerical, and logical thoughts. The right side of the brain is the center for art, music, and other creative endeavors.

Dr. Mary Ann Block, author of *No More Ritalin: Treating ADHD without Drugs*, believes that children with ADHD are usually right-brain dominant in their information processing and learning styles. They show a tendency to be kinesthetic learners, which means they learn best while using their hands. Most school activities accommodate left-brain learners, who are typically logical thinkers and auditory and visual learners. She believes the right-brain dominant child may be diagnosed as learning disabled even though they are often bright.

Children with ADHD and highly creative individuals are thought to have differences in the left brain compared to right-brain relationship. Howard Gardner, creator of the idea of multiple intelligences, speculates that these differences can be traced to specialization in the right and left hemispheres of the brain. A Web site http://www.borntoexplore.org lists several of these left-right brain differences.

Right Brain Traits

- Is intuitive following hunches or feelings and proposes ideas that sound illogical
- Has little awareness of time; does not fit well into schedules
- Arranges events and actions haphazardly
- Deals with information on the basis of need or particular interest at the time

- Relates to things as they are commonly known; may be identified as a concrete thinker
- Sees the big picture of things
- Likes visual imagery and may respond to pictures, colors, shapes
- Responds well to music, body language, touch
- Is visual and spatial and uses this to estimate and perceive shapes
- Likes music
- Interest in ideas and theories and may react imaginatively
- Has suspicious judgment of people or a situation until it feels right
- Learns through exploration

Left-Brain Traits

- Is methodical organizing information, classifying, and categorizing
- Keeps track of time and thinks in terms of past, present, and future
- Arranges events and actions in sequence
- Thinks in terms of sequence, one thought at a time
- Likes details, and the particulars of a thing
- Is verbal and uses words to name, describe, define things
- Processes information methodically in a well-planned way
- Learns through systematic plans

The idea of laterality and left-right brain dominance has not been proven in scientific tests using imaging but is an interesting psychological speculation and has some support especially among psychologists and educators. Some of the ideas of brain-based learning are built on these premises of hemispheric dominance.

However, if people look at children with ADHD, they see many of the behaviors dubbed right-brain traits. This speculation has led to the idea of handedness. The speech centers in the brain are related to handedness, with the left speech center controlling the right side of the body and the right speech center side relating to the left side.

A number of studies have found a higher than expected rate of nonrighthandedness—either ambidexterity or left-handedness—in the ADHD population. Norvilitis and Reid (2005) investigated this issue with two studies: one with clinically assessed children with ADHD and a second with college students that was based on responses to the Wender Utah Rating Scale. In the first study, teachers and parents reported greater attention deficits among children who were not only nonrighthanded but also described cross-dominance in the use of a foot, ear, or eye. For example, a boy may write with the right hand but use the left foot to kick a football. Thus the condition may not only be related to the hand the individual uses but may be indicative of use of one particular side. They also suspect that only a subset of handedness is associated with ADHD.

Another difference in lateralization is visuo-spatial attention. An association between ADHD and a reduction in attention in the left visual hemisphere is accepted. One study examined this occurrence by tracking eye movement of children with and without ADHD in response to a target

Children without ADHD responded more quickly in the leftward direction; those with ADHD did not show this response. The authors concluded that children with ADHD exhibit a consistent perceptual bias away from information presented in the left visual field.

Experts disagree on the number of people who are left-handed. Some researchers believe that up to 30 percent of the population has left-handed tendencies; others estimate that between 4 and 8 percent are left-handed. Questions of ambidexterity, the ability to use both hands, complicate the issue. Children who are left-handed have not been treated well in history. They have been considered clumsy, inferior, and even evil. It was not until the middle of the 20th century that educators accepted the idea of not trying to change with children who try to write with the left hand. A child's favored hand may become apparent as early as 8 months, and by age 3 the preference usually is well developed.

The question of why children are left-handed is still a puzzle, but it appears to be tied up with the same type of brain research that determines learning disabilities and ADHD. In most individuals, the left hemisphere of the human brain is usually dominant, but the nervous system is so constructed that the left hemisphere controls the right side of the body. Each hemisphere processes different kind of information. The left hemisphere is the center for language, science, mathematics, and logic. The right side is the source of dreams, fantasies, music, art, and emotion. This two-brain theory might assume that the left-hander will be right-brained and exhibit those characteristics more. Other scientists claim this is a bogus presumption and states that academic abilities are more related to intelligence, talent, and background, than to handedness.

Related to brain dominance theories is the notion that left-handedness is produced by a brain abnormality and that brains of left-handers are organized in a different way from right-handers. Many left-handers are adept at mirror writing, or writing backwards. The most famous example was the famous left-handed artist and scientist Leonardo da Vinci, who produced notebooks full of mirror writing. An added note of interest is that Da Vinci was noted for his impulsivity and nonmethodical way of working. The question is: Are the brains of left-handers organized differently from right-handers or does brain damage cause the person to be left-handed.

Some researchers pursue the idea that a neural defect causes left-handedness, and some type of brain damage caused them to be left-handed. One theory states that the blood supply to the left hemisphere was diminished during fetal growth. Another relates to birth traumas, such as premature birth, prolonged birth, breech birth, or other problems. The late Norman Geschwind (1982) theorized that the male hormone testosterone might be responsible for handedness. This hormone slows the left hemisphere development in the male fetus and possibly leads to dyslexia, attention deficit disorders, learning disabilities, and mental retardation. All these problems occur in greater numbers among males than females. Other researchers do not support this idea.

Stanley Coren (1992), a professor of psychology at the University of British Columbia, extensively investigated handedness. In his book he summarized the following basic pattern:

- Nine of 10 people are right-handed.
- Eight of 10 people are right-footed.
- Seven of 10 are right-eyed.
- Six of 10 are right-eared.

Individuals that have mixed dominance may experience more learning difficulties than those with total congruence or if all the functions are right-sided. Although 47 percent of women are totally congruent; only 41 percent of men are. Coren also stated in his book that being left-handed is related to a number of physical illnesses, such respiratory problems, arthritis, alcoholism, and early death. He also remarked that there was an inordinate number of left-handed criminals, such as Billy the Kid, Jack the Ripper, John Dillinger, and the Boston Strangler. This book caused quite a stir with its pessimistic conclusions, and further studies (1992) from the National Institutes of Health and Harvard Medical School found no risk of early death among a group of 3,774 left-handed people.

In applying some of these ideas to school difficulties, learning to read and write, children who are left-handed appear to have more difficulties, although no difference may exist in their intelligence. The problem may be that the way of English text reads from left to right. The natural progression of the hands and eyes is from the middle of the body outward. Right-handed people will naturally look and move to the right, and left-handed people to the left. Enstrom and Enstrom (1971) point out that most letters turn to "read right." For example, L, E, F, and C all open to the right. Left-handers may reverse the letters when writing and reading. The left-to-right progression is an essential skill in learning to read, but for left-handers, it is not a natural progression and may come slower.

Although no definite connection between laterality and ADHD has been established, the coincidences occur often enough to make valid studies and proposals.

Further Readings: Block, Mary Ann. 1997. *No more Ritalin: Treating ADHD without drugs.* New York: Kensington; Coren, Stanley. 1992. The left-handed syndrome: The causes and consequences of left-handedness. New York: Macmillan; Geschwind, Norman, and P. Behan. 1982. Lefthandedness association with immune disease, migraine, and developmental disorder. *Proceedings of the National Academy of Sciences USA* (August 1982):5097–100; Good news for south paws: Mortality of left-handed people. 1992. *University of California-Berkeley Wellness Letter* 8(February):2; Enstrom, E. A., and Doris C. Enstrom. 1971. Reading help for lefties. *The Reading Teacher* 25(October):41–44; Kelly, Evelyn B. 1996. *Left-handed students: A forgotten minority.* Bloomington, IN: Phi Delta Kappa Foundation; Norvilitis, Jill, and Howard M. Reid. 2005. Laterality and perceptual bias in ADHD. In *Attention Deficit Hyperactive Disorder Research*, edited by Michelle Larimer. New York: Nova Science Publishers; "The Intuitive Brain." http://www.borntoexplore.org/addint.htm. Accessed 2/3/2008.

Laws for People with Disabilities and ADHD

If children with ADHD have certain conditions, such as learning disabilities, conduct disorder, or oppositional defiant disorder, they may qualify under the Individuals with Disabilities Education Act (IDEA). Just being diagnosed with ADHD does not mean one will qualify. The condition must be such that it interferes with the education of the individual. For example, students who respond to behavior modification or medication may not qualify if the treatment aids their classroom performance. For those with defined disabilities that impair educational progress, they qualify to receive a custom-designed Individualized Education Plan (IEP); those without academic impairment can still benefit from the Rehabilitation Act (1973), Section 504.

At one time many children with disabilities were isolated and placed in separate homes and facilities. Children with ADHD or ADD were considered dumb and incorrigible; often they were encouraged to drop out of school. Some early advocates sought to improve the lot of students with special needs, but attitudes began to change when some people began to realize that soldiers from the World Wars needed counseling and vocational opportunities. The legal decision of *Brown v. Topeka Board of Education* (347 U.S.483 1954) for the desegregation of schools had implications; demanding the rights of all black children for access to equal education also included those with disabilities. In the 1970s advocates sought to change the old attitudes and provide all students with an equal opportunity for the best free and appropriate education. In 1971, a Pennsylvania court determined that retarded children are entitled to a free, public education when ever possible in the regular classroom. The *Mills v. Board of Education of the District of Columbia* (348 F.Supp.866 D.C. 1972) decision included all children with disabilities. The case mandated the three following provisions:

- A free appropriate public education (FAPE)
- An individualized education plan (IEP)
- Due process procedures.

The language of these two cases was included in the Education for All Handicapped Children Act (EAHCA) in 1975.

The following chronology describes the progress of the laws through time:

- **1954.** *Brown v. Board of Education.* Gave equal opportunity for black children including those with disabilities.
- **1972.** *Mills v. Board of Education of the District of Columbia.* Established due process procedures and an IEP.
- **1973.** The Rehabilitation Act. Section 504 introduced the first rules for addressing needs of children with disabilities. Children in school who cannot qualify under IDEA can qualify if they have a disability that impairs academic performance. *See also* Section 504.
- **1975.** Educating All Handicapped Children Act (EAHCA). This legislation became know as PL 94-142. It determines that disabled children should be mainstreamed or sent to regular schools, as much as possible. Implementation requires changes in school equipment and curriculum.
- **1990.** Americans with Disabilities Act (ADA). This law prohibits any discrimination based on disability.

- **1990.** Individuals With Disabilities Education Act (IDEA). As part of ADA, this law addressed children's rights to an appropriate education. Each student has an IEP developed by parents, teachers, and education specialists. *See also* Individuals with Disabilities Education Act (IDEA).
- **1997.** IDEA was amended to include more court cases and new regulations that strengthened the involvement of parents in developing the IEP.
- **2001.** No Child Left Behind Act. Signed into law on January 8, 2001, this sweeping reform included improved education and funding to support many initiatives, such as the inclusion of children with disabilities in regular classrooms. *See also* **No Child Left Behind Act.**
- **2004.** Individuals with Disabilities Education Act (IDEA). Changes how many services are provided but does not change the basic obligation to provide FAPE.

Further Reading: Kelly, Evelyn B. 2006. *Legal basics: A handbook for educators.* 2nd ed. Bloomington, IN: Phi Delta Kappa International.

Lead

The association between lead and ADHD is unknown. Although some studies have addressed the problem, the question is related to amount and type of exposure. H. L. Needleman of the University of Pittsburgh Medical School has conducted scores of studies over the last 20 years that do establish a link between children and specific hyperactive and attention deficit behavior traits. He has found that nutritional deficiencies and toxic accumulations of certain heavy metal can cause hyperactivity. Because bodies are smaller and their nervous systems are still developing, children are vulnerable to element imbalances. He found a common misconception is that lead exposure is only for urban children of low socioeconomic background, but contaminated soil, dust, food, and water may begin with prenatal exposure.

According to the American Academy of Child and Adolescent Psychiatry (1997), one out of every six children in the United States has blood levels in the toxic range. Other researchers believe that the amount of lead necessary to produce central nervous system problems is far lower than previously realized. Follow up studies indicate that the effects often persist into adulthood.

Braun et al. (2006) investigated studies that were contradictory. Many of them stated that the correlation between ADHD and lead was inconclusive. However, their recent findings from data obtained from the National Health and Nutrition Examination Survey 1999–2002 was that exposure to environmental lead is a risk factor for ADHD in U.S. children.

Adding to the correlation of lead levels and ADHD was a study by Michigan State University researchers who found that very low levels of lead in the blood that were thought to be safe could be contributing to ADHD. The study included 150 children who had some lead in the blood but none with the levels of 10 micrograms per deciliter, the current levels considered to be unsafe. Joel Nigg, the lead researcher found that children with ADHD had higher levels of lead in the blood than those without the disorder. Some scientists are calling for the "safe" level in the blood to be dropped from 25 mcg/dl to 5 mcg or lower.

Nigg did not study the source of the lead but speculates that lead dust came from old houses and schools. Obviously no one can eliminate all the dust and lead from those houses, but parents can carefully sweep up the dust, filter tap water, remove chipped paint, and watch what children put in their mouths, according to Nigg.

Further Readings: American Academy of Child and Adolescent Psychiatry. 1997. *Facts for families: Lead exposure.* American Academy of Child and Adolescent Psychiatry. 2004. *Facts for families: Lead exposure in children affects brain and behavior.* http://www.aacap.org/cs/root/facts_for_families/lead_exposure_in_children_affects_brain_and_behavior. Accessed 6/18/2009; Braun, Joe et al. 2006. Exposures to environmental toxicants and attention deficit hyperactivity disorder in U.S. children. *Environmental Health Perspectives* 114(12):1904–09; "MSU Researchers Link Low Lead Exposure to ADHD." 2007. http://news.msu.edu/story/963/&topic_id=11. Accessed 8/8/2008; Needleman, H. L. 1994. Childhood Lead Poisoning. *Current Opinion in Neurology* 7(2):187–90; Steele, Robert. "Can Lead Exposure Cause ADHD?" http://parenting.ivillage.com/baby/bsafety/03q63-p,00.html. Accessed 5/20/2009.

Learning Disabilities (LD)

Some children with ADHD may be considered to have learning disabilities (LD). There are many misconceptions about LDs. One myth is that the child is just refusing to do his or her work in school. Actually an LD is defined as a significant discrepancy between one's intelligence or general mental abilities and academic achievement in some area, such as reading, math, spelling, handwriting, or language. The prevalence rates can vary greatly depending on how significant the difference between the IQ and achievement is defined.

Several types of measures and formulas are used to define an LD. One of the most common uses standard deviation formulas derived from test scores on math and reading. A standard deviation is arrived at in this way. A large group of students will take the test, and the scores are charted on a bell-shaped curve. The average score of the students will be placed in the center of the curve. Statisticians have found that a certain percent of students will fall above and below the average. For example, if 34.13 percent fall above and below the average on that specific test, that range is called plus or minus one standard deviation and would contain 68.26 percent of all scores. A standard deviation of plus or minus two will represent the next 13.59 percent on either side of the scale, and those that fall within the range of plus or minus three in the standard deviation would be a small number at either end of 2.27 percent. IQ tests are based on the normal curve and are easy to diagram because the average score is 100. A person who scores 130 would be in the above normal range. All tests can be put on the normal curve. Standard deviation is a statistical calculation that takes all the scores and then calculates the average or mean. That score is put in the center of the curve. Then the difference between the score of each person who took the test and the mean is calculated. That deviation is squared and added up, and that sum is then divided by the number of raw scores of students who took the test. This is called a norm-referenced test and is based on many students who take the test at a given time. Over the years of giving the test, the numbers are adjusted and calculated to give the relationship of an individual's performance on the test. The term standard deviation may be used to describe to a parent the performance of the child on a given test.

The discrepancy formula compares scores on the IQ test with the reading and math norm-referenced achievement tests. A problem with the discrepancy formula is the tendency to overestimate the number of students with an LD. For example, a student is performing in an average manner in school but is intellectually above average or gifted according to the IQ score. If the number of a 10 percent discrepancy is used, one study found that 38 percent of children with ADHD had a reading disability and 55 percent had a math disability. Using a discrepancy of 20, Frick et al. (1991) estimated that 16 percent of students with ADHD had a reading disability and 21 percent had a math disability.

A second approach is to define an LD as having a score falling below 1.5 SDs from the mean on an achievement test, regardless of IQ. This removes the idea of discrepancy. Using this approach, Barkley (1990) found the following prevalence of LD in children with ADHD: 21 percent in reading, 26 percent in spelling, and 28 percent in math; for children without ADHD, they found 0, 2.9, and 2.9 percent, respectively.

Approximately 20 to 30 percent of children with ADHD also have a specific learning disability. In preschool years, these disabilities include difficulty in understanding certain sounds or words and/or difficulty in expressing oneself in words. In school age children, reading or spelling disabilities, writing disorders, and arithmetic disorders may occur. A type of reading disorder, dyslexia, affects up to 8 percent of elementary age children.

Children with both ADHD and LDs are the ones most in need of special education services. The term LD relates to a broad category of developmental disorders that include difficulties in reading, mathematics, and writing. Diagnosis is based on behavioral information and assumes normal intelligence, intact sensory systems, and absence of a handicap that might cause a person to have difficulty learning. Although interventions may be effective, the difficulties in learning may persist throughout the lifespan.

The most widely researched category of LD is the reading disability (RD) dyslexia. For most children with RD, the difficulty is in phonological processing or processing the sounds of words, orthographic response or recognizing letters, and speed or fluency. The deficits are presumed related to neurobiological abnormalities.

RD tends to run in families and research shows that about 50 percent of the variance in reading problems can be explained by genetic influences, possibly traced to chromosomes 6 and 15. More boys than girls have the condition, but some studies suggest that the number of boys and girls is equal and that the bias is in the selection process.

An LD occurs often with ADHD. The exact correlation is difficult to determine because of the difference in assessment criteria. Between 8 and 39 percent of children with ADHD meet the criteria for RD, 12–27 percent have a spelling difficulty, and 12–30 percent have a writing disability.

Further Readings: Barkley, Russell. 2006. *Attention-deficit hyperactivity disorder: A handbook for diagnosis and treatment.* 3rd ed. New York: Guilford Press; Frick, P. J. et al. 1991. Academic underachievement and the disruptive behavior disorders. *Journal of Consulting and Clinical Psychology* 59:289–94; Gozal, David, and Dennis L. Molfese, eds. 2005. *Attention deficit hyperactive disorder: From genes to patients.* Totowa, NJ: Humana Press; Popham, W. James. *Modern Educational Measurement.* 3rd ed. Boston: Allyn & Bacon, 2000.

Lefthandedness. *See* Laterality.

Legal and Ethical Issues

People working with individuals with ADHD should be aware of several legal and ethical issues. Children with ADHD often exasperate parents who have little skill in handling situations that may arise. Barkley (2006) outlines four issues that people who work with students need to be aware of. The following situations should be considered for those who provide mental health services and for educators:

1. Who is the guardian? A first issue involves custody or guardianship as to who can request the evaluation of the child who may be suspected of having ADHD or a comorbid condition. Many children with ODD, ADHD, and CD come from families that are divorced or separated or are in single-parent homes with another man or woman in the home. The mental health professional must be extra careful to determine who has the legal custody to request services on behalf of the child. In cases of joint custody, which is common in divorce/custody situations, the professional must determine whether the nonresident parent has the right to dispute the referral or to consent. Failure to do this investigation can lead to legal difficulties. Although these issues apply to all evaluation of children, they appear to be more common in families seeking assistance with children with ADHD.

2. Reporting of abuse or neglect. A second issue must be clarified with the parents at the beginning. Clinicians must forewarn that any suspected physical or sexual abuse or neglect must be reported to state authorities. Because of the stressful nature of dealing with children with ADHD, CD, or ODD, these children have a greater likelihood of being struck for punishment or that other types of abuse exists. Many parents themselves have psychiatric disorders, which might lead to abuse. The person dealing with the evaluation must be aware of these duties and of the laws of the state in dealing with child abuse.

3. Access to entitlements. Children with ADHD may qualify for access to certain governmental protections and entitlements. Children with ADHD in the United States are entitled to special education services under the "Other Health Impaired" category of the Individuals with Disabilities Education Act (IDEA; Public Law 101-475), provided that the ADHD is serious enough to interfere with the education of the child. Usually the term ADHD will not be applied and the comorbid terms of CD or OCD will relate to interference with the normal educational process of the child. If children come from families of lower economic means, they may be eligible for financial assistance under the Social Security Act. Clinicians need to

be aware of these laws and services that are available in order to be advocates for children with ADHD in their care. *See* Individuals with Disabilities Education Act (IDEA).

4. How accountable are children with ADHD for their actions? If ADHD is a developmental disability of self-control, how responsible are they children for their acts? Does having ADHD give these children an excuse to break the law? According to Barkley, although it is a developmental disorder, it is not like insanity in that the person is excused from responsibility. ADHD may explain why certain behaviors may occur, but it does not excuse legal accountability and should not be used as a defense for determination of guilt in criminal activities. ADHD is one of several predisposing factors for impulsive behavior, but is not a direct cause of criminal conduct.

Further Readings: Barkley, Russell. 2006. *Attention-deficit hyperactivity disorder: A handbook for diagnosis and treatment.* 3rd ed. New York: Guilford Press, 358–59; Latham, P., and R. Latham. 1992. *ADD and the law.* Washington, D.C.: JKL Communications.

Life Expectancy

Because of impulsive and lack of control of personal behavior, ADHD has an impact on life expectancy. The reduced regard for future consequences has an impact on health conscious behaviors such as exercise, proper diet, moderation in use of caffeine, tobacco, and alcohol, and use of illegal substances. Concern over life expectancy and ADHD is fairly well founded. Swensen in a 2004 study found that individuals with ADHD are twice as likely to die prematurely from their misadventures as their people without ADHD. Although longevity studies have not been done on identified children with ADHD, most of whom are now in their 40s, Friedman et al. (1995) did a follow-up of Terman's study of highly intelligent children when they were in their 70s. Friedman found that half of the "Termites" had died, and that impulsive, under-controlled personality characteristics were the most significant childhood personality traits predictive of reduced life expectancy by all causes. Individuals who had this set of characteristics lived an average of 8 years less than those who did not.

The following relationships between ADHD indicate a reduced life expectancy:

* Accident proneness in childhood
* Speeding and auto accidents in adolescence and young adulthood
* Crime
* Suicide attempts
* Use of and abuse of substances, primarily tobacco and alcohol
* A general pattern of risk taking.

Further Readings: Swensen, A. R. et al. 2004.. Incidents and costs of accidents among attention-deficit/hyperactivity disorder patients. *Journal of the American Academy of Child and Adolescent Psychiatry* 42:21415–1423; Friedman, H. S. et al. 1995. Psychosocial and behavioral predictors of longevity: The aging and death of the "Termites." *American Psychologist* 50:69–313.

Lisdexamfetamine Dimesylate

Lisdexamfetamine dimesylate is the generic name for Vyvanse, a trademark for Shire, Inc. Lisdexamfetamine dimesylate is a central nervous system stimulant prescription used as a treatment for ADHD. The medication may help increase attention and decrease impulsiveness and hyperactivity and is a federally controlled substance because it can be abused or lead to dependence. Selling or giving away lisdexamfetamine dimesylate is against the law. *See also* Vyvanse.

M

Magnetic Resonance Imaging (MRI)

Magnetic resonance imaging (MRI) has been used in the majority of studies investigating differences in brain anatomy between those with ADHD and healthy controls. Without subjecting the person to ionizing radiation, MRI can produce views from different angles. MRI is superior for detecting white-matter lesions and avoiding bony pictures associated with computerized tomography (CT).

The workings of the MRI are quite complicated. Images are produced when hydrogen nuclei in water molecules are magnetized. Atomic nuclei with an odd number of protons or neutrons have a spin, which creates a magnetic dipole moment. When the atoms of a subject's brain tissue are placed within a strong magnetic field, the nuclei have their lowest energy state and their magnetic dipoles are aligned in a parallel fashion with respect to the magnetic field. Within the magnetic field, the nuclei spin around the axis of the field—a process called precession—which causes a release of energy. The scanner localizes and detects this energy in the form of radio frequency electromagnetic waves. Then an external radio frequency pulse is added to affect the resonance of the nuclei and displace the dipoles from the plane parallel to the magnetic field. Upon removal of the external source, nuclei return to their lowest energy state and again become parallel to the magnetic field. The detected signals are then converted to an image. Some of the newer high-field MR scanners increase the resolution and thus the validity of studies quantifying brain structures clinically. Newer applications of MR technology include magnetic resonance spectroscopy (MRS), functional magnetic resonance imaging (fMRI), and diffusion imaging. These new processes have enabled investigators to explore the biochemical and physiological function basis of the brain and ADHD.

Further Reading: Gozal, David, and Dennis L. Molfese, eds. 2005. *Attention deficit hyperactive disorder: From genes to patients.* Totowa, NJ: Humana Press.

Magnetic Resonance Spectroscopy (MRS)

Magnetic resonance spectroscopy (MRS) measures directly the concentration of certain metabolites in the brain. The technique is used to gauge the relative concentrations of common biological isotopes such as hydrogen, lithium, carbon, sodium, and phosphorus. To be observable, a nucleus must have a nonzero spin property and be present in sufficient concentrations. MRS can measure specific neurochemical concentrations and composition within a brain region. For example, chemicals noted in the proton spectrum, including choline, N-acetylaspartate (NAA), creatine, and glutamate/glutamine-aminobutyric acid, can be quantified in this fashion.

Using MRS, certain neuroanatomical and neurophysiological abnormalities have been identified in children and adolescents with ADHD. Investigators have correlated regional brain structure and or function with performance on neurocognitive tests, including those measuring attention and inhibition to examine specific regions of brain abnormalities in youth with ADHD.

Further Reading: Gozal, David, and Dennis L. Molfese, eds. 2005. *Attention deficit hyperactive disorder: From genes to patients.* Totowa, NJ: Humana Press.

Manganese Exposure. *See* Industrial and Environmental Toxins.

Medicines. *See* Drug Interventions.

Memory, Working

Children with ADHD have not generally had difficulty on traditional measures of working memory, such as recall, long-term storage, and long-term retrieval. The problem does appear to arise with the executive function or putting things all together.

Working memory is defined as the ability to hold information accurately in mind that will be used to guide a subsequent response. This construct is divided into two basic types: nonverbal and verbal working memory. Researchers have developed a variety of tests that include tasks for recall, long-term storage, and short-term retrieval. Tasks involving nonverbal working memory typically involve delayed memory recall for objects and particularly for their spatial location.

Nonverbal working memory is subdivided into visual-spatial working memory, sequential working memory, and sense of time. Several tests have been designed to measure these constructs.

Visual-spatial memory is that which enables one to locate things or designs. This type of memory is used in finding where one has put things or whether one has a meeting at a certain time. Research in this area with children with ADHD is rather limited. Among children of preschool age, some tests have shown that those with ADHD have impaired memory for spatial location, whereas other studies did not find these results. Use of visual-spatial working memory might seem to be involved in the organization and reproduction of complex designs. However, Frazier et al. (2004) in a metaanalysis (a study of all the studies that have been done) found that accuracy of design copying may not be a problem for children with ADHD, although the copies of their designs may lack organization.

A second type of nonverbal memory is sequential working memory. This type shows the capacity to hold a sequence of information in mind. This capacity would seem to be involved in the ability to imitate the complex and lengthy behavioral sequences that would be new to a child. An example would be whether the child can imitate increasingly lengthy and novel sequences of three simple motor gestures such as fist, palm on side, palm down. These tests may not measure a problem with memory but more motor coordination. The evidence from other studies is not convincing that children with ADHD have a sequential working memory deficit.

The sense of time is also a part of nonverbal working memory. Aspects of the sense of time are mediated through the prefrontal cortex, basal ganglia, and cerebellum, areas that are also involved in people with ADHD in the following six areas:

1. Time perception. Tests for time perception involves the presentation of pairs of related short-duration items to a participant, who must make judgments about differences in the duration of these intervals. Children with ADHD had difficulty with discriminating very short intervals; however, another study did not find differences in intervals of short duration but made more errors of discrimination at the presentation of at intervals of longer duration.

2. Motor timing. Motor timing reflects the ability of a person to either freely reproduce a repetitive motor response at a regular interval or to mach a repetitive motor response to a brief repetitive stimulus. Neuropsychiatrists have found this type of timing to involve the basal ganglia and cerebellum. Given that these structures are implicated in ADHD, children with the condition may have difficulty in short-term motor timing.

3. Time estimation. Time estimation is the person's ability to accurately perceive the duration of a time or temporal interval. Children who are defined as impulsive may have more difficulty in performing these tests. Two factors may come into play during these tests. If there is a distracter, children with ADHD are more prone not to do as well as control children, and those with poor sustained attention may not score well on these tasks.

4. Time production. Time production is the ability to generalize at verbally specified clock time interval. In these tasks, individuals were asked to turn a flashlight on and off for a defined time interval, such as 5 or 10 seconds. General research did not find this to be a problem either in children or adults unless distracters were present.

5. Time reproduction. For all people time reproduction tasks are the most difficult of timing tasks, placing heavy demands of working memory. In this test a flashlight is turned on and off during a period of time, but not told the duration of time. The subject is then asked to replicate the time. To use the working memory, the person must watch the sample interval, hold the duration in mind, and then generate an equivalent duration of time using the flashlight. Teenagers with ADHD made greater errors on this time reproduction task, when compared to control subjects. Also, the longer the duration time, the greater the reproduction error.

6. Use of time management in natural setting. Researchers used rating sheets from parents and teachers to study time management in a natural setting. They used 25 items related to how often the children got ready for deadlines on time, did homework on time, completed chores on time, and talked about time and their past. Children with ADHD had significantly more problems than the control group.

In the area of verbal working memory, a greater number of studies have been performed. These tasks unusually involve retention and oral repetition of a group of numbers usually in reverse order and mental computation in arithmetic. Children with ADHD have been found to be significantly less proficient in performing in the area of numerical memory than control groups.

Children with ADHD are generally not impaired with storage and recall of simple information relating to verbal memory. However, when long complex amounts of verbal information must be held in mind, especially if the length of time is tested, then people with ADHD may show deficits. When the subjects must organize material or information, they appear less proficient than those matched controls. When viewing television for recall of a story, children with ADHD appear less proficient, especially if toys are present as a distracter. Other elements related to working memory are hindsight, forethought, and planning.

Adam Baddeley defined the idea of working memory as a psychological construct of simultaneously storing and processing information. He suggested that working memory is made of four systems:

- A phonological loop for verbal and acoustic information
- A visuospatial sketchpad for visual and spatial information
- An episodic buffer that integrates information from the central system and from different modalities.
- A central executive system that oversees the above functions.

Rapport and colleagues use a similar definition of working memory as a set of memory processes that serve to construct, maintain, and manipulate cognitive representations of incoming stimuli. They propose that working memory is a primary deficit in children with ADHD that results in disorganized behavior and a need to seek additional stimulation.

Memory Training Programs

Cogmed, a company founded in 2001 in Naperville, Illinois, is a leading company in the field of neurotechnology. Based on the work of Karolinska Institute in Sweden, a new study from the ADHD clinic of Southern California demonstrated the effectiveness of the Cogmed Working Memory Training to improve attention and executive processing in children with ADHD. The study found significant improvements in working memory, mental stamina, and inhibition and decreases in ADHD symptoms. The Cogmed Working Memory Program used video game software to perform verbal and spatial working memory tasks 5 days for 5 weeks. Thirty-five ADHD children raging in age from 7 to 17 were trained in the Cogmed Working Memory Program. Each student had been screened positively for ADHD based on a battery of neuropsychological tests, which were applied to all 35 children before training and then again 4 weeks after training. More than 90 percent showed improvement. The same tests were given to 17 of the children 6 to 8 months after training. Eighty percent had improved significantly.

In addition, parents' check lists showed significant improvements in impulsivity, task initiation, working memory, and planning. The children were assessed while not taking their medications.

Further Readings: Baddeley, D. 1986. *Working memory.* Oxford: Oxford University Press; Barkley, Russell. 2006. *Attention-deficit hyperactivity disorder: A handbook for diagnosis and treatment.* 3rd ed. New York: Guilford Press; Frazier, T. W. et al. 2004. Meta-analysis of intellectual and neuropsychological test performance in attention-deficit/hyperactivity disorder. *Neuropsychology* 18:543–55; Gozal, David, and Dennis L. Molfese, eds. 2005. *Attention deficit hyperactive disorder: From genes to patients.* Totowa, NJ: Humana Press; Medical News Today. "Boston Researchers Present Study Showing Working Memory Training in School Can Help Students with Attention Deficits." http://www.medicalnewstoday.com/articles/89527.php. Accessed 5/27/2009; Rapport et al.

Mercury Poisoning. *See* Industrial and Environmental Toxins.

Methylin

The active ingredient in Methylin is methylphenidate, a stimulant drug. The FDA approved MethylinER 10- and 20-mg tablets in May 2000 as a treatment for ADHD. MethylinER adds two more options to help physicians provide control and greater flexibility in treating ADHD. MethylinER has an 8-hour duration of action, although behavioral efficacy is assessed most accurately on an individual bases. The extended release formulation helps children when dosing schedules are problematic at school or other functions.

There is also a Methylin oral solution of 5 and 19 mg/5ml. The oral solution can be stored at room temperature.

MethylinER and Methylin oral solution are federally controlled substances CII because they can be abused or lead to dependence. Selling Methylin may harm others and is against the law. Tell you doctor if you or your family have a history of or have abused or been dependent on alcohol, prescription medicines, or street drugs. *See also* Methylphenidate (MPH)

Methylphenidate (MPH)

Methylphenidate (MPH) and dexmethylphenidate are prescription medications that have proven effect in the treatment of ADHD in children, adolescents, and adults. The drugs increase effective utilization of dopamine and norepinephrine in parts of the brain that regulate attention and behavior to control symptom and improve functioning. Researchers have shown that stimulant medications are the most effective treatment options for ADHD. The American Academy of Pediatrics and the American Academy of Child and Adolescent Psychiatry consider these medications the best treatment options; however, behavioral interventions and lifestyle modifications are also recommended.

MPH is available as the following compounds:

- Ritalin and Methylin (MPH) immediate release 5-, 10-, and 20-mg tablets, 3- to 4-hour duration; chewable 2.5-, 5-, and 20-mg tablets.
- Metadate ER and Ritalin SR (MPH, extended release, wax matrix) 10- and 20-mg tablets with variable absorption and 3- to 8-hour duration.

- Methylin ER (MPH extended release with methylcellulose base) 10- and 20-mg tablets; a grape-flavored oral solution, 5 mg/5 ml and 10 mg/5 ml doses and 3- to 8-hour duration.
- Ritalin LA (MPH long-acting) 10-, 20-, 30-, and 40-mg capsules that can be opened and sprinkled on food; 8- to 12-hour duration.
- Metadate CD (MPH controlled delivery) 10-, 20-, and 30-mg capsules that can be opened and sprinkled on food; 8- to 12-hour duration.
- Concerta (MPH once daily18-, 27-, 36-, and 54-mg bullet-shaped caplets that cannot be opened or crushed; tablet shell may appear in stool; 12-hour duration.
- Daytrana (MPH patch) 10-, 15-, 20-, and 30-mg patch; apply to clear hairless area in the morning and remove after 8 hours; duration coincides with the time the patch is worn.
- Focalin (dexmethylphenidate) immediate release 2.5-, 5-, and 10-mg tablet; twice as potent as MPH; 3- to 5-hour duration.
- Focalin XR (dexmethylphenidate extended release) 5-, 10-, and 20-mg capsules; can be opened and sprinkled on food; 12-hour duration.

Even though MPH and dexmethylphenidate are available as different brand names and formulations, these drugs still have the same active medicine when they are absorbed in the blood stream. For example, when swallowing Ritalin LA, Metadate CD, or Concerta, the person will have the active ingredient MPH in the blood stream. When swallowing Focalin or Focalin XR, the person will have dexmethylphenidate in the blood stream.

Concerns About MPH

Both MPH and dexmethylphenidate should not be taken by individuals with schizophrenia, schizoaffective disorder, bipolar disorder, or other psychotic disorders because the condition may worsen. Women who are pregnant or trying to be pregnant should avoid these drugs. People with heart defects such as structural abnormalities, uncontrolled high blood pressure, persistent rapid heart beat, any disorder of the blood vessels, overactive thyroid, glaucoma, or uncontrolled seizures are at a greater risk for these adverse cardiac/cardiovascular effects. However, those without structural cardiac abnormalities are also at risk. In 2006 the FDA warned of serious cardiac and cardiovascular risk including sudden unexplained death (SUD) with MPH or dexmethylphenidate use and abuse in children, adolescents, and adults. Studies have shown that adults taking the drug have higher rates of heart attack and stroke compared to those who do not take stimulants, and therefore the risk compared to the benefit of taking the drug needs to be considered. In addition, psychiatric adverse events including hallucinations and increased aggression have been reported in individuals taking MPH and dexmethylphenidate. The risk of these effects is greater in those with existing psychiatric illness. *See also* Concerta; Ritalin.

Neither of the drugs should be taken together or within 14 days of a drug called a monoamine oxidase inhibitor (MAOI) used to treat depression. The medicines taken together can result in dangerously high blood pressure that can be fatal.

Both MPH and dexmethylphenidate carry a risk for abuse to get "high," thus the U.S. government's Drug Enforcement Agency (DEA) considers each a controlled substance. Pharmacies must closely regulate the storage and dispensing of these medications. Taking MPH and dexmethylphenidate to treat ADHD does not increase the likelihood of developing a substance abuse disorder, and it may prevent the individual from self-medicating with alcohol, marijuana, or other illicit drugs. However, if a person has an active substance abuse disorder, MPH and dexmethylphenidate are not good treatment options.

Taking MPH and Dexmethyphenidate

There are several points to remember about taking these drugs:

- With the exception of Concerta, MPH and dexmethylphenidate should be taken as prescribed on an empty stomach early in the day to minimize sleep disorders.
- Immediate release formulations should be given two or three times a day to provide symptoms relief throughout the day.
- Long-acting medications that last for 8 to 12 hours should be taken once a day in the morning. Capsules that have beads may be opened if a person has trouble swallowing; however, these beads should be swallowed whole without chewing. If they are chewed, they will be taken from the stomach directly to the bloodstream and the long-lasting action will no longer be in effect.
- Concerta has a tablet shell that is not changed in the intestine and may appear in the stool intact. Concerta should not be given to people who have narrowing of the intestine or those who have had stomach bypass surgery.
- The MPH patch should be applied to a clean hair-free area in the morning before school and removed approximately nine hours later.
- While taking MPH and dexmethylphenidate, one should not use alcohol or illegal drugs.
- Strong organic acids can affect the absorption of MPH and dexmethylphenidate. Avoid the following foods for at least one before and two hours after taking medications: citrus fruits and juices, soda/carbonated beverages, lemonade, Gatorade, vitamins and food supplements containing vitamin C.
- If one overdoses on MPH and dexmethylphenidate, treat it as a poison incidence and immediately call 911. Overdosing can cause high fiver, tremors or muscle twitching, large pupils, extreme agitation, abnormal heart rhythms, seizures, extreme high blood pressure, and in some cases, death.

The following are possible side effects of MPH and dexmethylphenidate:

- The most common side effects are loss of appetite and insomnia. Taking the medication on a full stomach or having the physician lower the dose may avoid these side effects.
- Loss of appetite and weight loss can be improved by serving the child small frequent meals of favorite foods when the stimulant effects are low. This could occur in the morning before taking the medication or at night when the medication's effects have lessened.
- Insomnia can be avoided by giving the medication as early in the day as possible. Some doctors may prescribe sedating medications, such as clonidine,

guanfacine, or trazodone at night. Melotonin has been found effective to manage insomnia associated with ADHD medication use in children.

- Children may experience abnormal tics such as eye-blinking, nose scrunching, or shoulder shrugging. This may indicate the medication is too strong or that the medication needs to be changed.
- Mild anxiety or restlessness can be managed with dosage reduction or changing the prescription.
- The MPH patch can cause irritation such as a rash and discomfort at the patch site. Rotating the patch may help; however, if the irritation continues, the patch should be discontinued.
- Severe anxiety, panic attacks, mania, hallucinations, paranoia, and delusions are all possible. If they occur, the health care provider should be contacted immediately for discontinuation and evaluation.

Further Readings: Food and Drug Administration. "Label Insert for Ritalin" http://www.fda.gov/; National Alliance on Mental Illness. http://www.nami.org. Accessed 5/27/2009.

Modafinil

Modafinil (Provigil; Cephalon, Inc.) is a novel agent that is indicated to improve wakefulness in patients with excessive sleepiness, narcolepsy, and other conditions related to sleep disorders. A study suggests that the drug inhibits the sleep-promoting neurons by blocking norepinephrine reuptake. Some medications for narcolepsy has been useful in ADHD when the following conditions are prevalent:

- An unsatisfactory response to stimulant or antidepressants after trials of two or three different agents
- Inability to tolerate treatment-emergent side effects such as insomnia or loss of appetite
- Presence of risk because of moderate-to-severe side effects or a history of cardiac problems
- Development of tolerance to the benefits of stimulants or antidepressants
- ADHD symptoms in populations with special problems such as psychoses, schizophrenia, or other developmental disorders
- Presence of severe mental retardation
- Inadequate response to monotherapy
- Use in combination with a stimulant or antidepressant to treat a comorbid diagnostic condition

Modafinil is labeled for use in patients 16 years or older with sleep disorders and is not presently labeled by the FDA for use in ADHD. It is generally well tolerated, with common side effects including insomnia, abdominal pain, depression, headache, nervousness, and nausea.

Multimodal Interventions

A number of interventions are encouraged for treating ADHD. The treatments may include one of more of the strategies. See each one of the treatments under the specific heading. Treatments include parent education and support, dietary intervention, neurofeedback such as EEG, biofeedback, and functional neuromuscular stimulation, psychophysiology, educational and behavioral interventions, behavioral modification, psychostimulant medication, SAMONAS sound therapy, exercise for inhibition of primitive reflexes, Bowen therapy, craniosacral therapy, relaxation training and hypnosis, social skills training, energy therapy (EFT), Reiki, Bach flower essences, aromatherapy, meditation/prayer, stress management, and discovering and nurturing a talent.

Multimodal Treatment Study of Children with ADHD (MTA)

The National Institute of Mental Health sponsored a large multiple-site study called the Multimodal Treatment Study of children with ADHD (MTA). This massive study of 579 elementary school children, both boys and girls, was presented by Dr. Peter Jensen at the 2000 Academy of Pediatrics meeting, in Chicago.

The children were assigned to one of four treatment programs:

- Medication management alone
- Behavioral treatment alone
- Combination care
- Routine community care

In each of six study sites containing from 95 to 98 children, three groups were treated for the first 14 months in a specified protocol and the fourth group was referred for community treatment of the parents' choosing. All the groups were reassessed regularly through the study period. An essential part of the program was the cooperation of the schools, including principals and teachers. Both parents and teachers rated the children on hyperactivity, impulsivity, and inattention, and the symptoms of anxiety and depression, as well as social skills. The children in two groups of medication management alone and combination treatment were seen monthly for one-half hour at each medication visit. Also, during this treatment, the physician spoke with each parent, met with the child, and sought to determine any concerns that the family might have regarding the medication or the child's ADHD-related difficulties. The physicians also sought input from the teachers on a monthly basis. The doctors in the medication-only group did not provide behavioral therapy but did advise the parents when parents or children asked concerning any problems the child might have.

In the behavior treatment only group, families met ups to 35 times with a behavior therapist, mostly in group sessions. The therapies also consulted the children's teachers at school and supervised a special aide assigned to each child in the group. Also, children attended a special 8-week summer treatment program where they worked on academic, social, and sports skills and intensive therapy were provided to help each child improve behavior skills.

Children in the combined groups received both therapies. They received all the counseling with medication meetings and also the behavioral therapy. Those children who were in routine community care saw the doctor of the parents' choice one or two times a year for short periods of time. These sessions would be what the physician would normally give to patients. The doctor did not have any interaction with teachers.

The researchers found that those in long-term combination treatments and the medication-management alone were superior to intensive behavioral treatment and routine community treatment. In some areas such as anxiety, academic performance, oppositional behavior, parent-child relations, and social skills, the combined treatment was usually superior. Another advantage of the combined treatment was that children could be successfully treated with lower doses of medicine, compared to the medication-only group.

Further Readings: Jensen, P. S. et al. 2001. Findings from the NIMH multimodal treatment study of ADHD (MTA): Implications and applications for primary care providers. *Journal of Behavior Pediatrics* 22:60–72; MTA Cooperative Group. 1999. A 14-month randomized clinical trial of treatment strategies for attention-deficit/hyperactive disorder (ADHD). *Archives of General Psychiatry* 56:1073–86.

N

National Attention Deficit Disorder Awareness Day

The U.S. Senate declared September 7, 2004, as the first National Attention Deficit Disorder Day. Senator Maria Cantwell (D-Washington) introduced the resolution and Senator Richard Durbin (D-Illinois) cosponsored the initiative. The resolution recognized ADHD as a major public health concern and hoped to draw attention to the dearth of information about the disorder. The document also stated that the hope of identifying this day would encourage an honest discussion about ADHD and its impact on children and adults in schools, in the workplace, and in relationship and would encourage sufferers to seek relief. The thrust of the day was to give information and to counteract misinformation that is often inaccurate and misleading.

Several items were contained in the resolution:

- To designate a specific day as National Deficit Disorder Awareness Day
- To recognize ADHD as a major health concern
- To encourage people of the United States to find out more about ADHD and its supporting mental health services and seek treatment if appropriate
- To express the sense of the Senate that the Federal Government has a responsibility
- To endeavor to raise public awareness about ADHD
- To continue to improve access to and the quality of mental health services dedicated to improve the quality of life for children and adults
- To request the President issue a proclamation calling of federal, state, and local administrators to observe the day with appropriate programs and activities

In the 109th Congress, Senators Cantwell and Durbin in presented Resolution 544 for National Attention Deficit Disorder Awareness Day on September 20, 2006. This resolution emphasized how ADHD is the most extensively studied mental disorder in children and affects an estimated 3 to 7 percent of 400,000 school age children. Supporting organizations included National Mental Health Organization, American Counseling Association, American

Psychiatric Association, Children and Adults with Attention Deficit/Hyperactive Disorder, and the Federation of Families for Children's Mental Health.

Further Reading: ADDers. "USA 1st Official ADD Awareness Day." 2004. http://www.adders.org/news87.htm. Accessed 5/27/2009.

Neurofeedback

Neurofeedback, a type of biofeedback, is designed to help people control brain wave patterns using electroencephalography (EEG).This approach for treating ADHD has been studied and practiced for a number of years. By placing electrodes on the scalp, the EEG measures the waves of electrical activity and brain wave pattern of the brain. The individual is not aware of these involuntary brain processes and through the information provided in neurofeedback can become aware of his own biological state and gain some control over it.

Neurofeedback works in this way. Everyone has the following five major types of brain wave patterns:

- Delta waves, a very slow wave of one to four cycles per second seen mostly during deep sleep
- Theta waves, slow brain waves of five to seven cycles per second, seen during daydreaming or almost to the point of falling asleep
- Alpha waves of eight to twelve cycles per second, seen during relaxed states
- Sensorimotor rhythm waves (SMR) of twelve to fifteen cycles per second, seen during focused relaxation to prepare a person for a physical challenge
- Beta waves fast waves of thirteen to twenty-four waves per second, seen during concentration or mental work states.

When a normal person tries to read or concentrate, he increases the amount of beta waves in certain parts of the brain. In people with ADHD, these waves are not seen. Instead of the increase of beta waves, the children increase the theta or daydreaming waves. This indicates that other children are concentrating to complete a task, but the children with ADHD are drifting off. The children have a high theta/beta wave ratio.

Neurofeedback seeks to increase the beta/theta ratio. Over a series of forty or more sessions the child works to increase the ratio using various activities and games.

Dr. Joel Lubar and colleagues of the University of Tennessee have reported effective of neurofeedback in the treatment of people with ADHD. In studying more than 1,200 children, Lubar found that the basic issue for these people is the inability to maintain beta concentration states for sustained periods of time. He also found these children have excessive theta daydreaming feedback. Through the use of neurofeedback, the patients were taught to increase the amount of beta waves and decrease the amount of theta waves. In other words, they learned to make their brains more active.

The format of the neurofeedback is like a game. The patient's brain is hooked up to the equipment with electrodes, and the computer feeds back the activity of the brain to the person. Sitting in front of the computer monitor, patients watch their brainwave activity as they respond to games. Many are able to gradually shape brainwaves to appear normal. NASA has developed a technique that blends biofeedback with video games. Neurofeedback gives the patient control over the process, and some have reported success.

David Rabiner, Duke University, divided 100 children diagnosed with ADHD into two groups for treatment: both groups received stimulant medication, parent counseling, a program of school academic support; however one group received neurobiofeedback in addition to the regular treatment. The study lasted for 12 months. Children in the neurofeedback group had attention training sessions lasting 30 to 40 minutes and were tested periodically with QEEG scans to determine effectiveness. A QEEG scan is a technique to identify the pattern of the cortical brain region under activity in children with ADHD. Training continued until the patients no long exhibited abnormal cortical slowing. The results showed that incorporating neurofeedback can yield important benefits. Only those participants whose attention training included biofeedback showed benefits after medication was discontinued. Their results indicated that gains from neurofeedback training cannot be just attributed to the placebo effect but reflect meaningful changes in EEG activity.

However, neurofeedback is still considered controversial. Russell Barkley, a noted ADHD researcher, claims little evidence exists that neurofeedback works at all. He considers some of the research is faulty and that use of technology in a medical environment has a placebo effect. Long-term effectiveness needs to be established. Another critic is neurophysiologist Sam Goldstein who believes also that the older studies were flawed but would like to see more research into the technique. Obviously, on the use of neurofeedback for ADHD, diverse ranges of viewpoints exist.

Further Readings: Amen, Daniel. 2001. *Healing ADD: The breakthrough program that allows you to see and heal the 6 types of ADD.* New York: Berkley Books; Rabiner, David. "The Role of Neurofeedback in the Treatment of ADHD." http://www.add.org/articles/TheRoleofNeurofeedbackintheTreatmentofADHD.html. Accessed 5/27/2009; "The Role of Neurofeedback in ADHD Treatment." http://www.add.org/articles/TheRoleofNeurofeedbackintheTreatmentofADHD.html. Accessed 6/18/2009.

Neuroimaging

Neuroimaging is a technique using high technology devices that take pictures of the brain. The pictures reveal the function of different parts of the brain.

In 1990 Alan Zametkin and colleagues at the National Institute of Mental Health published a landmark article that evaluated brain metabolic activity in 25 adults with ADHD who had a childhood history of the disorder. The authors used positron emission tomography or PET scans to detect states of brain activity and found reduced metabolic activity in the frontal and striatal regions of the brain. Although, there was difficulty in replicating the exact study, this article with its demonstration that reduced brain activity in particular regions became a seminal idea for other investigators to pursue.

Since that time, a number of neuroimaging studies have concentrated on the brains of people with ADHD. Some studies concentrate on the anatomy and physiology, and other studies focus on blood flow and the physiological functions of the central nervous system. The following are several neuroimaging techniques that provide different looks at the brain:

- Computerized tomography (CT). Used for more than 30 years to examine the CNS
- Magnetic Resonance Imaging (MRI). Used in a majority of studies to investigate the differences in the anatomy of people with ADHD compared with healthy controls
- Single-photon Emission Computed Tomography (SPECT). Used to study the function of the brains
- Positron Emission Tomography (PET). Used to measure metabolism and neurotransmitters
- Functional Magnetic Resonance Imaging (fMRI). Used to study anatomy as well as changes in blood flow
- Magnetic Resonance Spectroscopy (MRS). Used to study chemicals in the brain.

These study tools are valuable in studying what is happening in ADHD and possible interventions.

A new biological evaluation tool has been in clinical trials in four sites in the United States. This test uses the chemical agent Altropane which lights up certain areas of the brain when the patient is put into a brain scanner. Altropane measures the number of dopamine transporters and the natural brain chemicals, which most physicians believe are increased beyond normal levels in ADHD. This is consistent with the fact that the most commonly prescribed medication Ritalin blocks these dopamine transporters. Boston Life Sciences, a biotechnology company, holds the patent for Altropane, which is manufactured by Alseres Pharmaceuticals. *See also* Computerized Tomography (CT); Functional Magnetic Resonance Imaging (fMRI); Magnetic Resonance Imaging (MRI); Magnetic Resonance Spectroscopy (MRS); Positron Emission Tomography (PET Scans); Single-Photon Emission Computed Tomography (SPECT).

Further Readings: Medical News Today. "Boston Life Sciences, Inc. Announces The Issuance Of A U.S. Patent Licensed To BLSI By Harvard Et Al That Covers Methods For The Diagnosis Of ADHD." 2006. http://www.medicalnewstoday.com/articles/49349.php. Accessed 5/26/2009; Gozal, David, and Dennis L. Molfese, eds. 2005. *Attention deficit hyperactive disorder: From genes to patients.* Totowa, NJ: Humana Press; Zametkin, A. J. et al. 2009. Cerebral glucose metabolism in adults with hyperactivity of childhood onset. *New England Journal of Medicine* 323:1361–66.

Neurons

About 100 billion neurons, tiny cells of about one-millionth of an inch across, are in the brain and nervous system. Each neuron has a similar pattern: a cell body, which has tens of thousands of tiny branches called dendrites. Dendrite literally means "little tree" because the structures look like limbs of small trees on the cell body. The dendrites receive messages from other neurons. Each neuron also has a long extension, called an axon, which sends information to other cells. Axons can range in length from less than a millimeter to over a meter long. The axons of one neuron never touch the dendrites of another because a tiny gap called a synapse exists between the two. The electrical message or impulse is helped across the gap by a neurotransmitter. Also the impulse only flows in one direction: from the dendrite of one neuron through the cell body through the axon across the synapse to the dendrite of the next neuron. Every neuron makes from 1,000 to 10,000 synapses with surrounding neurons. It is interesting to imagine a piece of brain the size of a grain of sand that would contain 100,000, 2 million axons, and 1 billion synapses, all talking to each other.

Further Readings: Brown, Thomas E. 2005. *Attention deficit disorder: The unfocused mind in children and adults.* New Haven: Yale University Press.

Neurotransmitters

Neurotransmitters are chemicals in the brain that help transmit the electrical impulses in the brain from one neuron to another. There are about fifty different neurotransmitter chemicals. These chemicals are manufactured in the brain and stored in tiny bubbles called vesicles, located near the back end of each neuron. When a message comes through a neuron, the vesicles release small amounts of the neurotransmitter to help carry the electrical impulse across the synapse or the gap between neurons. The action is very quick. Each molecule of a transmitter stays on the receptor for only about 50 milliseconds (one thousandth of a second). Twelve messages can be carried across the synapse in 1 millisecond.

Any transmitter not used in the process is pumped back into the vesicle by specialized cells called transporters. This movement allows the system to reload for more action in a fraction of a second. At any one given time, vast numbers of messages are surging through millions of circuits in the brain all supported by neurotransmitters. Two neurotransmitters, dopamine and norepinephrine, are important in ADD and ADHD.

Dopamine plays an important role in signaling possible reward situations and in registering reward as it is experienced. Dopamine is produced deep in the midbrain in the ventral tegmental area at rates and in amounts that vary according to the brain's needs. The main pathways of the dopamine system extend throughout the prefrontal cortex and into limbic centers to release dopamine in response to perceived danger or reward. As the brain registers pleasure, more dopamine helps to sustain the rewarding action. Critical for motivation is the dual role that dopamine circuits play in mobilizing the effort to get what the individual needs. What happens when dopamine is not released? The brain does not experience motivation to work, even for rewards that otherwise might be pleasurable. Roy Wise in a 1989 study of rats, monkeys, and humans showed that when the effects of dopamine are blocked, motivation and pleasure are also blocked. Dopamine itself does not create the pleasure but establishes the conditions where sensations are recognized as pleasurable.

Norepinephrine is the primary neurotransmitter produced in the reticular system and locus coeruleus. When the locus coeruleus fires, it distributes norepinephrine through its broad network of connections, alerting and increasing excitability in its many neural networks. Lack of such firing is associated with inattention, increased drowsiness, and sleep.

J. A. Owens in the book *Conn's Current Therapy* distinguishes between the two neurotransmitters in this way: Abnormal dopamine levels play a role in attention and hyperactivity, whereas low levels of norepinephrine may contribute to inattention and the inability to control impulsive behavior. Research suggests that persons with ADHD manufacture dopamine and norepinephrine just like everyone else, but their brains do not release and reload these neurotransmitters. As a result many messages that need to get carried along are not transmitted effectively and efficiently.

Further Readings: Brown, Thomas E. 2005. *Attention deficit disorder: The unfocused mind in children and adults.* New Haven: Yale University Press; Owens, J. A., and Dalzell, V. 2004. Attention deficit and hyperactivity disorder. In *Conn's current therapy*, 56th ed., edited by R. R. Rakel and E. T. Bope, 947-958. St. Louis, MO: Elsevier.

No Child Left Behind Act

Children with ADHD are not addressed in the No Child Left Behind Act (NCLB). Provisions of the act are complex and controversial. In calculating the formula for NCLB, the data about groups of children are disaggregated, or figured separately, rather than just left with the group from the entire school. Schools are given quotas for improvement in each one of the disaggregated areas.

Generally just the diagnosis of ADHD that can be helped with medication or other strategies do not qualify for disability designation. However, if the is so severe as to impair educational performance, the child may qualify. Generally these children would qualify for designation as a comorbid condition such as a learning disability, conduct disorder, or oppositional defiant disorder.

NCLB was enacted in 2002 as part of the reauthorization of the Elementary and Secondary Education Act of 1965. The purpose of the act is "to ensure that ALL children have a fair, equal, and significant opportunity to obtain a high-quality education and reach, at a minimum, proficiency on challenging state academic achievement standards and state academic assessments." (20 U.S.C. Section 6301).

The following are provisions of the act:

- Each state must set aside at least 2 percent of NCLB grants for it lowest-achieving schools with the greatest needs.
- State plans must be coordinated with IDEA and other federal programs.
- States must adopt standards of what children are expected to know and be able to do. Courses must contain coherent and rigorous content and encourage the teaching of advanced skills.

- States must develop and implement a single statewide accountability system that uses sanctions and rewards to ensure adequate yearly progress (AYP).
- AYP requires schools to apply the same high standards of achievement to all public schools. All students must make continuous progress on measurable objectives for each subgroup. Children with disabilities, including ADHD, are one of the subgroups. Each state defines AYP with measurable objectives.
- States must ensure that not later than 12 years after the end of the 2001–2002 or the 2013–2014 school year all students in each subgroup, including those with ADHD, will meet or exceed the proficient levels of academic achievement on statewide tests.
- At least 95 percent of students in each group are required to take the statewide assessments in reading, math, and science. Failure to test at least 95 percent of children with disabilities automatically results in failure to make AYP.
- Students with disabilities will receive "reasonable adaptations" and accommodations to measure children's achievement toward their appropriate academic standards. These reasonable adaptations have been a source of contention.
- What are the adaptations for children with ADHD? Possibly, giving them more time on tests. However, the test for students with disabilities cannot be "watered-down" and must have the same standards.
- Parents have a right to know. At the beginning of the school year, the local education agency (LEA or school district) must notify parents about the professional qualifications of teachers.
- All districts must implement scientifically based, empirically validated instructional programs, and parents should be in on the choice of these programs.

The consequences for failing to comply with NCLB are drastic. If a school fails for two consecutive years to make AYP as defined by the state, then all students have the option to transfer to another school. Priority is given to the lowest-achieving schools and students from low-income families. After the fifth year of corrective actions, the following actions may be taken:

- Give up Title I grants
- School choice is continued, and parents may choose another school.
- Reopen as a charter school.
- Replace all or most of the staff.
- Contract with a private agency to run the school.
- Turn the LEA over to the state.
- Other major restructuring strategies.

NCLB is undergoing reauthorization in 2008. Some provisions will probably be changed. NCLB has received lots of criticism for not considering individual children but lumping their progress in a group. Another area of criticism involves that different states have different standards.

Further Reading: Kelly, Evelyn B. 2006. *Legal basics: A handbook for educators.* 2nd ed. Bloomington, IN: Phi Delta Kappa International.

Norepinephrine

Norepinephrine (NE) is one of two neurotransmitters that are important in ADD and ADHD. The other neurotransmitter is dopamine. As a neurotransmitter norepinephrine is packaged after manufacture in the brain into chemicals that help transmit electrical impulses in the brain from one neuron to another. The chemical is stored in tiny bubbles called vesicles, located near the back end of each neuron. When a message comes through a neuron, the vesicles release small amounts of the neurotransmitter to help carry the electrical impulse across the synapse or gap between neurons. The action is very quick. Each molecule of a transmitter stays on the receptor for only about 50 milliseconds (one thousandth of a second).

Both NE and dopamine (DA) play essential roles in attention and thinking. Both agents contribute to maintaining alertness, increasing focus, and sustaining thought, effort, and motivation. NE and DA are structurally similar and differ only in the presence of a hydroxyl group; DA is a precursor or forerunner to NE synthesis in the brain. However the difference in the behavioral effect and actions in the brain show these chemicals have distinct complementary roles.

NE arises from the locus coeruleus (LC), a small area in the basal brain located near the pons in the midbrain. Here, cell bodies generate NE. From this region NE projects and diffuses widely in the brain. Floyd Bloom, a pioneer of functional research on NE, called it a "neuromodulator" because of its generalized effect that differs from a neurotransmitter that is more localized.

NE has a role in the following processes:

1. Maintaining and increasing overall arousal
2. Regulating excitability and response to danger or opportunity
3. Contributing to memory storage and retrieval, especially emotionally intense events
4. Assisting in emergency response
5. Maintaining basal or tonic alertness; for example, when reading a book at night, the effort to remain alert and stay on task is partially mediated by NE.

Aston-Jones et al. (1999) suggests a picture to describe the functional role of NE. One is walking through the woods at dusk and suddenly hears an abrupt crack of the sound of a stick being broken some yards away. The senses burst alive as the person turns the head in the direction of the sound, the heart begins to race, and the mind frantically rushes to determine the source of the noise. Your thoughts race to determine if this is danger. The increase in pulse rate is from epinephrine arising in the adrenal glands, but NE mediates the cognitive mental component of alerting and reasoning. Here one decides whether to run, drop to the ground, or stand perfectly still. Experience also has a role in NE modulation.

Alteration of the NE system disrupts cognitive and arousal function that is part of several disorder, including ADHD. The hypothesis that led to measuring NE, epinephrine, and DA in ADHD and in normal situations is understood in the context of neuroimaging and animal studies. A role for all three neurotransmitters exists in ADHD. The neurotransmitters affect attention, alertness, and arousal through a crucial balance. Simply too much or too little of a single neurotransmitter does not explain the diversity or complexity of ADHD symptoms. Imaging does show that NE contributes to generalized alertness and to acute activation; NE is also critical to executive functioning involved in reasoning, learning, and problem solving.

Further Readings: Aston-Jones G. et al. 1999. Role of locus coeruleus in attention and behavioral flexibility. *Biological Psychiatry* 46:1309–20; Berridge, C. W. et al. 2003. The locus coeruleus-noradrenergic system: Modulation of behavioral state and state-dependent cognitive process. *Brain Research Review* 42:33–84; Hunt, Robert D. 2006. "Functional Roles of Norepinephrine and Dopamine in ADHD." *Medscape Medical Psychiatry and Mental Health*, 11(1). http://www.cme.medscape.com/viewarticle/523887. Accessed 5/27/2009.

Nutrition

Food does more than just keep us from being hungry. What one chooses to eat can have a direct effect on feelings and behavior. The science of nutrition is gaining attention, because studies are appearing to show these connections. Scientists have recognized the importance of food in treating certain metabolic condition. For example, children with the condition phenylketonuria (PKU) can consume nothing that has the amino acid phenylalanine and must have a specific diet to control the disorder.

The study of nutrition and its role in ADHD is based on correlational studies. In a correlation study, the researcher has shown that statistically there has been a connection or statistical correlation between the ADHD and the entity of study. Correlation studies do not show cause and effect. It should be emphasized that the reader should take these studies for what they are- someone has shown a connection or correlation between two things. Correlation studies do not show cause and effect.

The following nutritional deficiencies have been correlated to learning disabilities and ADHD:

- Calcium deficiency.
- High serum copper.
- Iron deficiency can cause irritability and attention deficits.
- Magnesium deficiency may lead to fidgeting, anxiety, restlessness, psychomotor problems, and learning difficulties.
- Malnutrition in general is related to learning disabilities; the child does not have to look malnourished, a forgotten fact in affluent countries.
- Dyslexic children appear to have abnormal zinc and copper metabolism: low zinc and high copper.
- Iodine deficiencies have been linked to learning difficulties.

Likewise, the role of nutrition in treating ADHD is controversial. The mainstream medical community is ambivalent about the role of nutrition and generally does not regard nutrition as viable in reducing symptoms. However, a number of individuals promote the idea that if food contributes to ADHD, eliminating certain foods from the diet may relieve the symptoms.

Food as medicine dates back to Hippocrates who said, "Let your food be your medicine, your medicine be your food." The proposition of the intake of food as being significant has basis in some scientific studies. Several studies indicate that children with ADHD are metabolically different from other children, and thus diet modification plays a role in the management. Several nutritional programs include the Feingold Diet; elimination of certain food additives; elimination of flavor enhancers, soft drinks, and sugar; safety issues with water; addition of certain essential fatty acids; herbal remedies; and keeping a balance of amino acids and proteins.

Perhaps the best know of dietary alternatives is the Feingold Diet, which involves removing salicylates (aspirin derivatives), artificial colors and flavors, and certain synthetic preservatives from children's diets. Benjamin F. Feingold, M.D., was Chief of the Allergy unity at Kaiser Permanente Medical Center in San Francisco when he treated a belligerent patient with a severe case of hives. Suspecting that she was aspirin sensitive, he told her to eliminate aspirin and all foods that had additives similar to aspirin. Not only did the child's hives go away but her attitude also improved. This experience led him to eventually become convinced that diet and nutrition were important in treatment. He taught that if a person is sensitive to something, there could also be a behavioral effect. The Feingold Association of the United States provides information about this diet.

The second area that some researchers have connected to ADHD is that of food additives. The Department of National Health and Welfare defines a "food additive" as any substance or its byproducts, the use of which may affect the characteristics of foods. These additives are usually chemicals and are not spices, seasoning, and flavorings. About 10,000 additives are approved in the United States. They are usually connected with foods that have been highly processed and consequently are in nature high in calories and of less nutritional value. If a person is sensitive to such chemicals, behavior can be affected. A proponent of eliminating additives is Dr. Michael Lyon, author of *Healing the Hyperactive Mind: Through the New Science of Functional Medicine*. He points out that these are true sensitivities resulting from the reduced ability of the liver or other systems to detoxify the body. Eliminating manmade pesticides and food additives may reduce this toxic load on the brain.

Salt, pepper, and glutamic acid are the three most important flavor boosters in the United States. The popular form is monosodium glutamate (MSG). Although classified as a food additive, it has drug-like effects on some people. Glutamates and aspartate are closely related and are considered by some as powerful free radicals or substances that cause damage to the body. Eliminating food with MSG from the diets of some ADHD children who are sensitive has resulted in improvement in many problems.

Overconsumption of soft drinks may cause problems when these drinks replace healthy drinks such as low-fat milk and water. One of the problems identified here is the presence of phosphoric acid, which leaches calcium from bones and causes health problems. Excess sugar intake creates all sorts of problems including elevated cholesterol and triglyceride levels.

Water contaminated with arsenic, mercury, asbestos, aluminum, chlorine, fluorine, and *Escherichia coli* may be related to behavior problems.

Plants are probably one of our oldest forms of food and nutritional supplements. These include oat straw, gotu kola, yellow jasmine, hops, St. John's wort, wild lettuce, German chamomile, passion flower, kava kava, and valerian.

Amino acids are considered the building blocks of life. They are nitrogenous organic acids that make the proteins that are part of the peptides and proteins of the body. Eight amino acids are essential for life: isoleucine, leucine, lysine, methionine, phenylalanine, threonine, tryptophan, and valine. A deficiency of an amino acid in a child or adult may cause problems such as ADHD.

In the 1980s vitamin B6 was promoted as a helpful remedy for children with learning difficulties including inattentiveness. In 2006 a study showed that children with autism had significantly lower magnesium than control subjects and that the correction of this deficit was helpful. Later zinc and multivitamins have been promoted as cures, and currently the addition of certain fatty acids such as omega-3 has been proposed as beneficial.

Mild stimulants such as caffeine and theobromine may improve the function of some children who have ADHD. *See also* Feingold Diet; Food Additives; Herbal Medicine; Sugar.

Further Readings: Ali, Elvis et al. 2001. *The all-in-one-guide to ADD and hyperactivity.* Niagara Falls, NY: AGES Publications; Lyon, M. 2000. *Healing the hyperactive mind: Through the new science of functional medicine.* Calgary, AB, Canada: Focused Publishing; Hersey, Jane, and Robert C. Lawlor. 1996. *Why can't my child behave?: Why can't she cope? Why can't he learn?* Alexandria, VA: Pear Tree Press.

O

Obesity

Some recent studies have connected obesity and ADHD. According to Bazar et al. (2006), obesity and ADHD are both increasing in prevalence. At one time researchers thought that ADHD and the activity involved would keep students from gaining weight. However, several new studies show that childhood exposure to television may link ADHD and obesity. ADHD is related to dysfunctional cognitive overstimulation, and obesity is related to changed patterns of diet and exercise. Bazar and colleagues contend that ADHD and obesity are comorbid and propose that the two represent different manifestations of the same underlying dysfunction. They call the happening "environmental oversampling syndrome," which occurs when there is an oversupply of information both in the form of food and sensory content. Thus, the person may independently be predisposed to both obesity and ADHD.

The pathologic mechanisms may overlap so that overeating contributes to ADHD and hyperstimulation contributes to obesity. The emerging association between psychiatric and metabolic disorders such as overeating suggests a possible biologic link between the two. Environmental oversampling syndrome may represent the various metabolic, inflammatory, and behavioral conditions. Conditions that seem very different, such as insulin resistance, diabetes, hypertension, syndrome X, obesity, ADHD, depression, psychosis, sleep apnea, inflammation, autism, and schizophrenia may operate through common pathways. Treatments that are beneficial to one condition may benefit the others.

Waring and Lapane (2008) found that children with ADHD are at a 50 percent higher risk for being overweight if they are not taking medication for the condition. However, those who are medicated have an increased risk of being underweight. The researchers from Brown University, Providence, Rhode Island, collected data from 63,000 children ages 5 to 17 from the 2003–2004 U.S. National Survey of Children's Health. Children with ADHD should be monitored for overweight/underweight issues

Further Readings: Bazar, K. A. et al. 2006. Obesity and ADHD may represent different manifestations of a common environmental oversampling syndrome: A model for revealing mechanistic overlap among cognitive, metabolic, and inflammatory disorders. *Medical Hypotheses* 66(2):263–69; Reinberg, Steven. "ADHD Might Raise Kids' Obesity Risk." http://health.usnews.com/articles/health/healthday/2008/07/07/adhd-might-raise-kids-obesi. Accessed 7/19/2008; Waring, M. E., and Lapane, K. L. 2008. Overweight in children and adolescents in relation to attention-deficit/hyperactivity disorder: Results from a national sample. *Pediatrics* 122(1):e1-6.

Obsessive Compulsive Disorder (OCD)

Children and adults with obsessive compulsive disorder (OCD) have certain behaviors that are repeated over and over. It may be that they wash their hands constantly or are overly conscious about germs. They may have to do certain things or certain movements in a certain way. Sometimes tic disorders and OCD are grouped together.

Peterson et al. (2001) has performed the largest study to date following 976 children into early adulthood and examining the relationship among ADHD, tic disorders, and OCD. The study found that OCD declined initially by adolescence but then increased by 3.3 percent in early adulthood. Tics and OCD were significantly related to each other at adolescence and again in young adulthood, whereas OCD was associated with ADHD at both time points. The Peterson study suggested some relationship between childhood ADHD and adult OCD, but most of the children with ADHD did not develop tic disorders or ADHD. The risk among children with ADHD of having OCD is not a clear one and may be at most 3–5 percent. However, Brown (2000) found the inverse relationship may be true and suggests that 6–33 percent of children with OCD may have ADHD.

Further Readings: Brown, T. E. 2000. Attention-deficit/hyperactivity disorders with obsessive-compulsive disorder. In *Attention-deficit disorders and comorbidities in children, adolescents, and adults,* edited by Thomas Brown, 209–30. Washington, D.C.: American Psychiatric Press; Peterson, B. S. et al. 2001. Prospective, longitudinal study of tic, obsessive-compulsive and attention-deficit/hyperactivity disorder in an epidemiological sample. *Journal of the American Academy of Child and Adolescent Psychiatry* 40:685–95.

Oppositional Defiant Disorder (ODD)

Children with Oppositional Defiant Disorders (ODD) are those that display significant problems with stubbornness, defiance and refusal to obey, temper tantrums, and antisocial behavior. Studies have shown that more than 65 percent of those who are referred to clinics may have this disorder, and 45 to 84 percent of those with ADHD may meet the full diagnostic criteria for ADD either alone or with conduct disorder (CD). ODD may occur by itself in the absence of CD; CD rarely occurs alone in children with ADHD and almost always occurs being seen in the context of ODD.

Bird et al. (1993) found that 93 percent of their Puerto Rican children with ADHD also had either ODD or CD. The most common types of conduct problems found in these studies are lying, stealing, truancy, and to a

Table 13 ODD Behaviors in ADHD and Normal Children

Behavior	Hyperactive Children, %	Normal Children, %
Argues with adults	72.4	21.1
Defies adult requests	55.3	9.1
Deliberately annoys others	51.2	13.6
Blames others for own mistakes	65.9	16.7
Is easily annoyed by others	70.7	19.7
Spiteful or vindictive	21.1	0
Swears	40.7	6.1

Source: Barkley, Russell et al. 1990. Does the treatment of ADHD with stimulant medication contribute to illicit drug and abuse in adulthood: Results from a 15-year prospective study. *Pediatrics* 111:109–21.

lesser degree physical aggression. Children with comorbid ADHD and CD/ODD have higher levels of impulsivity than children with only ADHD. This implies that the presence of ODD/CD implies a more serious form of ADHD. However, in the United States, the difference between ADHD and ODD are defined. Symptoms of hyperactivity do not mean the child is defiant. ODD by itself appears to decline significantly with age, which CD increases with age.

Barkley et al. (1990) studied behaviors in a group of hyperactive children compared to a normal group. All the differences were significant except "is spiteful or vindictive." The prevalence of these behaviors in ODD is shown in Table 13.

Disrupted parenting may be more a correlate of CD than ODD and may reflect antisocial characteristics of the parents. One form of CD may be genetic, existing in spite of family environment. *See also* Conduct Disorder (CD).

Further Readings: Barkley, Russell. 2006. *Attention-deficit hyperactivity disorder: A handbook for diagnosis and treatment*. 3rd ed. New York: Guilford Press; Barkley, Russell et al. 1990. Does the treatment of ADHD with stimulant medication contribute to illicit drug and abuse in adulthood: Results from a 15-year prospective study. *Pediatrics* 111:109–21; Bird, H. R. et al. 1988. Estimates of the prevalence of childhood maladjustments in a community survey in Puerto Rico. *Archives of General Psychiatry* 32:361–68.

Osteopathy

Dr. Andrew Still (1828–1917) founded osteopathy in 1878. Osteopathy differs from traditional medicine because it asserts that rather than expose the body to outside treatments like drugs, doctors should seek to regulate the body's functions by natural means.

An osteopath may have additional training in cranial osteopathy or study of the skull or cranium. The brain is covered by a tough membrane, called the meninges. The outer layer of the meninges is called the dura or dura mater. Osteopaths believe that the meninges are constantly under tension, which may create pressure in the head. When this occurs, the individual cannot concentrate or may lost control and have temper tantrums. According to their beliefs, all children with ADHD display this tension. Other organs may be affected. For example, the diaphragm, the muscle lying between the chest and abdomen may become very tight. A number of factors can contribute to the increased tension:

- Prenatal shock or physical trauma, which causes increased release of stress hormone that affect the fetus
- Drugs, cigarettes, and medications (including those used at birth)
- Shock to the infant, such as a lack of oxygen at birth
- Chickenpox

The treatment involves very slow release of membrane tension by manipulating the membranes to where they should be.

Further Reading: Cooper, Paul, and Katherine Bilton. 1999. *ADHD: Research, practice and opinion.* London: Whurr Publishers.

P

Parenting the Child with ADHD

ADHD can tear families apart, no matter what the age of the person with ADHD. Families in general have tremendous power both to help and to hinder. If the family is willing to be a partner in working with the person with ADHD, then helping will be more effective than all the medications, behavior modifications, and alternative therapies ever devised. However, if the family focuses on the person' problem behaviors, it will continue to be a war zone. For the family to use its considerable power to heal, it must be willing to accept the challenge of change.

Here are tips for the management of ADHD within the family (Hallowell 1994):

1. Get an accurate diagnosis. The importance of the diagnosis as a starting point is exceedingly important. Insist on taking time to get this diagnosis and do not accept the first physician who will give medication as a quick bandaid. ADHD is a neurological disorder that needs thoughtful evaluation.

2. Educate all family members. Everyone must learn the facts about ADHD as a first step for treatment. The entire family must have information about the condition and make sure that all questions from everyone are answered. Many of the helpful sources are listed in Appendix B. The attitude of the family is of utmost importance; having information is the beginning of the change in the family's attitude.

3. Try to reinvent the reputation of the family member with ADHD to one of respectability. Reputations within the family can be just like reputations within a town or an organization, keeping the individual in the model of negative expectations. Try to develop the positive aspects of that person, and try to convince the family to accept these positive aspects. This person can bring something special to the family: energy, creativity, and humor. The person with ADHD usually livens up any gathering that he or she attends. He may be irreverent and impulsively speaks his mind. Try to accept the positive contributions that he can make to the family.

4. Be sure to recognize that no one is to blame for ADHD. It is not Mother's or Dad's fault, nor is it the fault of a distant relative. All members of the

family must understand that no one is to blame. Such lingering thoughts may give the person an excuse for irresponsible behavior.

5. Make it clear that ADHD is a family issue. Some medical problems may affect only one family member, but not ADHD. Its effects begin in the morning and continue through dinner. It affects vacations and quiet times. Each member can become a part of the solution to the family's problem.

6. Take care to balance the attention among members of the family. The child with ADHD cannot be the only one who gets the attention, even if it is negative. He or she cannot run the show. Other siblings also need to have attention; parents must organize their lives so that the children without ADHD can express their feelings and feel they are important too.

7. Try to avoid the big struggle that may pit family members against each other. This struggle is especially common in families where ADHD is not diagnosed or where it is not properly treated. Without care, this struggle can eat away at a family and consume them.

8. Once a diagnosis is made, learn to negotiate. One of the best books on negotiating, which is written for business but also applies to the psychology of family living, is *Getting to Yes: Negotiating Agreement without Giving In* by Roger Fisher and William Ury. The following four principles are given in this book:

   • Negotiate on the principle and on the merits. Separate people from the problem. Attack the problem without attacking the person. When the person is attached to the problem, he or she may never give in because of losing face.

   • Focus on interests and not positions. Negotiating should never be debating but instead look at mutual interests that need to be satisfied. Teenagers especially may become entrenched on a position that they do not even believe in to save face.

   • Generate a list of options before deciding what to do. Do not think everything must be wrapped up in one meeting. Give the people who are involved an opportunity to think about the options. People with ADHD may impulsively want to close options and have a quick solution. Guard against closing too soon.

   • Base the results on some objective criteria. Such criteria might include: What do other families do about the problem? What does the school recommend? What does the medical community recommend? Is there a set of religious or personal values that enters in?

9. If the family cannot be successful in negotiations, consider bringing in a family therapist or professional.

10. Role playing can be extremely helpful in helping members see themselves as others see them. The person with ADHD is not usually known for being perceptive about their effect on others. Videotaping scenarios may also help.

11. When you sense the big struggle coming, try to disengage from it. Once it has started, it is hard to get out of. The best way to handle it is not to get engaged in it in the first place.

12. Make sure everyone in the family is heard. Sometimes the quiet ones are neglected and will not speak up.

Successful People with ADHD: Clarence Page (1947–), Prize-winning Journalist and Commentator

Clarence Page found out he had ADD when his son Grady, a bright verbal boy, had so much difficulty in school. When his teachers suggested that Grady may have a learning difference, he was surprised when they asked if others in the family had the same difficulty and suggested he attend a lecture "Fathers of Sons with ADD". Clarence began to think of himself: disorganized, waiting until the last minute to write stories, and thriving in the chaotic environment of the newsroom. He drank a lot of coffee and chain-smoked, two habits that calmed him down and helped him focus. He began to think of himself in school and the difficulty that he had focusing long enough to read long books. He described his life as fifty TV sets going on in his mind.

At first he was in denial about both Grady and himself, but the more he studied and talked to people, he realized that he had ADD. He began taking Ritalin and found that he was indeed able to focus without smoking and drinking coffee. Clarence was an example of a parent who was diagnosed with adult ADD because of his son. Taking Ritalin has enabled him to turn off forty-nine of the TV sets in his brain, and he now focuses only on one.

Source: Corman, C. A., and E. Hallowell. 2006. *Positively ADD: Real stories to inspire your dreams.* New York: Walker and Company.

13. When there is success, be sure to applaud it. Try to get everyone focused on positive goals rather than gloomy negative expectations.
14. Be sure to clearly outline the family expectations, rules, and consequences.
15. Avoid the pattern of loving the child one day and hating him or her the next. Although all children may be demons one day and little angels the next, keep your feelings on an even keel.
16. Parents must present a united front. Make time to confer with your spouse about the progress being made. Such conferences will keep one parent from being the ogre and the other taking the side of the child. Children delight in playing one parent against the other; regular conferences will keep this from happening.
17. Do not keep ADHD from other member of the family. It is nothing to be ashamed of.
18. Find the problem areas. Such times may include study time, morning, bedtime, dinnertime, times of transition, and vacations. Negotiate with each other on how to make it better, and ask each other for specific suggestions.
19. Have family brainstorming sessions, when a crisis is not occurring. Figure out how the situation could be better handled. Be willing to try new solutions.
20. Listen to people from the outside, such as teachers, pediatricians, therapists, and other parents and children. Sometimes a source from the outside my help when family members will not listen to each other.

21. Make the effort to accept ADHD in the family just as you would any other condition. Try to normalize it as much as possible.
22. Keep a sense of humor. ADHD can drain a family's energy; try to look at various situations in a humorous way.
23. Enlist support groups. There are on-line sources for support as well as community-based supports. Find these sources and use them. You will find you are not alone.
24. Encourage members of the family to cultivate their own interests. This is very important for parents of children with ADHD. They are so overburdened by dealing with the difficult child that they forget themselves.
25. Be sure to let your child know that you care about him or her. Demonstrating love and affection will develop self-esteem in children. When a child must be corrected, do it in a way to instruct them and not punish.
26. Children with ADHD can try the patience of parents. However, remember that you are the adult and must remain calm. When you are calm, the child, who is upset, will calm down too.
27. Children with ADHD respond better to routine. Organize your life and the life of the child. That may mean regular schedules for meals and bedtime. Calendars are helpful in keeping track of events and activities.
28. Give your child only one direction at a time. Simplify instructions. Tell the child exactly what you want him or her to do.
29. If you believe that the child's disability may interfere with learning, investigate using a computer or a simple writing computer like Alphasmart (Renaissance Learning, Atlanta, GA) in the classroom. Handwriting may be a problem, and such devices can help. You should be able to get these accommodations simply by asking.
30. Keep the hope. Hope is the best medicine in maintaining a positive outlook.

Further Readings: Fisher, Roger, and William L. Ury. 1991. *Getting to yes: Negotiating agreement without giving in.* New York: Penguin Books; Hallowell, Edward M., and John J. Ratey. 1994. *Driven to distraction: Recognizing and coping with attention deficit disorder from childhood through adulthood.* 141–47. New York: Touchstone Press.

Parent Training Programs (PT)

Parent training programs are considered as one of the prongs of treating children with ADHD. Numerous research studies have established its efficacy and effectiveness for the management of the disruptive child in the home. There are many way to conduct PT programs for children with ADHD. Arthur Anastopoulos in "Counseling and Training Parents" in Barkley (2006) established an eight- to twelve-session program that can be used for training and consists of the following ten steps:

1. Program overview. The parents are given an orientation to ADHD, its causes, risks, and effective and ineffective treatments.
2. Understanding parent-child relations. Parents are taught about causes of child's disruptive behavior and the principles of behavior management.
3. Improving positive attending skills. Parents are taught the power of positive attending in human relationships and assigned to practice with catching the "child being good."

4. Extending positive attending skills and improving child compliance. Parents are taught to give effective commands and increase parent monitoring.
5. Establishing a home token/point system. Parents are shown how to create a token system, setting the system up for 8 weeks.
6. Adding response cost. Parents introduce fines for misbehavior.
7. Using time out. Parents learn how to use time out.
8. Managing behavior in public places. Parents are taught to discuss public places and set up three rules and establish incentives and penalties.
9. School issues and preparing for termination. Parents are taught the nature of school behavior problems and are assigned to meet with teacher.
10. Booster session. Parents are given encouragement on how to continue what they have learned in the training.

Several community-based programs for parent training have been designed. Barkley (2006) established a model called Community Parent Education Program (COPE). The workshops are an integration of principles, techniques, and goals of social-learning-based parenting programs, social-cognitive psychology, family systems theory, and models for larger support groups.

Further Reading: Barkley, Russell. 2006. *Attention-deficit hyperactivity disorder: A handbook for diagnosis and treatment.* 3rd ed. New York: Guilford Press.

Pemoline. *See* Cylert.

Pharmaceuticals. *See* Drug Interventions.

Phytotherapy. *See* Herbal Medicine.

Porphyria Disease

Porphyria is a hereditary enzyme-deficiency disease that can lead to behavior changes, depression, and hallucinations. Sometimes the behaviors will mimic those of attention deficit and hyperactivity. The disease is caused by abnormalities in the production of heme, a substance that makes up the red blood cells. Porphyria causes both skin and neurological complications. Because many enzymes are required for the production of heme, abnormality of even one can cause the disease.

The diagnosis of this disease is very difficult because the range of symptoms is very common to many disorders, and interpretation of the tests is very complex. A person with porphyria must avoid sunlight, fasting, consumption of any alcohol, dehydration, and supplement that contain iron.

Further Reading: "Porphyria Disease." http://www.depression-guide.com/porphyria. htm. Accessed 8/11/2008.

Positron Emission Tomography (PET Scans)

Positron emission tomography (PET) is an imaging technique that measures regional cerebral blood flow, oxygen and glucose metabolism, cerebral blood volume, and the extraction of water actors the blood-brain barrier.

PET may also examine neurological receptor binding, with specific radio-tracers designed for such targets as D2dopamine, 5-HT2 serotonin, gluta-mate, histamine, and opiate receptors. Images are based on the tracer's ability to emit a short-lived particle called a positron. However, in order to make positron-emitting radioisotopes, a cyclotron is necessary to generate isotopes of carbon, nitrogen, oxygen, or fluorine. During the process, posi-trons collide with nearby electrons and produce two photons that travel in the opposite direction. The detector creates the image by using a "coinci-dence circuit" that recognized the simultaneous ionization.

The energy of the g-photons detected in PET is higher than those created in single-photon emission computed tomography (SPECT), thereby creating higher sensitivity. PET also produced cross-sectional images inherently. Although PET is a powerful and promising technique, it is very expensive and has limited availability. The positive-emitting isotopes live only a few hours and must be manufactured near the site of usage.

Further Reading: Gozal, David, and Dennis L. Molfese, eds. 2005. *Attention deficit hyperactive disorder: From genes to patients.* Totowa, NJ: Humana Press.

Posttraumatic Stress Disorder (PTSD)

Posttraumatic stress disorder (PTSD), a relatively new disorder that was introduced in DSM-III, can be the result of both victimization and nonvic-timization trauma. Several studies have shown that there are no meaningful differences between the group with ADHD and a control group in trauma exposure of PTSD. According to a study by Wozniak et al., approximately 12 percent of the group with ADHD had been exposed to some type of traumatic event, compared to 7 percent of those in the control group; the statistics were not significantly different. The authors of the study found there was no meaningful association of ADHD with trauma, but that child-hood bipolar depression was an antecedent for later trauma.

Further Reading: Wozniak, J. et al. 1999. Antecedents and complications of trauma in boys with ADHD: Findings from a longitudinal study. *Journal of the American Academy of Child and Adolescent Psychiatry* 38:48–55.

Preschool ADHD Treatment Study (PATS)

The preschool ADHD treatment study (PATS) is the first major effort to examine the safety and efficacy of the stimulant methylphenidate (MPH) for ADHD in the preschool age group. The 70-week PATS study uses a random-ized, placebo-controlled, double-blind design with children ages 3 to 5 who had severe and persistent symptoms of ADHD that impaired their function-ing. To avoid using medications at such an early age, all children who entered the study were first treated with behavioral therapy. Only those who did not show sufficient improvement were considered for the medica-tion part of the study. The study was conducted at the New York Psychiat-ric Institute, Duke University, Johns Hopkins University, New York University, the University of California, Los Angeles, and the University of California at Irvine.

The study enrolled 303 preschoolers ranging in age from 3 to 5 years. According to the National Institute of Mental Health (NIMH) report, "only those with the most extreme ADHD symptoms who did not improve after behavioral therapy and whose parents agreed to have them treated with medication were included in the study. In the first part of the study, the children took a range of doses from a very low amount of 3.75 mg daily of methylphenidate, administered in three equal doses, up to 22.6 mg/day. By comparison doses for older children usually range from 15 to 30 mg/day. The study compared the effectiveness of methylphenidate to placebo. It found the children taking methylphenidate had a more marked reduction of their ADHD symptoms compared to children taking a placebo and that different children responded best to different doses."

The study was governed by a strict set of ethical standards and additional review to ensure the safety of the very young children. Their health was closely monitored throughout the duration of the study. The teacher rating of the children who attend preschool at various stages also was reviewed. Similar to the 1999 NIMH MTA study, and other studies of school-aged children, PATS found the medication did appear to slow the preschoolers' growth rates. The children grew about half an inch less in height and weighed about 3 pounds less than expected.

About 89 percent of the children tolerated the drug well, but 11 percent or about 1 in 10 had to drop out because of side effects. Weight loss of more than 10 percent was considered a severe side effect resulting in investigators' discontinuing the medication. Other side effects included insomnia, loss of appetite, mood disturbances such as feeling nervous or worried, and skin-picking behaviors.

The study did show that preschoolers with severe ADHD symptoms can benefit from the medications.

Further Readings: Wilens, T. E. et al. 2003. Does stimulant therapy of attention deficit/hyperactive disorder beget later substance abuse? A meta-analytic view of the literature. *Pediatrics* 111:179–85; "Preschoolers with ADHD Improve with Low Doses of Medication." http://www.nimh.nih.gov/press/preschooladhd.cfm?Output=Print. Accessed 4/12/2007.

Preschoolers

With the added emphasis on preschool education and the number of preschools that are available to children, the diagnosis and consideration of ADHD is not just in school-aged children. ADHD has become the most common mental health diagnosis for children ages 3 to 5. According to the September 2007 issue of the *Harvard Mental Health Letter*, researchers have begun to explore the use of drugs and other treatments for preschoolers.

When children are such a young age, it is quite difficult to determine whether the behavior is a problems or is just "kids being kids." How does one tell? Behaviorists are specialists who study children of similar age and determine a range of normal behaviors. For example, a child who is so hyperactive that he consistently squirms while belted in the car seat and always ends up with the belt around his neck is obviously deviating from the norm. Comparing this child with others the same age would assist in determining whether the symptoms are inconsistent with the developmental level.

Such behaviors in preschoolers with ADHD indicate they are not just inattentive and overactive; they are a real danger to themselves and others. In spite of instruction and warnings, they may play with matches or rush into traffic. They are noisier than other children and appear to have no concern when corrected. Obviously, they cause havoc in both home and school.

Although the Food and Drug Administration (FDA) has not approved stimulant drugs for children under age 6, a large controlled trial of methylphenidate (Ritalin) and other drugs in children ages 3 to 5 found that giving the medication is not as effective as in school-age children.

Parent training is the most popular alternative. This training is based on the belief that assisting parents to develop positive skills is important. If a parent is negligent or intrusive, it might trigger hyperactive behavior in a child who has such a tendency. If cruel or harsh discipline is used, it may evoke stubbornness and unusual resistance. Parents are shown how to set appropriate limits and use moderate rewards and punishment. The researchers encourage parents and physicians to be slow to make the diagnosis and to consider parent training and even specialized day dare before resorting to stimulant drugs.

Limited research is also a major problem in dealing with preschool children. Clinical practice guidelines are lacking. Child mental health professionals from the Bradley Hasbro Children's Research Center, one of the first psychiatric hospitals exclusively for children, and eleven other institutions have developed recommendations for clinicians who are considering medications for children ages 3 to 6.

Programs to assist preschool children with ADHD are being developed and researched. One such innovative curriculum program called Tools of the Mind hopes to improved academic performance, reduce diagnoses of ADHD, and close the achievement gap between children from poor families and those from wealthier homes. Dr. Adele Diamond, University of British Columbia, led the first evaluation of Tools program (2007). This program focuses on executive functions (EFs) or the ability to put things together, which is located in the prefrontal cortex area of the brain. Functions include resisting distraction, considering responses before speaking, mentally holding and issuing information, and mental flexibility to think outside the box. Diamond noted how these skills are rarely taught to the preschooler, but can provide a huge advantage, especially for disadvantaged children. Diamond attributes part of the recent explosion in ADHD in preschoolers to some children's never learning to exercise control, attention, and self-discipline. She believes that some of the children are simply deficient in these skills because they have never been taught. Tools encourage out-loud instruction and dramatic play. In today's school climate of high-stakes testing, children in preschool are pushed into areas, such as reading and writing, before many are physically able. This puts pressure on teachers and gives little time for the child to learn these important EF skills. Diamond believes that preschool teachers must limit play and spend more time on instruction; however, "social-pretend" play may be more critical to academic success.

Physcian Guidelines for Treating Preschoolers with ADHD

Although there is limited research and few guidelines, use of stimulants, antidepressants, and other psychiatric drugs is on the rise with preschool-age children. A group of mental health professionals from the Bradley Hasbro Children's Research Center, the first psychiatric hospital exclusively for children, and 11 other institutions have developed recommendations to help clinicians who are considering medications for children ages 3 to 6.

Preschool Psychopharmacology Working Group, a consortium of researchers in early childhood psychiatric disorders, psychopharmacology, general and behavioral pediatrics, neurodevelopmental processes, and clinical psychology developed the guidelines. The results were published in the December 2007 *Journal of the American Academy of Child and Adolescent Psychiatry*, with the lead author Dr. Mary Margaret Gleason of Bradley Hasbro. Treatments were recommended for ADHD, disruptive behavior disorders, major depressive disorder, bipolar disorder, anxiety disorders, posttraumatic stress disorder, obsessive-compulsive disorder, pervasive developmental disorders (such as autism), and primary sleep disorders. Many of these disorders are comorbid conditions with ADHD.

The study developed the treatment algorithms (procedures that guide through recommended assessment and treatment steps) based on a review of existing literature on the use of psychiatric medications in preschoolers, knowledge about preschooler's development, available data on school-age children and adolescents, and expert clinical experience.

Step one is a comprehensive diagnostic assessment, considering the child's emotional and behavioral symptoms, relationship patterns, medical history, and developmental history and status. If a psychiatric condition is diagnoses, the study authors recommend beginning with family-focused psychotherapy. Parent management training or parent-child (dyadic) psychotherapy must be considered before ordering medication. Even if medication is deemed necessary, it should be used in conjunction with psychotherapy. Dr. Gleason said that the guidelines are not intended to promote medications, but that they may actually reduce the number of preschoolers who are taking psychiatric drugs.

Here are the guidelines for the physician:

- At every decision point reassess the diagnosis and formulation. These steps are critical because preschoolers develop and change so rapidly.
- Psychotherapeutic interventions are essential and must be continued.
- Each step must be marked by a preponderance of evidence that supports the recommendations; this allows clinicians to consider the evidence and anecdotes of behaviors, and apply it to the individual patient.
- If a child is responding to medication, have a period of discontinuance; this trial period will enable the physician to reassess the child's symptoms and appropriate treatment.

- If the child at the end of the regimen of treatment still has ongoing impairment and distress, consult with an expert in child psychiatry.
- The researchers emphasize that ongoing research must be continued in this unknown area.

One effort for study is the Preschool ADHD Treatment Study (PATS). This is an ongoing multisite study sponsored by the National Institute of Mental Health. PATS is the first major effort to examine the safety and efficacy of a stimulant for ADHD in this age group. *See also* Preschool ADHD Treatment Study (PATS).

Further Readings: Gleason, M. M. et al. 2007. Psychopharmacological treatment for very young children: Contexts and guidelines. *Journal of the American Academy of Child and Adolescent Psychiatry* 46(12):1532–72; Diamond, Adele et al. 2007. Preschool Program improves cognitive control. *Science* 318(5):1387–88; Medical News Today. "How Best to Treat Preschoolers with ADHD: The Harvard Medical Letter Discusses the Options." 2007. http://www.medicalnewstoday.com/articles/81498.php. Accessed 5/27/ 2009; Research Matters. "Preschool Program Improves Cognitive Control." December 10, 2007. http://www.nih.gov/news/research_matters/december2007/12102007kids.htm. Accessed 5/27/2007; Wilens, T. E. et al. 2003. Does stimulant therapy of attention deficit/hyperactive disorder beget later substance abuse? A meta-analytic view of the literature. *Pediatrics* 111:179–85.

Public Awareness and ADHD

In history people with ADHD did not fare very well. The public in general considered the traits of a child with the disorder as coming from bad seed: being disrespectful or willfully choosing to be disruptive and disorderly. Before the 1980s, there were a handful of ADHD organizations that developed, but during this decades more than 100 were organized into national networks and political action organizations. In 1987 a group of parents and two psychologists in Plantation, Florida, frustrated by what to do and where to turn, formed a group for children with attention deficit. Now the group Children and Adults with Attention-Deficit/Hyperactive Disorder (CHADD) has more than 20,000 members worldwide. The Attention Deficit Disorder Association (ADDA) was formed in 1989. Greater interest in the conditions evoked this great public/parent activism. Initiatives were taken to have state and federal laws studied and evaluated to include ADHD as an educational disability in need of special services in public schools.

When the Education for All Handicapped Children Act of (PL 94-142) was passed in 1975, the intent was that children who were classified with minimal brain dysfunction (MBD) under the category of learning disabilities would be eligible for special educational services, but children with hyperactivity, attention deficit, or ADHD were not included because of the impact it would have on learning or behavior disorders for mandated special services. Thus, many school districts denied these students special services.

When parents began to win lawsuits for services to children of ADHD, in the 1990s the U.S. Department of Education reinterpreted PL 94-142, and the reauthorization is known as Individuals with Disabilities Education Act (IDEA) includes ADHD under "Other Health Impaired" because of the

Successful People with ADHD: Scott Eyre, Relief Pitcher Chicago Cubs (1972–)

When Scott Eyre was in elementary school, he had no idea that forgetting his homework and feeling confused in math class was part of having ADD. School was difficult for him but because of the encouragement of his mother, he built his strength of character and worked doubly hard and was allowed to play baseball, a game that he loved. He made it through high school and went to a junior college in Idaho. The Texas Rangers offered him a job and sent him to the Instructional League in Florida, where he had a terrible injury to his right elbow. After recovering, he worked very hard and signed with the major leagues to pitch.

He still did not know that he had ADD but noticed that one of his teammates took a pill each day. He found out that the friend had ADD and the pill helped him focus. That led to his diagnosis of ADD and medication. He now speaks freely about his ADD and how it just made him try harder when people tried to put him down. He diligently takes his medication and hopes that if his example can help one child to take medication, he has had success.

Source: Corman, C. A., and E. Hallowell. 2006. *Positively ADD: Real stories to inspire your dreams.* New York: Walker and Company.

impact of attention and alertness. Under this provision, children with ADHD could be considered for special services, provided that the disability impaired educational attainment. *See also* Individuals with Disabilities Education Act (IDEA); Legal and Ethical Issues.

As a reaction to the federal impetus for children and the increased attention to medication for people with disabilities, several groups began to question the scientific basis for treatment and the use of federal funds in education. One of the leaders was the Church of Scientology and its Citizens Commission on Human Rights (CCHR). In 1987 in a publication called *Ritalin: A Warning to Parents*, the group claimed that Ritalin was a dangerous and addictive drug often used by intolerant educators and parents and by money-hungry psychiatrists as a chemical straightjacket to subdue normally exuberant children. They claimed that use of Ritalin could frequently result in violence or murder, suicide, Tourette's syndrome, permanent brain damage or emotional disturbance, seizures, high blood pressure, confusion, agitation, and depression. The publication also claimed that the increasing production of Ritalin was leading to increased abuse of these drugs by the general public. A group of scientologists picketed scientific meetings and public conferences on ADHD and distributed leaflets to parents and students. CCHR focused on rare cases of adverse reaction to stimulants to make the effort to persuade the public that overprescribing these drugs was a threat to schoolchildren. They proposed that ADHD was a myth and decried the evils of Ritalin.

According to Barkley, great controversy was generated in the media and in some lay groups, but no evidence was presented in these articles and no widespread controversy existed in professional or scientific fields about the disorder. However the explosion of parent and professional support groups counteracted the scientology groups and with their emphasis on education neutralized some of the information from the group.

Further Readings: Barkley, Russell. 2006. *Attention-deficit hyperactivity disorder: A handbook for diagnosis and treatment.* 3rd ed. New York: Guilford Press; Citizens Commission on Human Rights (CCHR). 1987. *Ritalin: A warning to parents.* Los Angeles: CCHR.

R

Reading Disability (RD). *See* Learning Disabilities (LD).

Reflex Inhibition

Dr. Stephen Clarke at the Center for Developmental and Learning Difficulties in Berkshire, England, has developed a technique based on the theory that learning difficulties, such as dyslexia, hyperactivity, and autism, are cause by immature neurological reflexes. He believes that these children have not completed their normal developmental sequences, beginning in the fetal life. Because of this abnormal development, the child is impaired in some way.

Clarke's treatment uses a small, soft, dry paintbrush to gently stroke certain lines of the body, face, hands, and feet. Thus it becomes possible to either inhibit or stimulate a reflex. The brushing is repeated morning and evening using 40 strokes per session for a period of 4 to 6 weeks.

Further Reading: Cooper, Paul, and Katherine Bilton. 1999. *ADHD: Research, practice and opinion.* London: Whurr Publishers.

Reflexology

This ancient theory of healing using the body's natural healing mechanisms has many variations. The practice relies on the premise that parts of the body are linked by flows of energy. In acupuncture, these flows were called meridians, but in reflexology there are 10 energy zones from head to toe. There are longitudinal zones, one for each foot and one linking the great toe to the brain and to the thumb. Also transverse zones go across the body and feet. There is a relationship between hands and feet called crossed reflexes.

To treat hyperactivity, firm pressure is applied gently to the soles of the feet, and then movement is applied to the other zones of the body. As the child becomes accustomed to the treatment, he or she may apply the pressure.

Further Reading: Cooper, Paul, and Katherine Bilton. 1999. *ADHD: Research, practice and opinion.* London: Whurr Publishers.

Reframing ADHD Behavior

Reframing is a technique of finding new and positive ways of thinking about a child's problems and behavior and considering how the parent and teacher can help find ways to help. With so much negativity and problems associated with ADHD, it is easy for both parents and teachers to become fed up with the condition and the person who has it. Children with ADHD can become locked into these cycles of negativity. Parents and teachers may find themselves perpetuating the cycles.

At first this approach appears to defy common sense because it stresses the importance of framing all the child's behaviors as positively as possible. This is not the same as condoning unwanted or undesirable behavior, but to help understand and develop ideas about positive ways to look at the behavior. Reframing behaviors in positive ways helps students believe that the adult in their lives like them and cares about them.

The reframing technique should be used where it has a chance to be effective and productive. Sometimes it may involve mild disapproval of current behavior and done in a way to provide positive reframing of the unwanted behavior; the reframer then indicates that there are situations other than the present one in which these qualities are more appropriately displayed. However, some behaviors, such as those that are violent or harmful to other students, may not lend themselves to reframing.

For reframing to be successful it must be

- convincing, in that it fits the facts of the situation as adult and child see them;
- done in a genuine way without sarcasm;
- be congruent with your way of behaving toward the student.

These practices were adapted from clinical setting by Molnar and Lindquist in the United States and applied to behavioral problems in the United Kingdom by Cooper and Upton.

Further Reading: Molnar, A., and Lindquist, B. 1989. *Changing problem behavior in schools.* San Francisco: Jossey-Bass.

Reiki

Reiki has been mentioned as a complementary treatment for ADHD. Reiki is a Japanese technique for stress reductions and relaxation that also promotes healing. Administered by the laying on hands, Reiki is based on the idea that an unseen "life force energy" flows through us and causes us to be alive. If this energy is low, one is likely to get sick and feel stress; if it is high, one may be happy and healthy.

A Reiki master seeks to treat the whole body, including the mind and spirit by transferring the life force energy during an attunement. The force is available to everyone. The founder of the system was Dr. Mikao Usui, who promoted that one must practice simple ethical ideals to promote peace and harmony. It is not a religion but requires meditation and active commitment to improve one's self.

Further Reading: The International Center for Reiki Training. http://www.reiki.org. Accessed 5/27/2009.

Reuptake

Reuptake occurs when a substance that a cell produces is reabsorbed by that cell. For example, a neurotransmitter transporter or carrier of the neuron just before the synapse may experience reuptake before the neurotransmitter has a chance to act. Some of the neurotransmitters are lost and not reabsorbed. Reuptake is necessary for normal functioning because it allows for recycling of neurotransmitters and regulates normal levels of neurotransmitter present in the synapse and how long a signal last. Because neurotransmitters are too big to diffuse through the membrane, special transport proteins are necessary for the reabsorption of the neurotransmitters. In ADHD certain deficits in the neurotransmitters dopamine and epinephrine are noted.

Drugs used in ADHD are grouped in two major categories: stimulants and nonstimulants. Both work by affecting specific neurotransmitters, dopamine and norepinephrine, within the brain. Low levels of dopamine appear to play a role in inattention and hyperactivity, whereas low levels of norepinephrine may contribute to inattention and the inability to control impulsive behavior:

1. Stimulants block the reuptake of both dopamine and norepinephrine (dual reuptake inhibitors) and enable more of the neurotransmitters to exert effects in the frontal cortex of the brain to help with organization.
2. Nonstimulants block the reuptake of norepinephrine more selectively than they do other neurotransmitters.

Further Reading: Medicine Net. "Definition of Reuptake." 2003. http://www.medterms.com/script/main/art.asparticlekey=25240. Accessed 5/27/2009.

Ritalin

Ritalin hydrochloride and Ritalin-SR methylphenidate hydrochloride sustained-release tablets are the registered trademarks of Novartis Pharmaceutical Corporation, East Hanover, New Jersey. Ritalin is a mild central nervous system (CNS) stimulant, available as 5-, 10-, and 20-mg tablets for oral administration. Ritalin SR is available in 20-mg tablets. Methylphenidate hydrochloride is methyl-a-phenyl-2-piperineacetate hydrochloride with the structural formula: $C_{14}H_{19}NO_2 \cdot HCl$.

The actual method of action in humans is not completely known, but it presumably activates the brainstem arousal system and cortex to produce its stimulant effect. Ritalin is indicated for ADHD as a part of an integral total treatment program that includes other remedial measures such as psychological, educational, and social interventions. It is indicated for people with the following group of inappropriate symptoms: moderate-to-severe distractibility, short attention span, hyperactivity, emotional lability, and impulsivity.

Several warnings are included in the package insert:

- Ritalin should not be used in children under 6, because safety and efficacy in this age group have not been established.
- Sufficient data on long-term use of Ritalin in children are not yet available. Although a causal relationship has not been established, suppression of weight gain and height has been reported with long-term use of stimulants in children.
- Ritalin should not be used for severe depression or in psychotic children, and it may worsen the condition.
- The drug should not be used for the prevention or treatment of normal fatigue states.
- Some clinical evidence exists that Ritalin may lower cause seizures in people with a prior history of seizures.
- Patients with hypertension should be monitored if using Ritalin.
- Symptoms of blurring of vision and other visual disturbances have been reported in rare cases.
- Ritalin should not be used with coumarin or other anticoagulants, drugs for depression, or anticonvulsants such as phenobarbital.
- Ritalin should not be prescribed for women of child-bearing age unless the physician determines the benefits outweigh the risks.

Ritalin can be used as effective treatment in some patients; however, the person must be constantly monitored for adverse side effects.

S

Samonas Auditory Intervention

Samonas is an alternative or complementary treatment for ADHD. An acronym for specifically activated music of optimal natural structure, the Samonas system is a tool for auditory intervention based on neurobiological research using experiencing classic music therapy. The therapy provides direct stimulation to the middle ear, cochlea, auditory nerve, and cerebral cortex. It also provides indirect stimulation to the entire central nervous system.

Based on some of the work of Alfred Tomatis, German scientist and musician Ingo Steinbach developed the idea that music's overtones (high-frequency sounds) profoundly energize and invigorate the ears, brain, and total body. The music must be enjoyable, euphonic, and a fine quality because he found that the brain is more responsive to pleasant sounds. At his laboratory he developed special technology that records music and nature sounds with high frequencies and bass overtones.

Samonas sound therapy teaches an individual to listen and trains the auditory system so that the full range of sound can be processed without distortion, hypersensitivity, and frequency loss. Using headphones and top-quality equipment, the participant listens every day for 4 weeks to 7 months or more to classical music that is specially recorded. This provides massage to the middle ear and stimulation to the inner ear and results in the specific input the brain needs to process the full range of sound necessary for brain development.

Section 504

Section 504 is a federal law that is part of the Rehabilitation Act of 1973. It guarantees rights to people with disabilities, including access to a free and appropriate education. If ADHD symptoms create a substantial limit in the child's ability to learn, the individual may qualify under Section 504. Section 504 prohibits districts that receive federal funds from discriminating in the delivery of school programs and activities. The section differs from the Individuals with Disability Education Act (IDEA) in that it is broader and is intended to prevent discrimination against students with disabilities. The definition of a disability under Section 504 has three parts:

1. The student has a physical or mental impairment. This is not limited to the eleven classifications under IDEA. ADHD is one of the classifications, but sometimes parents will not want to go with the IDEA. For Section 504 eligibility can be provided by a medical diagnosis and by qualified school personnel with appropriate training.
2. The impairment must limit a major life activity. Unlike IDEA, the limitation is not just to learning. Courts have interpreted the meaning in global terms and require that the student have a history of such impairment. Students with communicable diseases, diabetes, ADHD, asthma, or allergies may qualify.
3. The frame of reference is the average student in the general population. The limitation is considered "substantial" if the child cannot do things that the average child of the same age can do. Norm-referenced standardized test data may be useful in determining this relation to the average student.

Usually the accommodations in the classroom include the use of assistive technology, such as computer-aided instructions, and access to therapy. No legal requirements exist for making a 504 plan, but parents do need to be involved. The following are examples of issues and possible accommodation under Section 504:

- Teachers will not let an elementary student go on a field trip because of disruptive behaviors that are part of his ADHD. An accommodation would be to hire a behavior specialist or management person to accompany the child on the trip.
- A high school student with ADHD receives a failing grade for schoolwork that is not finished within the allotted class time. It would be reasonable to shorten the assignment or provide extra time without penalty.
- A youth is removed from the soccer team for failing grades. If the failing grade was determined to be part of ADHD, the team could amend the grade requirement or provide special instruction for him to meet the standard.
- A child is unable to copy work from the board because of the inability to focus on the task; an accommodation would be to provide print copies of all work on the board.

Reasonable accommodations will assure that children with ADHD will have the same opportunities to succeed as their peers.

Further Readings: "ADHD and Education." Texas Partners Resource Network. http://www.PartnersTx.org. Accessed 5/18/2009; Kelly, Evelyn B. 2006. *Legal basics: A handbook for educators*. 2nd ed. Bloomington, IN: Phi Delta Kappa International; "Know Your Children's Educational Rights." *ADDitude* August/September 2006. http://www.additudemag.com/adhd/article/1623.html. Accessed 5/19/2009; Zirkle, Perry A. 2005. *Section 504: Students issues, legal requirements, and practical recommendations*. Bloomington, IN: Phi Delta Kappa Educational Foundation.

Seizure Disorders

Seizure disorders and ADHD are often confused. Many conditions may cause seizures. High fever, brain trauma, and tumors may result in seizures.

Epilepsy is probably the most common cause. There are several types of epileptic seizures: grand mal, where the individual falls down and shakes all over; psychomotor, in which the individual may walk around but not be aware of the surroundings, or petit mal, called absence seizures.

Absence seizures are the ones most confused with ADHD. During an absence seizure, the brain's normal activity shuts down and the child stares blankly. These bouts may last only a few seconds, but during the time the individual may blink or jerk repeatedly and drop objects being held. The small voluntary movements are known as automatisms. The attack is over as rapidly as it begins; however, attacks may occur several times during the day. One can see how a teacher would confuse this type of seizure with daydreaming.

Goodman (2002) reported on a study at the annual meeting of the American Epilepsy Society that studied overlapping symptoms between ADHD and certain seizure disorders. The researcher Dr. Mary Griebel and colleagues interviewed parents of 153 children who showed symptoms of possible seizures to single out precise descriptors that distinguish seizure disorders from nonseizure events, such as ADHD. The descriptors included a checklist about the presence or absence of these behaviors at the time of diagnosis in parents of 82 children with new-onset seizures and 119 children with ADHD. The following are the 13 descriptors: glassy eyes, jerking/twitching, stiffening, failure to respond, inability to remember the event, changes in breathing, staring, drooling, unusual mouth movements, biting the tongue, mumbling, turning of eyes or head to one side, and fidgeting. In the study when parents rated positively that children had glassy eyes and changes in breathing but did not fidget, 96 percent of the patients were correctly diagnosed as having absence seizures. However, when parents did not rate glassy eyes and changes in breathing but did note fidgeting, 96 percent were correctly diagnosed as ADHD. Griebel concluded that the presence of four behaviors—glassy eyes, fidgets, jerking or twitching, and changes in breathing—can aid in the differential diagnosis between seizure disorder and ADHD.

Some parents worry that drugs (both stimulant and nonstimulant) for ADHD may lower the seizure threshold for children who have both seizure disorder and ADHD. Martin Hoffman, M.D., reviewed several studies and concluded that new-onset seizures appear to be a rare consequence of stimulant therapy. Worsening of seizures is also uncommon, and the stimulants appear to be safe. He does recommend close monitoring of children with preexisting seizure disorders. He did find that when combined with phenytoin, methylphenidate (MPH) may reduce the level of the phenytoin; when given with carbamazepine, MPH level may increase. Although the FDA has not approved bupropion for ADHD, some evidence exists that it is effective for ADHD. This drug does carry an increased risk of seizures and should not be taken by anyone who has a history of seizures, including fever seizures.

Further Readings: Goodman, Alice. 2002. Study offers suggestions for differentiating between pediatric seizures and ADHD. *Neurology Today* 2(2):36; Hoffman, Martin. 2006. "Treatment of ADHD in Children with Seizure Disorders." http://www.medscape.com/viewarticle/536122. Accessed 8/8/2008.

Sensory Integration Disorder (SID)

Sensory integration disorder (SID) sometimes is called an ADHD look-alike. The person may have easy distractibility, impulsivity, social problems, and developmental delays. However, SID results from a neurological disorder in which the brain's ability to integrate certain information received from the body's five basic senses is affected. A. Jean Ayers in the 1960s developed SID to explain the relationship between behavior and brain functioning. The senses send bits of information come to the brain, which them must organize and integrate these sensations for the person to function.

According to Sensory Integration, International, the following signs indicate SID:

- Oversensitivity or undersensitivity to touch, movement, sights, or sounds
- Tendency to be easily distracted
- Social and emotional problems
- Activity level that is unusually high or unusually low
- Physical clumsiness or apparent carelessness
- Impulsive, lacking self-control
- Difficulty in making transitions from one situation to another
- Inability to unwind and calm self
- Poor self-concept
- Delays in speech, language, and motor skills
- Delays in academic achievement

SID is treatable with occupational therapy, but some alternative therapies such as therapeutic body brushing or tactile stimulation have emerged. Music therapy promoted active listening. By providing treatment at an early age, SID may be managed successfully.

Further Readings: "Help for Sensory Integration Disorder in Kids." http://www.medicinenet.com/script/main/art.asp?articlekey=50348. Accessed 6/18/2009; Iannelli, Vincent. "Sensory Integration Disorder." http://www.pediatrics.about.com/od/weeklyquestion/a/94_sensory_intg.htm. Accessed 8/9/2008; Incredible Horizons. "Signs, Symptoms, and Background Information on Sensory Integration." http://www.incrediblehorizons.com/sensory-integration.htm. Accessed 5/27/2009.

Serotonin

Research into the role of serotonin, an important neurotransmitter, and ADHD has recently developed to answer questions relating to the complete picture of children with ADHD. Although the central premise of researchers has been that of dopamine (DA) dysfunction leading to the behaviors of inattention, hyperactivity, and impulsivity in ADHD, a number of limited studies have considered the activity of serotonin. A neurotransmitter is a chemical that occupies the gap between two or more nerve cells and allows tiny electrical currents into the adjacent cell. Each neurotransmitter fits into a unique receptor like a key fitting into a lock, allowing messages to be carried along nerve pathways. Chemically serotonin is known as 5-hydroxytryptamine or 5-HT.

The central premise of the catecholamine hypothesis—that dopamine transmitters are involved—is based in part on two things: the effectiveness of methylphenidate or Ritalin-type drugs and brain images indicating reduced activity in the frontal-striatal regions. Studies of psychostimulants indicate that between 70 and 80 percent respond, leaving about 20 percent that do not. Also, the MTA study indicated that clinical improvements may not extend beyond 25 to 30 percent and can deteriorate remarkably after 2 years. Recent thinking is that another system—perhaps the serotonin system—is coming into play.

Serotonin as a neurotransmitter conveys positive sensations of satiety by regulating the appetite, satisfaction, and relaxation. When converted to the substance melatonin, it helps us sleep. A deficiency of serotonin can cause depression, upset the appetite mechanism, or lead to obesity or other eating disorders such as anorexia or bulimia.

Serotonin is produced from an essential amino acid tryptophan, obtained from food and converted to serotonin in the presence of vitamin B6 (pyroxidine) and magnesium. The body does not produce tryptophan; it is obtained from food. The absorption of tryptophan competes with the absorption of other amino acids in the digestive tract; consuming refined carbohydrates such as sugar accelerates this absorption. Sugar then stimulates the production of insulin, a hormone that transpose glucose, fatty acids, and other amino acids into body cells. Insulin speeds up absorption of amino acids other than tryptophan. Thus, tryptophan is left for conversion to serotonin, and the person feels happy and satisfied. The person low in serotonin is inclined to consumer greater amounts of sugar in an attempt to increase serotonin production.

Scientists have advanced several reasons for the possible important role of serotonin in ADHD:

- Researchers developed a strain of knockout mice without the gene responsible for the dopamine transporter (DAT-KO); treating the mice with serotonergic drugs, they found a calming effect to their hyperactive and aggressive behavior.
- There is considerable evidence of interaction between dopamine and serotonin neurotransmitter systems; different subtypes mediate the regulation of serotonin over DA.
- Specific serotonin genes may be present as risk factors for ADHD.

Research into the role of serotonin and the possible use of drugs targeting serotonin is ongoing and probably will produce future treatment implications.

Further Readings: Lombroso, Paul J. et al. 2001. Genetics of childhood disorders: XXIII. ADHD, Part 7: The serotonin system. *Journal of American Academy of Child Adolescent Psychiatry* 40(2):253–57; Oades, Robert D. 2007. The role of the serotonin system in ADHD: Treatment implications. *Expert Reviews of Neurotherapy* 7(10):1357–74; "The Serotonin Connection." http://www.hypoglycemia.asn.au/articles/serotonin_connection.html. Accessed 8/6/2008.

Single-Photon Emission Computed Tomography (SPECT)

One of the most widely used functional neuroimaging techniques for studying ADHD is single-photon emission computed tomography (SPECT). SPECT can measure regional cerebral blood flow (rCBF), as well as localize and determine the densities of various receptors in the living being. Also, rCBF is considered to be an indirect measure of the activity of neurons and the metabolism of glucose in corresponding brain areas. The SPEC study begins with injecting a flow tracer joined with a radionuclide (for example, ^{99m}Tc) into the veins of the subject. The flow tracer is then localized to a receptor or to where there is increased blood perfusion. Fleeting γ-rays or photons, which are emitted as the radioisotope decays, capture the image by detecting the concentration of the bound nucleotide. The amount of uptake of the tracer can be quantified accurately. Various molecules are used to localize specific receptor such as TRODAT for the dopamine transporter (DAT1).

SPECT is relatively affordable because it does not have to use the cyclotron for radioisotope product. The radioactive decay half-life of most SPECT isotopes is long, so the compounds may be manufactured in one location and shipped to another. SPECT is not used in the diagnosis of people with psychiatric disorders but is used clinically in assessment of brain tumors, seizures, and other anomalies. It is not typically used for research purposes in children because it requires ionizing γ-radiation. *See also* Neuroimaging.

Further Reading: Gozal, David, and Dennis L. Molfese, eds. 2005. *Attention deficit hyperactive disorder: From genes to patients.* Totowa, NJ: Humana Press.

Sleep Disorders

Sleep-cycle problems are frequent for people with ADHD. These difficulties can interfere with relationships, work, school, and overall energy level. Chronic sleep deprivation can make ADHD worse. According to Dr. Daniel Amen, people with ADHD may feel groggy or fuzzy-headed in the morning. Parents complain that they may have to wake up a child many times, and then it becomes a hostile battle, starting off the day with everyone in a bad mood.

Likewise diagnosis of ADHD is complicated because some children who are hyperactive or inattentive actually may have sleep problems and not ADHD. Two sleep disorders in general, snoring and sleep apnea, may lead to hyperactivity and inattention.

Sleep apnea is very serious. In this condition, the person stops and starts breathing, sometimes dozens of times, during sleep. Researchers do not completely understand the link between sleep apnea and hyperactivity, but when children are treated for the disorder, their hyperactivity often disappears. Children with true ADHD do not often experience sleep apnea, but they may have disturbances in the REM stage, which is the dream stage of sleep, which may affect behavior. If a child snores and has trouble sleeping, a pediatric sleep specialist or an ear, nose, and throat physician should be consulted.

Doctors are not sure why people with ADHD appear to have more sleep problems than others. Some researchers posit that it has to do with serotonin, the neurotransmitter that is possibly tied to inattention and impulsivity. People need serotonin to fall asleep, and if the chemical is deficient, getting to sleep may be difficult.

A 2006 study reported in *Michigan Medicine* linked tonsils to behavior and sleep problems. Dr. Ronald Chervin reported that children who have surgery to remove their tonsils are very likely to behave and sleep better

1 year later. Previously, there have been findings of a link between children's behavior and sleep-related breathing problems. The 78 children in the study who had their tonsils out were much more likely than a comparison group of 27 children to have had behavior and sleep problems at the start of the study, but at the end of the study, tests showed little difference between the two groups. Eleven of twenty-two children who were diagnosed with ADHD no longer had the condition after the tonsillectomy. The results suggest that sleep and breathing problems are part of the ADHD problems, but according to Chervin treating them is not a cure-all. The study does suggest that a child who has breathing problems when sleeping and behavior problems at school could possibly benefit from the surgery.

The following ideas from Dr. Amen may assist the child in going to sleep:

- Watching television 1 to 2 hours before bedtime may be overstimulating. The news especially is full of bad things that happen, which may cause the person with ADHD to reflect on the bad things that happened during the day.
- Eliminate active play such as wrestling, tickling, or teasing at least1 to 2 hours before bedtime. Try to substitute quieter activities such as reading or drawing.
- If you are going to read yourself to sleep, try boring books not action-packed thrillers.
- Try a warm, quiet bath before bedtime.
- Some people respond to sounds such as nature tapes or the sounds of fans.
- A mixture of warm milk with a teaspoon of vanilla and sugar may increase the serotonin in the brain.
- Learn self-hypnosis. Follow the procedure: focus your eyes on a spot and count slowly to 20 and let your eyes feel heavy as you count; close them as you get to 20.
- Dr. Amen has a sleep tape that is a sound machine that produces sound waves the same frequency as a sleeping brain. The tape "brain train" is found at http://www.mindworkspress.com.
- Sleep control therapy includes going to bed when sleepy and using the bedroom only for sleep; when you are unable to sleep go to another room.
- Maintain a regular rise time in the morning regardless of sleep duration during the previous night.
- Avoid daytime naps.

Dr. Amen says that no one suggestion works for everyone. Calling in an expert sleep therapist may be essential for persistent problems.

Further Readings: Amen, Daniel. 2001. *Healing ADD: The breakthrough program that allows you to see and heal the 6 types of ADD.* New York: Berkley Books; Gavin, Kara. (2006). "Kids Behave and Sleep Better after Tonsillectomy, University of Michigan Study Finds." *Michigan Medicine* http://www.med.umich.edu/opm/newspage/2006/sleep.htm. Accessed 5/18/2008.

Smoking and ADHD. *See* Substance Use Disorders (SUDs).

Specific Learning Disability (SLD)

The term specific learning disability (SLD) refers to one of more of the basic psychological processes involved in understanding or in using language, spoken or written, which may show itself in an inability to listen, think, speak, read, write, or spell or to do math, and includes perceptual disabilities, brain injury, minimal brain dysfunction, dyslexia, and developmental aphasia.

The term does not include learning problems that are primarily the result of visual, hearing, or motor disabilities; of mental retardation; of emotional disturbance; or of environmental, cultural, or economic disadvantage. A high number of children with ADHD also have learning disabilities.

People may need specialized, supportive instruction to address their learning deficits, as well as strategies to learn to manage the behavior and inattention common to ADHD. Children with ADHD and SLD often have with problems with self-esteem. It is essential that young children see themselves as capable learners.

Further Reading: "ADHD and Education." Texas Partners Resource Network. http://www.PartnersTx.org. Accessed 5/18/2009.

Still, George

George Still, a British physician, was an early pioneer the study of children with ADHD. In 1902 at the Royal College of Physicians, he published three lectures that described 43 children in his practice that had serious problem with sustained attention. Acclaiming that these children lacked "moral control of behavior," he told how many were aggressive, defiant, resisted discipline, lawless, spiteful, cruel, and dishonest. He found the proportion of males to females was 3:1 and also noted that many of these had certain other conditions such as tics. A major hypothesis was that inhibition, moral control, and inattention were casually related to each other and that there was a possible neurological deficiency attributed to genetics or pre- or postnatal damage. *See also* History of ADHD.

Strattera

Strattera is the registered trade name of Eli Lilly and Company, Indianapolis, Indiana, for the generic compound atomoxetine. The drug is used to treat ADHD in children, teens, and adults but has not been studied in children less than 6 years old. There are other trade names for atomoxetine. Strattera comes in 10-mg (white), 18-mg(white and orange), 25-mg (blue and white), 40-mg (blue), 60-mg (blue and orange), 80-mg (brown and white), and 100-mg (brown) capsules.

Strattera is a prescription medication that is used to treat children over 6 years old, adolescents, and adults with ADHD. It is the first and so far only medicine that is not a stimulant that is approved by the FDA for ADHD. Strattera is less likely to cause tics than stimulant medication and may be effective in children with ADHD.

Strattera should be used as an adjunct to psychological, educational, social, and other interventions in the treatment of ADHD. Researchers have shown that Strattera is effective in decreasing inattention and hyperactive/

impulsive symptoms as measured on various rating scales. It is an option for those who do not tolerate stimulant drugs or who have not responded to them, as measured on various rating scales. Response to treatment with the drug has not been studied for more than 1 year in children and 2 years in adolescents. The safety and effectiveness have not been established for this medicine for children less than 6 years of age.

Strattera should be taken regularly exactly as the physician prescribes with 8 ounces of water, and no more than the prescribed amount in any 24-hour period should be taken. It may be taken with or without food and should be swallowed whole. This capsule should not be opened or sprinkled on food.

Important Facts About Strattera

The effect of Strattera may not be felt for several weeks but the person should not stop taking this medication without talking to the physician. Individuals taking Strattera should drink plenty of fluids and avoid becoming dehydrated because this reduction in fluids increases the risk of hypotension or low blood pressure. Strattera may cause dizziness and drowsiness. Therefore, individuals taking the drug should avoid driving, operating machinery, or performing other hazardous activities until they know how this medicine affects them. Strattera is not a stimulant and is not considered a controlled substance by the Drug Enforcement Agency (DEA). It does not have the same abuse potential as stimulant drugs.

People with several types of conditions should avoid Strattera. Those individuals with schizophrenia, schizoaffective disorder, bipolar disorder, or other brain disorder with psychotic symptoms should avoid this medication because it may make the symptoms worse. Any individual who has high blood pressure, blood vessels problems, blood disorders, heart disease, tachycardia or rapid heat rate, or the eye disease narrow-angle glaucoma should avoid Strattera because the medication may worsen the condition. Do not use Strattera within 2 weeks of taking a medication in a class called monoamine oxidase inhibitors (MAOIs) or MAOI-like medications used to treat depression. The interaction with these medications can be fatal. Strattera may increase the risk of suicidal thinking in children and adolescence with ADHD; close monitoring for signs of suicidality, such as increased aggression, hostility, agitation, irritability, and suicidal talk or behaviors is essential.

The common side effects of Strattera are as follows:

- Upset stomach, nausea, vomiting, decreased appetite, constipation, dry mouth, insomnia, decreased libido or sexual side effects, menstrual cycle changes, hot flushes, unusual tiredness, feeling of sluggishness, sedation, sleepiness, irritability, or mood swings.
- Allergic reactions such as difficulty breathing, closing of the throat, swelling of the lips, tongue, face, or hives, have occurred.
- In rare cases liver damage has occurred. These symptoms include dark urine, flu-like symptoms, persistent anorexia, itchiness, abdominal pain, or yellowing of the eyes or skin.

The following medications can interact with Strattera:

- Newer antidepressant such as Prozac (fluoxetine) and Paxil (paroxetine) can increase the effects of Strattera.
- Blood pressure medication can become less effective when used with Strattera; therefore, monitoring blood pressure closely is imperative.
- Heart medications such as Cardioquin or Dura-Tabs (quinidine) can increase the effects of Strattera.
- Albuterol, a medication taken for asthma or difficult breathing, can increase the risk of high blood pressure and heart rate.
- Medications that have stimulant effects, such as amphetamines, Dexedrine, Adderall, and methylphenidate, can increase the effects of Strattera and have serious side effects.
- Many medications interact with Strattera; the person should talk with the physician or pharmacist before taking any prescription or over-the-counter medications, including herbal products.

FDA Alert 9/2005: Suicidal Thinking in Children and Teens

In September 2005, the FDA issued a warning that Strattera increased the risk of suicidal ideation in short-term studies in children or adolescents with ADHD. Children or adolescents who are started on therapy with Strattera should be monitored closely for suicidality (suicidal thinking and behavior), clinical worsening, or unusual changes in behavior.

FDA Alert 12/2004: Severe Liver Injury

Strattera can cause liver damage in rare cases. The person should call the doctor right way if there is itching, dark urine, yellow color in the eyes, upper right-sided abdominal tenderness, or unexplained "flu-like" symptoms.

Further Readings: Eli Lilly and Company. http://www.lilly.com. Accessed 5/27/2009; Food and Drug Administration, "Atomoxetine (Marketed as Strattera) Information." http://www.fda.gov/Drugs/DrugSafety/PostmarketDrugSafetyInformationforPatientsand Providers/ucm107912.htm. Accessed 6/1/8/2009; National Alliance on Mental Illness. "Strattera." http://www.nami.org. Accessed 5/27/2009.

Streptococcus (Strep). *See* Beta-Hemolytic Streptococcus.

Substance Abuse. *See* Substance Use Disorders (SUDs).

Substance Use Disorders (SUDs)

A strong link exists between ADHD, cigarette smoking, and substance use disorders (SUDs). Both research and clinical evidence have shown that a person who has one disorder may have the other. Understanding the nature of the ADHD/SUD overlap, how substance abuse develops, and which youngsters are at greatest risk are important in avoiding the situation and effectively managing those with problems.

According to Timothy Wilens, professor at Harvard Medical School and director of the substance abuse program at Massachusetts General Hospital, ADHD is often a precursor to the full spectrum of substance use disorder, and to help patients avoid the hazardous combination, it is important to provide cautionary guidance throughout childhood, screen all adolescents for substance abuse, and treat ADHD. Wilens et al. (2003) believes that the risk of SUD in individuals with ADHD extends across the timeline of life. When a pregnant mother first visits a physician, this is an opportunity to make it clear that addressing substance abuse is part of well-child care. Here the physician can show how using any dangerous substances increases the risk of spontaneous abortion or miscarriage, placental abruption disorders, postnatal withdrawal symptoms, neurobehavioral abnormalities, and sudden infant death syndrome (SIDS). Estimated exposure of the fetus while the mother is pregnant is 11 percent for tobacco, 10–13 percent for alcohol, and 3 percent for illicit drugs. Every year 40,000 babies are born with fetal alcohol syndrome; 40 to 50 percent of confirmed child abuse cases involve a parent with substance abuse.

Guidance on the importance of avoiding substance abuse should continue during middle childhood. Programs in school like DARE are important to assist children in framing appropriate attitudes about drugs, cigarettes, and alcohol. When peer influence becomes stronger during adolescence, teenagers are more directly exposed to substance abuse and may start to experiment with drugs. Monitoring the Future (Johnston 2006), an annual nationwide survey of behaviors, attitude, and values among 50,000 8th, 10th, and 12th graders in the United States, showed in the 2005 survey that more teens drank alcohol than used tobacco. For example, 47 percent of high school seniors said they had consumed alcohol within the previous month and 23 percent reporting use of tobacco. The survey showed that 10 percent of 8th graders and 25 percent of 12th graders had used some illicit drugs within the previous month. Although substance abuse and dependence are defined in DSM-IV, all children do not fit the descriptions of the diagnosis; therefore Wilens et al. (2003) believes that all teens should be tested for substance abuse.

Smoking and ADHD

Cigarette smoking is a gateway to SUD. Biederman et al. in a 2006 study found that the association of smoking with subsequent onset of other substance use applies even more strongly to youngsters with ADHD than to those without the disorder. Studying 97 youngsters with ADHD and 297 controls, all of whom were under 12 years of age, the researchers found that the 15 youngsters with ADHD who smoked cigarettes were significantly more likely to use alcohol and illicit drugs and to develop SUD in later years than the 76 youngsters who did not smoke. It appears that in youngsters with ADHD, smoking is a marker of elevated risk of SUD. The study reinforces the importance of counseling teens about not smoking.

Several studies have shown that individuals with ADHD initiate tobacco use earlier, have a harder time quitting, and smoke more than their non-ADHD counterparts. Scott Kollins, director of the ADHD Program at Duke University, and colleagues (1995) examined smoking rates in young adults in 15,197 smokers at about age 22. They found a striking, near perfect linear relationship between the number of self-reported ADHD symptoms and the

Table 14 SUD and ADHD across the Lifespan

Adulthood	ADHD is linked to cigarette smoking.
	ADHD is linked to severe SUD.
Older adolescence/young adulthood	ADHD is linked to SUD but it is not comorbid.
Adolescence	Parental abuse of SUD leads to increased ADHD in offspring.
	Comorbid ADHD is linked to early onset SUD.
Prepubertal period	Treating ADHD may protect from later SUD.
During pregnancy	Genetic factors may link SUD and ADHD risk.
	Exposure to alcohol and nicotine in the mother's uterus increases ADHD risk.

Source: Wilens, T. 2004. Attention-deficit/hyperactive disorder and the substance abuse disorders: The nature of the relationship, subtypes at risk, and treatment issues. *Psychiatric Clinic North America* 27:283–301.

likelihood of being a regular smoke. Those with the highest number of symptoms began smoking about 1 year and 3 months earlier than those who reported no symptoms. Kollins believes this suggests that symptoms may drive the relationship between ADHD and smoking and that it might be an attempt at self-medication.

Alcohol and ADHD

Alcohol is the most commonly used substance among adolescence as well as in society at large; thus the link between alcohol and ADHD is important. The following are two important themes from research:

1. Conduct disorder increases the risk of alcohol use disorder. Molina et al. (2003) conducted an ongoing study of 350 people in their mid-20s in the Pittsburgh area who had alcohol abuse problems. They found that individuals with comorbid ADHD and conduct disorder consumed alcohol more frequently and in greater quantity. Conduct disorder is the most common psychiatric comorbidity of alcohol use disorders in adolescents.
2. ADHD persistence is a predictor of alcohol abuse/SUD. The Pittsburgh study of Molina also showed that persistence of ADHD is a better predictor of alcohol abuse than the original ADHD status. Even after controlling for conduct disorder, ongoing symptoms of ADHD are associated with repetitive drunkenness and daily cigarette smoking. The link between ADHD and alcohol abuse was most pronounced in people with behavior disorder. In the spectrum of ADHD symptoms, impulsiveness is most associated with greater alcohol use.

Adult ADHD and Substance Abuse

About 20 percent of adults who abuse substances have ADHD. Several studies have shown that 35 to 71 percent of adult alcoholics had childhood-onset

ADHD that had persisted into their adult years. In this ADHD/SUD overlapping population, several characteristics are common:

1. Other psychiatric comorbidities are common. About one-third of adolescents with ADHD and a diagnosis of substance abuse have other psychiatric disorders such as major depressive disorder, generalized anxiety disorder, and traumatic stress disorder. Girls with ADHD and substance abuse are more likely than their male counterparts to have psychiatric problems, and they begin abusing substances about a year and a half earlier than boys do. For example, studies in cocaine abusers who sought treatment showed a high proportion with ADHD and a history of conduct disorder or antisocial personality conduct disorder and persistent ADHD beginning in adolescence.
2. People with ADHD may seek to self-medicate. Upadhyaya et al. (2005) found in a study of 334 college students of whom 84 had been diagnosed with ADHD a relationship between the use of substances for relief and ADHD. Smoking has been associated with improvement in executive functions such as planning ahead, setting priorities, and controlling impulses, which are often impaired in ADHD. This study suggested the presence of self-medication and self-treatment.

Screening and Treatment for ADHD/SUD

Primary care physicians may screen adolescent patients for the use of alcohol and drugs. For those who do not use drugs or whose use is minimal, delivering a cautionary message may be sufficient. However, according to a study at a 2005 American Academy of Pediatrics meeting, fewer than half of pediatricians screen their adolescent patients for alcohol and drug use. Perhaps one of the reasons is the short time for a visit or graciously getting parents to leave the room so the physician may interview the patient. A questionnaire for screening is called the CRAFFT. This instrument has six orally administered questions, is widely accepted, easy-to-administer, and is free. According to a study by Knight et al. (2002), the CRAFFT is 80 percent sensitive with a specificity of 86 percent for abuse or dependence. Two or more answers of "yes" to the CRAFFT questions indicate a positive result, and points to a follow-up interview to discuss the substance abuse. The following are the CRAFFT screening questions for drug/alcohol abuse:

- C: Have you ever ridden in a CAR driven by someone (including you) who was high or had been using alcohol or drugs?
- R: Do you ever use alcohol to RELAX, feel better about yourself, or fit in?
- A: Do you ever use alcohol/drugs while you are by yourself, ALONE?
- F: Do you ever FORGET things you did while using alcohol or drugs?
- F: Do your FAMILY or FRIENDS ever tell you that you should cut down on your drinking or drug use?
- T: Have you ever gotten into TROUBLE while you were using alcohol or drugs?

Free copies of the CRAAFT questionnaire can be found at http://www.crafft. org or http://www.ceasar-boston.org/clinicians/crafft.php.

When considering treatment for ADHD or SUD, the physician must consider that both of these conditions may have accompanying disorders or comorbidities. Half of all adolescents with SUD have ADHD, and pharmacotherapy is the best treatment. However, conduct disorder is even more common, and pharmacotherapy is not the best answer. For depression, which is comorbid with SUD, psychosocial intervention, behavioral therapy, family-based intervention, and medication are more effective.

When treating ADHD/SUD patients, it is best to first stabilize the SUD. If that is not feasible, pharmacotherapy for ADHD along with an emphasis on SUD may be used. Several principles guide the treating of ADHD/SUD combination:

- Because youth with ADHD may start using drugs earlier than other children, they should be educated about the dangers of substance abuse before age 11. Schools should have a role in this education, as well as parents.
- Physicians will generally try to stabilize the drug addiction before treating ADHD.
- Other conditions such as depression, conduct disorder, and anxiety must be taken into consideration when prescribing a drug for treatment. The agents such as stimulants, antidepressants, and antihypertensives are most commonly prescribed.
- Stimulants have been shown to be effective for more that 70 percent but must be watched carefully. Extended-release formulations have less potential for abuse.
- As the child grows into adolescence, substance use should be monitored closely. Counseling about the hazards of driving under the influence of drugs or alcohol is essential.
- Depending on the age of the child and the laws of the state, the child's consent may be required before screening. It is wise to get the child's consent except in cases of medical emergency. Also, the parents need to know what to do if tests are positive.
- For those who do not use drugs or whose use is minimal, a motivational counseling session is necessary. Those who cannot stop using drugs should be referred to professional counseling.
- Students who are bound for college must be warned against binge drinking; they must know that because of their ADHD, they are at risk for long-term use of alcohol or illegal drugs.

The potential for abuse of these medications is always present. The Upadhyaya et al. (2005) study of 300 college students found that those with 22 percent of those taking medications for ADHD said they had used the medication to get high, and 29 percent said they had given or sold their medication to someone else.

Club Drugs

To know of the potential of "club drugs," people that work with clients with ADHD need to be aware that these drugs used at nightclubs or raves are a serious risk. These drugs vary according to the region and may have new names. Because the clubs cost money to enter and the drugs cost also, they are usually found among affluent groups. A few of the drugs and their names are listed below:

- Ecstasy. This is a cross between amphetamine and the hallucinogen mescaline and is taken as a tablet.

- GHB (gamma-hydroxybutyrate). This famous date-rape drug is taken as powder, tablet, or capsule in combination with alcohol.
- Ketamine. This drug is a human and veterinary injectable anesthetic used for psychedelic effects.
- 5-MeO-Dipt (5-methyl-*N,N*-diisopropyltryptamine). This synthetic psychoactive drug is similar to the hallucinogen psilocybin, found in mushrooms.

Teens need to be aware that even using these recreational drugs only once can have lasting negative consequences.

Genetic factors appear to play a significant role in the development of SUD. Many of the same genes and risk alleles associated with ADHD have also been associated with SUD. Studies on nongenetic factors indicate that poor parental monitoring, deviant peer affiliations, and other factors of temperament play an important role. Some have shown concern that stimulant drug treatment might increase the risk of SUD in people with ADHD. However, a metaanalysis found that treatment with stimulant drugs actually protects against the development of SUD. Wilens et al. (2003) found that individuals with ADHD when treated with stimulants are only about half as likely to develop problems with substance abuse as individuals with ADHD who are not treated with stimulants. However, nicotine was not studied.

Researchers at Cornell University and the University of Kentucky found a connection between cocaine use during pregnancy and ADHD in children. The study found that rat fetuses exposed to cocaine levels comparable to daily recreational use in humans showed lasting dysfunction, especially in the area of attention. Lead researcher Dr. Rosemary Strupp found that although prenatal cocaine exposure does not seem to affect most areas of cognitive function, the deficits in attention are consistent and lasting (Lang 2000). In humans, this type of dysfunction could significantly affect the lives of children as seen in ADHD. Although the use of prenatal use of cocaine does not appear to be as devastating as those cases reported in the media in the 1990s, the problem of inattention is prevalent. However, in the population, it is difficult to determine the exact effect because of other confounding factors such as prenatal malnutrition, maternal stress, pre- and postnatal medical care, and accompanying exposure to nicotine, marijuana, opiates, and amphetamines.

The American Academy of Pediatrics has suggested recommended steps for parents and teachers, as well as health professionals, to use with the person who has ADHD/SUD.

Further Readings: Biederman, J. et al. 2006. Is cigarette smoking a gateway to alcohol and illicit drug use disorders? A study of youths with and without attention deficit hyperactive disorder. *Biology Psychiatry* 59:258–64; Johnston, L. D. et al. "Monitoring the Future: National Results on Adolescent Drug Use." 2006. Bethesda, MD: National Institute on Drug Abuse. http://www.monitoringthefuture.org/new.html. Accessed 5/27/2009; Lang, Susan. "Study Suggests Link between Maternal Cocaine Use, Attention Dysfunction in Kids." June 15, 2000. http://www.news.cornell.edu/Chronicle/00/6.15.00/cocaine.html. Accessed 5/27/2009; Knight, J. R. et al. 2002. Validity of the CRAFFT substance abuse screening test among adolescent clinic patients. *Archives of Pediatric Adolescent Medicine* 156:607 14; Knight, J. R. et al. 2005. Barriers to Screening Teens for Substance Abuse in Primary Care. Poster presentation, Pediatric Academic Societies 2005 Annual Meeting, May 14, 2005, Washington, D.C; Kollins, ?S. H. et al. 2005. ADHD and

Table 15 Recommended Steps for Use with a Person Who Has ADHD/SUD

Recommended Steps	Tips
Develop a warm, trusting relationship with the person.	Enhance the person's strength by showing an interest in his or her interests; practice motivational interviewing.
Find out to what and whom the person is connected, such as a close parent, teacher, coach, or specific activity, and promote this connectedness.	Research shows that connectedness is a crucial factor for adolescents in overall success.
The physician should take a medical and psychiatric history, including behavior, legal issues, school record, and driving performance. A family history should include information about depression, suicide, anxiety disorders, bipolar, substance abuse, and alcoholism.	
The physician should investigate a careful history of sudden cardiac history as well as any events of sudden cardiac death, early heart attacks, congenital heart disease, and significant arrhythmias.	The family history of heart disease may be important in recommending pharmacotherapy.
The person should be screened for comorbidities as well as ADHD.	Knowing if other conditions exist along with ADHD is important for treatment.
Provide the person with information about what is ADHD and what it is not.	The person should know that this condition is genetic, is a mild disability, has no relationship to intelligence, but still may have serious consequences.
Be sure the parent and person understands medications.	The major concern is that the child does well. There are certain risks in taking any medications. If there are side effects, the medication is wrong and needs to be changed.
	Also, other options such as counseling, tutoring, parental help, and consulting a social worker can be considered at this time.
For the physician, the person needs to decide whether to take the medication while the parent is out of the room.	A computer may be used to take the screening tests to avoid the reluctance to talk to a health professional.
The physician should screen for substance abuse and also sexual history.	
If the person decides to take medication, discuss the medication options.	Make the person aware of the relative merits of short- and long-acting formulations and possible side effects; help the person know about the effects of using caffeine, over-the-counter drug decongestants, club drugs, and other prescribed medicines.
Develop a treatment plan with goals.	Parent, patient, and physician should work together on the goals and different definitions of success; the adolescent may have an different conception what success is.
Monitor the person closely.	Evaluate the goals, medication, and monitor drug use, smoking, sexual activity, and substance abuse.

Source: Wilens, T. 2004. Attention-deficit/hyperactive disorder and the substance abuse disorders: The nature of the relationship, subtypes at risk, and treatment issues. *Psychiatric Clinic North America* 27:283–301.

smoking: From genes to behavior. *Archives of General Psychiatry* 62:1142–47; Molina, B. S. et al. 2003. Childhood predictors of adolescent substance use in a longitudinal study of children with ADHD. *Journal of Abnormal Psychology* 112:497–507; Upadhyaya, H. P. et al. 2005. Attention deficit/hyperactive disorder, medication treatment, and substance use among adolescents and young adults. *Journal of Child Adolescent Psychopharmacology* 15:799–809; Wilens, T. 2004. Attention-deficit/hyperactive disorder and the substance abuse disorders: The nature of the relationship, subtypes at risk, and treatment issues. *Psychiatric Clinic North America* 27:283–301; Wilens, T. E. et al. 2003. Does stimulant therapy of attention deficit/hyperactive disorder beget later substance abuse? A meta-analytic view of the literature. *Pediatrics* 111:179–85.

Sugar

The relationship between sugar and ADHD and behavior is one of the most controversial discussions in medicine. Most studies in nutrition do recognize that excessive sugar may contribute to diabetes, heart disease, obesity, and immune system dysfunction. However, the exact role of sugar in relationship with ADHD is still unclear, and definitive and replicated studies are scare or have not shown consistency.

Actually, there are many kinds of sugars, and several sources of various kinds of sugar. Chemists define sugar as a class of edible crystalline substances that include sucrose or table sugar, lactose or milk sugar, and fructose or fruit sugar. Sugar is a basic food carbohydrate that appears in sugar cane and sugar beets but also in fruit, honey, sorghum, and maple syrup. Commonly, when people refer to sugar, they think of sucrose or table sugar. The average American consumes an astounding 2–3 pounds of sugar each week probably because there are many hidden sources in processed foods such as bread, breakfast cereal, mayonnaise, peanut butter, ketchup, and many prepared meals. Diets that seek to limit sugar must also consider intake of other types of sugar and hidden sources of sugar.

Physiologically, excess sugar, which breaks down into glucose in the bloodstream, stimulates the pancreas to secrete higher insulin levels to drop the blood sugar level. This rapid fluctuation is not healthy because it places stress on the body. Another problem with sugar is that it may depress the immune system.

The debate of the role of sugar in ADHD has two clear-cut sides. First are the anecdotes of mothers who declare that, after eating anything sugary, their children are bouncing off the wall with activity. These people are convinced that foods and drinks that include sugar cause their children to be hyperactive and less attentive. They may refer to a few studies that appear to correlate sugar and restlessness or simply repeat anecdotal evidence of people they know or have read about on-line. On the other side is the official medical opinion that claims numerous studies show that children do not react to sugar and that sugar does not play a role in ADHD.

First, many mothers of children with ADHD declare that when their children ingest foods and drinks with sugar, they become overactive, restless, and inattentive. The relationship of diet and behavior became popular with the Feingold Diet that eliminated many food products, including sugar. The ideas were well covered in the media and took hold during the 1970s when the movement for alternative methods, taking responsibility for one's own health, and natural foods became popular. According to Feingold, diets eliminating certain things could help improve concentration and reduce impulsiveness and other ADHD symptoms. In the 1982, the National Institutes of Heath held a scientific consensus conference to discuss diet and behavior. They did find that elimination and restriction diets did help about 5 percent of children, most of whom had food allergies.

A few studies appear to confirm the mothers' claims. Wender and Solanto tried to link an increase in aggressive behavior in ADHD children to sugar ingestion. To assess the effects of sugar ingestion, they compared 17 ADHD children with nine age-matched normal children. They found that sugar ingestion as part of a high-carbohydrate breakfast increases the tendency for inattentiveness in some children with ADHD.

Some research indicates that children with ADHD may have abnormal sugar metabolism. Researchers Langseth and Dowd found that 74 percent of 261 hyperactive children in their study had displayed hypoglycemia or low blood sugar after eating refined sugar. Therefore, they concluded that eating large amount of sugar moved the pancreas to release a large amount of insulin, causing a significant decrease in blood sugar levels and a surge in epinephrine levels. Girardi and a team at Yale found that sugar ingestion triggers other metabolic abnormalities. They gave standardized oral glucose or simple sugar to 17 children with ADHD and 11 control children and compared the results. The glucose levels were similar in both groups, and both groups showed deterioration on a continuous performance test. However the drop in test scores in children with ADHD was significantly greater, and those with ADHD displayed impulsive behavior. The study appears to show that children with ADHD have a general impairment of hormone regulation and sugar may accentuate the defect.

Another metabolic happening may occur when eating refined sugar. Some have described sugar as "empty calories". Although it does provide no nutritional benefits other than calories, sugar does require a lot of other nutrients to process it thereby depleting the person's nutritional base. Therefore, if the lack of nutrients is related to ADHD, having a high sugar meal may drain these nutrients and push the individual into a nutrient deficient state. Some studies show that children who do not eat breakfast do not perform as well in school. Also, some studies show that children who eat sugar with a high carbohydrate meal do poorly on tasks requiring concentration and are much more aggressive. According these studies, it appears that that sugar does have some effect of physiology of at least some children.

The second position is that of the medical establishment that has determined sugar plays no role in hyperactivity. Hoover and Milich (1994) conducted a study using parents' evaluations of how sugar affects their children. They looked at 35 children who were reported to be sugar-sensitive by their mothers. The children were randomly assigned to an experimental group and a control group. Mothers of the children in the experimental group were told that their children received a large dose of sugar. Mothers in the control group were told their children received a placebo. Actually, all received a placebo; none were given sugar. Mothers in the sugar-expectancy group looked at their children and criticized them more. When the mothers believed that their children consumed sugar, they behaved as if their children were in greater need of supervision. Another study provided children with sugar one day and a sugar substitute the next day. Parents, children, and staff did not know whether the children were receiving sugar or the sugar substitute. Half of the parents were told their children received sugar, and half were told they were given a substitute. On any given day of the study, parents who were told their children received sugar rated them as more hyperactive and restless. Milich concluded that the parental expectations about the effects of sugar are the cause of the perception that sugar makes children more hyperactive. These expectations influence the way the parents interact with their children. According to these studies, expectations of the parents have lots to do with perceived hyperactivity. In 1985 White and Wolraich examined sixteen hyperactive children for 3 days in a hospital setting. The researchers manipulated the sugar content of the diet but found no effects on behavior or learning. Both of these studies were with very small samples. They concluded that the few studies that have been done found the effects are just as likely that sugar improves behavior as making it worse.

In reality, there are few repeated studies on the relationship of sugar and ADHD, and several of them, like the experiment of White and Wolraich, were done in a hospital setting in an artificial setting. Some recent nutritional studies have shown that large amounts of sugar can have a numbing effect on children and can actually induce tiredness. A study from George Washington University found that children with ADHD who ate a high-protein diet performed as well or better afterward than children without ADHD. Foods high in protein are meat, fish, yogurt, beans, peanut butter, and eggs. A study from Oxford University found that adding omega-3 fatty acids will moderate ADHD symptoms. Omega-3 fatty acids, which are contained in salmon, mackerel, sardines, and flax oil, are not a normal part of most diets.

There is no concrete evidence that sugar causes ADHD, and no major study has confirmed this fact; however, evidence that sugar does cause hyperactivity is not strong either. Scientists do have some idea that children with ADHD frequently have abnormal sugar metabolism, but normal children may also experience situations when sugar drains the body's reserves of vital nutrients.

Most nutritionists recommend that eating balanced meals from all food groups is the best strategy. Removing as many simple and refined carbohydrates from the diet as possible could have a positive effect not only on ADHD, but also on the health of people in general. These types of carbohydrates include candy, cake, white bread, potatoes, white rice, and pasta. These foods are quickly broken down in the body, often causing surges and dips in energy. The balance of eating green vegetables, fruits, whole grains, proteins, and healthy fats promotes general well-being and eliminates the possibility of a nutritional deficiency that might affect the child's behavior.

Further Readings: "ADHD and Diet: Is there a Link Between Sugar and Hyperactivity?" http://www.healthguidance.org/entry/1563/1/ADHD-and-Diet-Is-There-a-Link-Between-S. Accessed 7/30/2008; "Dr. X's Free Associations: Sugar and ADHD." http://drx/

typepad.com/psyhotherapyblog/2008/06/sugar-and-adhd-html. Accessed 7/30/2008; Hoover, D., and Richard Milich. Effects of sugar ingestion expectancies on mother-child interactions. *Journal of Abnormal Psychology* 22 (4):501-15; Kane, Anthony. "The Role of Sugar in ADHD." Mhtml:file://C:\Documents and Settings\Evelyn\My Documents\The Role of Sugar in ADHD. Accessed 7/15/2007; ADHD Central. "Myth: Sugar and Food Additives Cause ADHD." 2007. http://www.healthcentral.com/adhd/c/1443/14464/myth-sugar-food-adhd/pf/. Accessed 7/30/2008; "Sugar: Does it Cause ADHD?" 2005. http://www.riversideonline.com/health_reference/Childrens-Health/AN00583.cfm. Accessed 5/27/2009; White, J. W., and M. Wolraich. 1995. Effect of sugar on behavior and mental performance. *American Journal of Clinical Nutrition* 62(supple):242S-9S. http://www.ajcn.org/cgi/reprint/62/1/242S?ck=nck. Accessed 6/18/2009.

T

Teaching Children with ADHD

Many of the points that relate to good teaching apply to all children. Whether this is a school or home situation, key principles are important:

- Communicate with the child precisely and clearly. Tell the child exactly what to do. The focus must be very sharp and not lost in a fog of detail or ambiguity.
- Protect the child by reducing distractions, unwanted stimuli, and teach to the child's cognitive and personal strengths.
- Protect and nurture the child's self-esteem by maximizing opportunities for success, communicating with warmth and acceptance, and positive recognition in form of praise and rewards.
- Children with ADHD are likely to benefit from rules expressed to them graphically, with visual cues.
- They may not have the linguistic skills necessary to understand verbal rules, to discuss ethical issues or to deal with complex emotion. Teaching these skills should be part of the curriculum.
- Children with ADHD may be overwhelmed by a group situation. Instead, it may be wise to pair them rather than have a group activity.

Few educators are familiar with major finding from recent scientific studies of ADHD. For years most educators, physicians, psychologists, and parents have considered ADHD as a cluster of behaviors and as a label for students who are disruptive in class and who won't stop talking. Increasingly, scientists are realizing that it is a complex syndrome of impairments that affect the executive or management function of the brain.

A teacher's observing the following symptoms may indicate this complex syndrome:

- The student has trouble organizing and getting started on tasks. He may fumble around in his backpack; his notebook is an unorganized mass of papers.
- The student has problems attending to details and may be easily distracted and may do homework the night before and then fail to turn it in. This

common happening with these students irritates parents who may observe the student working the night before.

● The person varies in alertness, sometimes appearing to pay attention and other times staring out in space. Processing speed also varies.

● She may have problems sustaining and shifting focus when it is necessary. This student may be the one that is still working on an English worksheet when it is time for math.

● The student may have trouble using short-term working memory and accessing recall. He may be the student who flails his hand and gets out of his seat asking to be called upon, but when he is called upon, he says, "I forgot." Even more problematic is when parents work with him for a test the next day, and he knows the answers, but when he takes the tests, he forgets them and fails the tests.

● This student has difficulty maintaining motivation to work. He brings little toys the play with or draws unrelated pictures in his notebook. Parents will tell you that they know he is "smart" but is just being a lazy boy.

● The student may have problems managing emotions properly.

Although many of these behaviors are common in growing children, the student with ADHD or ADD displays them fairly consistently to the interference with learning.

The teacher may observe these behaviors and think the student is just being difficult. Actually all of the above involve the executive function of the brain that includes activation, focusing, effort, emotion, memory, and action. In daily life these clusters of functions operate without conscious involvement, and none of us work at peak efficiency all the time. However, those students with executive function difficulties may lag behind those of the same age and developmental level. *See also* Executive Function.

Teachers are aware of the various developmental differences of students. The ability to exercise self-management function develops slowly from early childhood through adolescence into early adulthood. We have different expectations from 10-year-olds for following directions, paying attention, remembering information than from 5-year-olds. According to Thomas Brown (2005), these self-management networks are not completely developed until late teens or early twenties. Some students may not manifest their ADD impairments until middle or high school until they encounter overwhelming work.

Importance of Early Identification

When a student underachieves or misbehaves chronically, the teacher should consider having the student evaluated for ADD/ADHD. In order to do this, teachers, psychologists, and school administrators need to understand the new model for attention deficit disorders. Early identification can prevent student from becoming demoralized by repeated experiences with frustration and failure.

Dealing with Distraction

Then how do busy teachers deal with students who have the cluster of symptoms that impair performance in the classroom? Students with ADHD are often hypersensitive to distraction. They should be seat them in a place that is relatively free from distractions, if possible away from the doors and windows. Their seat should be in a place where the teacher can detect if the student is or is not paying attention and can intervene without embarrassment or disrupting the teaching of the lesson. Having an atmosphere of calmness and quiet is essential. This does not mean that it will always be completely quiet, but the situation must be calm. The person with ADHD may have a greater need for quiet and may need a special place to study away from the group.

All children benefit from clear, predictable, uncomplicated routine and structure. Having a routine for time and broad units and repeating that pattern is helpful to these students. However, although the structure may be the same, avoid repetitive, boring tasks. The work should be interesting and stimulating. Children with ADHD may require more frequent feedback.

Rewards and Consequences

Praise and rewards can be given when a child has achieved a desired target. Instead of giving sweets as rewards, use preferred activity time such as working on a computer or some neat game.

Joey Pigza Swallowed the Key

What is it like to think the thoughts of a kid with ADHD at home and in school? Jack Gantos created a character called Joey Pigza, who helps one get into the mind of what is happening when a person has attention-deficit/hyperactive disorder. In the book, *Joey Pigza Swallowed the Key,* Joey tells in his own words how at school they say that he is wired bad, or wired mad, or wired sad, or wired glad, depending on his mood and what teacher ended up with him. They had a big meeting about him at school and his mom came home with a big file. When his mother said that he needed extra help but no teacher wanted to put up with him, Joey blurted out that he did not understand how the teacher could think he was a pain because he was always in the principal's office, helping out in the library or cafeteria, or assisting the school nurse.

Joey describes his feelings as being like spring that was wound so tight that he was more like a rat in a maze without words or feeling but with the impulse to go, go, go. He goes to a gifted class but because of his behavior, he gets kicked out. He goes to a doctor whom he calls Special Ed who gives him some prescription meds that are no match for his mood swings. In the end he does find help in a special education center and feels calmness as he takes a new medication and settles down in the time-out chair to read his book.

Source: Gantos, Jack. 1998. *Joey Pigza swallowed the key.* New York: Farrar, Strauss, and Giroux.

Tips for Teachers

1. Have a designated quiet place where the child can go. It may be a carrel or screen in an ordinary classroom.
2. Delineate and focus the task for the student. Sometimes the student with ADHD is distracted by his or her own thoughts.
3. Give clear, concise instructions with as few subparts as possible. Have the student repeat the task requirements back to the teacher orally, preferable in their own words.
4. When giving a list of instructions, try to give one at a time. Give time to finish one instruction before the next one is given.
5. Give the instructions in writing so that the list will be there in case the student forgets.
6. Establish a clear, predictable, and uncomplicated routine and structure. It helps if the day is divided into broad units of time and this pattern is repeated daily. The idea will be to present the students with a routine that they will eventually learn and memorize.
7. Within each block of lesson time, break down tasks and activities into tasks and subtasks. However, avoid presenting the student with an enormous list of these tasks and subtasks. Complexities of timetabling and working structure may tend to confuse the student who is struggling with organization. However, once a daily timetable has been established, tape it to the student's desk or inside his or her daily planner.
8. Keeping a daily planner is important. This can be a vital tool for communication with parents. Some teachers agree to sign the planner daily to keep parents aware of homework and tests that are coming up. However, do not agree to accept this responsibility for initiating signing it. Students should bring it to the teacher, and the parents should understand this. Otherwise, teachers may be blamed for not upholding their end of the agreement.
9. Avoid repetitive tasks. Although the daily routine should be simple and predictable, tasks should be stimulating so the child will no be distracted and bored.
10. However, encourage children to tackle tasks of increasing complexity. Initially, these tasks should be short and only increased when the student has had success in the shorter assignments. This point is important not only in skill development, it is also valuable in enhancing student's self-confidence and self-esteem.
11. Academic products and performance, such as work completion, are always preferred targets for intervention rather than specific behaviors like staying in the seat. This stresses the need to focus on positive, desirable outcomes rather than the negative, unwanted behavior.
12. Children with ADHD often require more specific and more frequent feedback on their work performance than most pupils. This is partly due to their memory and attention problems, as well as being a byproduct of low self-esteem.
13. When a child has achieved a desired target, use praise and rewards. Small and immediate rewards are more effective than long-term or delayed rewards. Because the ADHD student may be easily distracted, rewards should not be overly elaborate or overshadow the task.

14. Negative consequences in the form of mild punishment can be effective. These consequences should be clearly focused and highly specific.

15. Remind the student in terms of the task requirement. For example, instead of saying "Please get to work," say "Please stop talking and get back to reading page three of your history booklet."

16. Be positive in your attitude toward the behavior of children. Children do not like to be reprimanded by teachers who hold them in high regard; however, students find it difficult to accept praise from teachers who treat them with contempt or disrespect.

17. Preferred activities, such as working on a computer, are more effective rewards than concrete things like sweets.

18. Reprimands should be given in a quiet, calm manner, accompanied by direct eye contact.

19. Previewing and reviewing the tasks helps students to know what is expected of them. Talk with the students about the likely rewards of successful completion. This is called "priming" and helps motivate the student with ADHD.

20. Use your best communication skills. Instead of saying, "I've told you a thousand times," address the issue and not the child. Sarcasm is not appropriate. Dialogue between teacher and student should be a daily occurrence.

21. Do not let the student take over the class or believe that you cannot handle that student. You do not have to feel sorry for the student or give in to the student. You are the adult in charge of the class.

Here are some behavioral interventions that may help enforce boundaries and requirement for students with ADHD:

- Time out. This is a place where the student who is misbehaving is sent for a short, specified time, where he or she will not receive stimulation or attention. The student should know: (a) why it is being done, with direct reference to the offense and (b) what it is intended to achieve (for example, a time for reflection and time to cool off.)

- Ignore-rules-praise. Ignoring the behavior may act as a reinforcement. This is not an act of rudeness and is directed at the behavior rather than then person. For example, in a group setting a student keeps yelling out the answer. The teacher can ignore the behavior and call on the student who does have his hand raised, saying, "I like the way Mary is raising her hand" or "Thank you for raising your hand, James." The student will get the idea that in order to be called upon, he or she needs to abide by the rules. Basically, this involves ignoring the misbehavior of child who is breaking the rules and praising those who are abiding by the rules. However, clear simple rules must be taught in the beginning of school.

- Behavioral contracts. This is a way of establishing expectations by discussing them with the child and then reinforcing them. An agreement is made that states the rules and how they are to be achieved. Rewards should be short term and low key.

- Token economies. This involves giving tokens in the form of points, stickers, or other currency as rewards for positive behavior. These tokens are then exchanged for a more concrete reward

Dialogue should be an ongoing aspect. Show a personal interest in student by asking them questions or sharing personal interest by asking them questions or sharing humor with them. This dialogue helps the teacher in the following ways:

- To monitor mood, state, and feelings about the success of a program
- To learn about personal, family, and social factors that may influence the child's performance
- To detect learning difficulties to develop positive relationships with the child
- To model positive role models of interaction for the child and other children

Using good communication strategies provides the best means of meeting the child's needs. It will also create a sense of being valued and accepted. Reframing of the ways to think positively about ADHD is a venerable goal for parents and teachers. *See also* Reframing ADHD Behavior.

Further Readings: Brown, Thomas E. 2007. A new approach to attention Deficit disorder. *Educational Leadership* 64(5). http://www.ascd.org/publications/educational_leadership/feb07/vol64/num05/abstract.aspx#A_New_Approach_to_Attention_Deficit_Disorder. Accessed 5/18/2009; Brown, Thomas E. 2005. *Attention deficit disorder: The unfocused mind in children and adults.* New Haven: Yale University Press.

Teenagers. *See* Adolescence.

Thyroid Disease

An imbalance of metabolism that occurs from either an overproduction or underproduction of thyroid hormones may be connected to behaviors of ADHD, especially inattentiveness and disorganization. The thyroid is a small butterfly-shaped structure located low in the front of the neck. This small gland controls the growth and metabolism of almost every organ in the body by producing two hormones: thyroxine, called T4, and triiodothyronine, called T3 . The pituitary gland located at the base of the brain triggers the release of these hormones when it secretes a substance called thyroid-stimulating hormone (TSH). If the thyroid produces too much of the hormone, the TSH level drops to zero.

In 1997 two University of Maryland scientists speculated that thyroid hormones may play a role in the hyperactive and impulsive symptoms of ADHD. Reporting in the February issue of *Psychoneuroendocrinology,* Hauser and Weintraub found a positive correlation between elevated levels of certain thyroid hormone and ADHD symptoms in a selected group of patients. Resistance to thyroid hormone is a condition when serum levels of T3 and T4 are elevated. Psychologists and psychiatrists, who did not know the patient had thyroid resistance, identified ADHD symptoms in interviews. High levels of T3 and T4 were correlated with ADHD. The findings only showed a correlation and did not imply that the thyroid was the cause of the ADHD behaviors.

Kidd (2000) studied people with ADHD to determine if integrated therapy would help. He found that many items contributed to ADHD, including responses to food additives, molds, fungi, and toxins. He also found that thyroid hypofunction may be a common denominator in linking toxic insults to ADHD behavior. He believes that this condition can be treated without the use of stimulant drugs and with supplementation, diet modification, detoxification, and other integrative/holistic techniques.

However, Spencer et al. (2006) determined that they did not find this relationship of ADHD and thyroid abnormalities including the syndrome of generalized resistance to thyroid hormone. They reviewed the thyroid function of 132 children and failed to find this connection. A minority of the people did have mild abnormalities of the thyroid, but they were not different from rates reported in the literature for normal children.

Further Readings: Donovan, Jennifer. 1997. "Hyperactivity Linked to Thyroid Hormones. http://sciencedaily.com/releases/1997/03/970312165626.htm. Accessed 8/7/2008; Hauser, Peter et al. 1997. Thyroid hormones correlate with symptoms of hyperactivity but not inattention in attention deficit hyperactivity disorder. *Psychoneuroendocrinology* 22(2):107–14; Kidd, P. M. 2000. Attention deficit/hyperactivity disorder (ADHD) in children: Rationale for its integrative management. *Alternative Medicine Review* 5(5):402–28; Spencer, T. et al. 2006. ADHD and thyroid abnormalities: A research note. *Journal of Child Psychology and Psychiatry* 86(5):879–85.

Tic Disorders

Tic disorders may make the emotional, social, and academic difficulties associated with ADHD worse. Limited clinical trials have analyzed the risk of first-onset tics in stimulant-treated patients with ADHD and found that first-onset tics had no elevated risk, although a close temporal relationship exists between stimulant treatment, and tic onset was seen in a small number of cases. Roessner et al. (2006) examined 22 studies that looked at a possible relationship between the use of psychostimulant medication to treat ADHD and the onset of tics or the worsening of preexisting tics in patients with Tourette's syndrome. The data found no significant increase although there were a few increases among individual children. Stimulant medications carry a warning about vocal and motor tics and Tourette's syndrome.

Further Reading: Roessner et al. 2006. First-onset tics in patients with attention-deficit-hyperactive disorder: Impact of stimulants. *Developmental Medicine in Child Neurology* 48:616–21.

Tonsils

Tonsils are structures located in the back of the throat whose function is hotly debated. Most people think tonsils act to absorb and filter some of the materials that individuals breathe and function as part of the immune system. Years ago, children had tonsils removed routinely or if they often got sore throats.

Tonsillitis refers to the inflammation of the tonsils and can be caused by viruses or bacteria. The viral infection usually resolves with treatment including rest, fluids, and pain medication. The most common bacteria causing tonsillitis is Streptococcus, commonly referred to as strep throat, which must be treated immediately with antibiotics. If not treated, the condition may develop serious conditions such as scarlet fever and rheumatic fever, which can damage the heart.

Today, surgery is usually performed only if a child is troubled by repeated ear infections or obstructed breathing, especially when sleeping. The most common symptom of obstructive sleep disorder or sleep apnea, which occurs when breathing stops and starts at intervals during the night, is snoring. Snoring occurs when the throat is narrowed or blocked and air does not get into the trachea or lungs. This lack of sleep may cause the child to be restless and inattentive, manifesting some of the same symptoms of ADHD.

Some recent studies have indicated that tonsillectomies may result in behavioral changes in children. Two studies in 2006, one from the University of Michigan and the other from the University of Kansas Medical Center, showed that when enlarged tonsils and adenoids are removed, the behavior changed dramatically. About half of those with ADHD before surgery no longer qualified for the diagnosis 1 year later. The researchers concluded that the result was the positive effect of more quality sleep. However, the physicians cautioned that taking out the tonsils and adenoids is not the cure for ADHD in every case. However, it is one that should be considered when there are breathing problems at night and behavior problems during the day.

Further Readings: "Study: Tonsil, Adenoid Removal Could Aid in ADHD Treatment." 2006. http://www.10news.com/health/9948935/detail.html. Accessed 5/27/2009; "Tonsil Removal and ADHD: Connected?" 2006. http://www.globalrph.healthology.com/main/article_print.aspx?content_id=3485 Accessed 5/27/2009.

Tourette's Syndrome

Many children with Tourette's syndrome (TS) have symptoms of ADHD, but only rarely is ADHD considered a comorbid condition. Tics are common in childhood. According to Peterson et al. (2001), tics occur in between 4 and 18 percent of children and adolescents, but have a high degree of remission by adolescence. TS is a rare but more serious condition occurring in one to five cases in 1,000 individuals. Compulsive muscular or vocal tics characterize this neurological disorder. The person may have various involuntary movements, such as eye blinks, facial twitches, or grimacing. Others may clear their throats frequently, snort, sniff, or bark out words. These behaviors can be controlled with medications.

A very small proportion of people with ADHD have TS. However, no evidence appears to point to a higher than normal frequency of TS among children with ADHD. However, as the severity of tic disorders increases, it is likely that these disorders may be seen with ADHD. According to a study by Comings (2000), about 61.5 percent of individuals with TS do have ADHD, and it appears there is a one-way connection between the two: children with TS may develop ADHD, but for children with ADHD there is little if any elevated risk of TS.

Several medications have been implicated in the development of tics. Parents of children who are taking medications for ADHD should watch carefully for the development of this side effect and consult the physician if the symptoms occur.

Further Readings: Peterson, B. S. et al. (2001). Prospective, longitudinal study of tic, obsessive-compulsive and attention-deficit/hyperactivity disorder in an epidemiological sample. *Journal of the American Academy of Child and Adolescent Psychiatry* 40:685–95; Comings, D. E. 2000. Attention-deficit/hyperactivity disorder with Tourette syndrome. In *Attention-deficit disorders and comorbidities in children, adolescents, and adults,* edited by T. E. Brown, 363–92. Washington, D.C.: American Psychiatric Press.

Tredgold, Arthur

Along with Dr. George Still, Dr. Arthur Tredgold is recognized as one of the pioneers in the field of attention disorders. In 1908 he built on Still's ideas of early, mild, and undetected damage to the brain to account for developmentally late-arising behavioral and learning deficiencies. He speculated that treatment could be accomplished by changes in the environment and possibly by medications. They also promoted the idea of special educational environments for these children. The ideas of Still and Tredgold would take hold about 70 years later. *See also* History of ADHD.

Turner Syndrome

Some mild forms of genetic disorders go unnoticed in children who are diagnosed with ADHD. Turner syndrome may be one of these mild disorders. Females have two X chromosomes in all the body's cells. Girls with Turners have only one or part of another X chromosome. Because the ovaries are not developed, the girl is always sterile and will not begin puberty or have menstrual periods without hormone therapy. She may have heart defects, kidney problems, high blood pressure, diabetes, thyroid disorders, and vision or hearing problems. Although the condition cannot be cured, many of the symptoms may be treated.

ADHD sometimes affects behavior in childhood. In general, the girls have normal intelligence, but they may have learning differences that make verbal learning easier and math difficult. They have difficulty with visual-spatial skills such as reading maps; memory and motor coordination may also present difficulties.

A questionnaire of parents conducted by the Turner Syndrome Society of the United States revealed some common threads of behavior. As an infant or child, the baby never slept or had difficulty sleeping. She was always on the go and had mood swings. The parents noted the girls were intense or spirited and had no middle mood. They had difficulty in dealing with new situations and needed help adjusting to novel situations. Some parents described the girls as oppositional, strong-willed, or stubborn. At the same time, they could be smart, articulate, kind, sweet, gifted in some areas, and big talkers. McCauley et al. (2002) published a study of behavior and self-esteem with Turner girls. She found statistical differences in the following three areas: social competence, behavioral problems, and anxiety.

Some of the same attributes are seen in children with ADHD. Mild cases of Turners syndrome are confused and misdiagnosed as ADHD and ADHD medications are prescribed.

Further Readings: McCauley, E. et al. 2002. Self-esteem and behavior in girls with Turner syndrome. *Journal of Developmental and Behavioral Pediatrics* 16(2):82–88; Michigan Department of Community Health. "What is Turner Syndrome?" 2006. http://www.michigan.gov/documents/Turner_factsheet_160406_7.pdf. Accessed 5/27/2009; "Turner Syndrome." http://movingmounainsforkids.com/turnersyndrome.asp Accessed 5/827/2009.

V

Vision Problems

If a child cannot see properly, school and daily activities are nearly impossible, which may cause ADHD-like symptoms, especially in educational settings. According to the Optometrists Network (2007), approximately 20 percent of school-aged children may have some learning-related vision disorders. When the special education, learning-disabled, and remedial populations are taken into consideration, about 70 percent of students have a visual component to their learning problems. This figure includes those with diagnosed learning disabilities, developmental delays, dyslexia, attention deficit disorder, and double vision.

The eye tests that are given on the Snellen eye chart at a distance of 20 feet does not assure that a child has the proper vision to perform close work in school for reading and writing. In fact, the child may have 20/20 vision at least in one eye but have a problem with eye alignment, eye teaming, focusing, and visual endurance.

In 2000 Dr. David Granet, director of the Children's Eye Center in San Diego, found that many of his patients that he was treating for convergence insufficiency (CI) also were being treated for ADHD (Schram 2000). CI means that the person cannot focus the eyes at close range. They noted that kids with ADHD, which is marked by inattentiveness, impulsive behavior, and hyperactivity, were having trouble sitting, focusing, and controlling their impulses. He reviewed the charts of 266 patients and found that nearly 16 percent with ADHD had CI problems, which is more than three times as many as would be statistically expected.

The puzzling correlation actually posed more questions than it answered and warns that the following situations may explain the relationship:

- CI may be diagnosed as ADHD making the numbers skewed.
- ADHD may be causing the CI.
- CI and ADHD may actually be caused by the same problem in the brain.
- Drugs that children take for ADHD may have a side effect causing the CI.
- The actual kind of patient (all eye patients) may cause the figures to be skewed.

Vision therapy may help not only students but also adults. However, the critical age for therapy is up to 7 or 8 years, although effective treatment of conditions like amblyopia or lazy eye can be treated at any age. Vision therapy can effectively treat "turned" or crossed eyes (strabismus) and is preferred to surgical intervention. State-of-the art technology and software allows vision therapists to offer challenging programs for enhancing eye teaming, focusing, binocularity, fusion and convergence skills, and perceptual skills.

Further Readings: Optometrists Network. "Attention Deficit Disorder." 2007. http://www.add-adhd.org/vision_therapy_FAQ.html. Accessed 8/7/2008; Schram, Thomas D. 2000. "The Eyes Have It in Attention Disorders: Visual Focus May be Affecting Mental Issues." http://www.add-adhd.org/textonly/convergence_insufficiency.html. Accessed 8/7/2008.

Vitamin B Deficiencies

Some nutritionists believe that lack of B vitamins is a main cause for inattention, hyperactivity, impulsivity, temper tantrums, sleep disorders, forgetfulness, and aggression.

The following are the effects of not having adequate B vitamins:

- Insufficient B vitamins in general can cause mood changes, insomnia, changes in appetite, sugar craving, and impaired drug metabolism. This group alleviates depression and relieves anxiety and restlessness.
- B1 is essential for nerve stimulation and for metabolism of carbohydrates to give both brain and body energy.
- B2 deficiency produces adverse personality changes and aggressive personalities.
- B3 is active in the formation of the neurotransmitter acetylcholine, which involved in depression.
- B5 is used as an antistress factor.
- B6 is important is regulating mood disorders and is especially implicated in treatment of depression.
- B12 deficiencies can cause difficulty in concentrating, remembering, mental fatigue, and low-level moods.

Further Reading: Depression Guide. "Vitamin B Deficiency." 2005. http://www.depression-guide.com/vitamin-b-deficiency.htm. Accessed 8/9/2008.

Vyvanse

Vyvanse, or lisdexamfetamine dimesylate (CII), is a central nervous system (CNS) stimulant prescription medicine used for the treatment of ADHD. Vyvanse may help increase attention and decrease impulsiveness and hyperactivity in patients with ADHD. Vyvanse should be taken as part of a total treatment program for ADHD that may include counseling or other therapies. Vyvanse comes in three different strengths and should be taken exactly as prescribed: once a day in the morning with or without food. This medication is a federally controlled substance (CII) because it can be abused or lead to dependence. Selling or giving away Vyvanse may cause harm to other and is against the law.

As a stimulant medication, it is important to know there are two major risks associated with Vyvanse:

1. Heart-related problems such as sudden death in patients who have heart problems or heart defects, stroke and heart attack in adults, and increased blood pressure and heart rate.
2. Mental or psychiatric problems. Note in all patients if there are new or worse behavior and thought problems, new or worse bipolar illness, or new or worse aggressive behavior or hostility. If children and teenagers experience new psychotic symptoms such as hearing voices, believing things that are not true or suspicions, or if there are new manic symptoms.

Vyvanse should not be taken if you or your child has the following symptoms:

- Have heart disease or hardening of the arteries
- Have moderate to severe high blood pressure
- Have hyperthyroidism
- Have glaucoma, an eye condition
- Are anxious, tense, or agitated
- Have a history of drug abuse
- Are taking or have taken within the past 14 days an antidepression medicine that is a monoamine oxidase inhibitor (MAOI)
- Is sensitive or allergic to or had a reaction to other stimulant medicine
- Has tics or Tourette's syndrome
- Has liver or kidney problems
- Has a history of seizures or abnormal brain wave tests (EEG)

Possible side effects of Vyvanse include the following:

- Slowing of growth both height and weight in children
- Seizures, mainly in patients with a history of seizures
- Eyesight changes or blurred vision
- Upper belly pain
- Dizziness
- Irritability
- Nausea
- Decreased appetite
- Dry mouth
- Trouble sleeping
- Vomiting
- Affecting the person's ability to drive or do other dangerous activities

Vyvanse should be stored in a safe place at room temperature and be protected from light. Sometimes medications are prescribed for purposes other than those listed. However, Vyvanse should not be given to other people even with the same condition; it may harm them, and it is against the law.

The FDA approved Vyvanse for children ages 6 to 12 in July 2007 and for use with adults on April 24, 2008. In the double-blind, placebo-driven trial with 414 adults that led to the FDA approval of Vyvanse, people with ADHD experienced significant improvements in ADHD symptom control within 1 week of treatment with once-daily Vyvanse. Treatment with Vyvanse at all doses, 30, 50, and 70 mg, was significantly more effective that placebo, resulting in a reduction in the score on the ADHD Rating Scale (ADHD-RS-IV), which is based on the 18 items provided in the DSM-IV-TR manual.

Further Readings: Shire US Inc. "Medication Guide: Vyvanse." 2009. http://www.vyvanse.com/pdf/medication_guide.pdf. Accessed 5/27/2009; "FDA Approves VYVANSE, The First and Only Once-Daily Prodrug Stimulant to Treat ADHD in Adults." 2008. http://www.medicalnewstoday.com/printerfriendlynews.php?newsid=105131. Accessed 5/8/2008.

W

Wellbutrin. *See* Bupropion.

Wender, Paul

Known by his colleagues as the "Dean of ADHD," Paul H. Wender, MD, has been a pioneer in identifying and treating ADHD. Wender obtained his under-graduate degree at Harvard and his medical degree at Columbia University College of Physicians and Surgeons and had special training in child, adoles-cent, and adult psychiatry at Harvard, Johns Hopkins, and St. Elizabeth Hospi-tal. For more than 38 years, he has been involved in psychiatric research.

Wender is known for being one of the main leaders of a school of thought followed since the 1970s, which uses many of the ideas of George Still, and describes the characteristic cluster of six symptoms in children with minimal brain dysfunction (MBD):

1. Motor behavior. The essential features are noted to be hyperactivity, poor motor coordination, excessive speech, colic, and sleeping difficulties. Although found in children with only attention problems, he argues this was a type of ADHD.
2. Short attention span. The most striking deficits include short attention and poor concentration. Distractibility and daydreaming are also included.
3. Learning. Most of these children are doing poorly in their academic per-formance. A large percentage is described as having specific difficulties such as learning to read, handwriting, and poor organization.
4. Impulse control. Wender describes low frustration tolerance, inability to delay gratification, antisocial behavior, lack of planning, forethought, and judgment. Sometimes the individual may have problems with bedwetting or defecation control. The child may also display disorderliness and reckless-ness when it comes to bodily safety.
5. Interpersonal relations. Extroversion, excessive independence, obstinacy, stubbornness, negativism, disobedience, sassiness, and imperviousness to discipline are some of the problems relating to interpersonal relations.
6. Emotion. The children display outbursts of the temper, depression, low self-esteem, and anxiety.

In 1971 he wrote his first monograph titled *Minimal Brain Dysfunction in Children,* in which he advanced the idea that the disorder was genetic in origin and mediated by the decreased activity of the dopaminergic system in the brain. In 2000 he added information about adults with ADHD.

Wender is Distinguished Emeritus Professor of Psychiatry at the University of Utah Medical Center. He has been a lecturer in psychiatry at Harvard Medical School and a senior consultant in the Developmental Biopsychiatry Research Program at McLean Hospital.

Further Reading: Wender, Paul H. 1971. *Minimal Brain Dysfunction in Children.* New York: Wiley.

Women

Only in recent years have a few studies begun to focus on the possibility that women have ADHD. Females with ADHD are often overlooked when they are young girls, and some believe that the symptoms present in a different manner. However, according to Michael Manos (2005), symptoms of inattention, distractibility, impulsivity, and hyperactivity in women are the same as symptoms of ADHD in men. Because ADHD is a biogenetic, the condition does not distinguish itself in symptoms that differ by sex.

In a 2004 study Biederman and colleagues compared women and men on the 18 DSM-IV symptoms of inattention, hyperactivity, and impulsivity, in which only one symptom, "talks excessively," was reported to be significantly different in women.

According to Barkley (2006), in childhood boys are three times more likely to have ADHD than girls and five to nine times more likely than girls to be seen by physicians. Brown et al. (1989) found that girls were more socially withdrawn and had the internalizing symptoms of anxiety and depression than did boys but had similar evaluations on clinical measures of their symptoms. Girls probably showed fewer aggressive and impulsive symptoms and had lower rates of conduct disorders. The age at diagnosis for girls tends to be much later. However, in adulthood, just as many women are diagnosed and treated as men. The difference appears not to be in the symptoms; the varied expression of symptoms in the daily lives of men and women is quite different. Researchers suggest that the brain function is the same in both males and females but the actual behavioral expression of brain functioning is very different.

One of the areas of differing expression is in the idea of locus of control, the place from which people feel they manage their daily activities. If one has an internal locus of control, the individual believes that he or she determines the happenings and events in life and that it is under control. She operates on the premise that she makes decisions that affect her environment. External control means that the individual things happens to her and that she has no control over life and her own efforts are not effective. Personal initiative makes no difference because of a "poor me—everything just happens to me." In general people with an external locus of control do not use or appreciate their talents and do not meaningfully contribute to the lives of others.

Rucklidge and Tannock (2001) found that girls with ADHD lose a sense of internal locus of control sooner than those without ADHD. In adulthood, their difficulties may be magnified in a sense of self-ineffectiveness and low self-regard. For example, a young woman with an IQ of 140 decided to work in her mother's nail salon because she thought that she was stupid and could do nothing else; years of failure in school because of inattention led her to the conclusion that she was not capable. She had come to the conclusion that in her life nothing that she could do would make the difference; she had an external locus of control.

Rucklidge observed the following in her study of women with ADHD:

- Women with ADHD are more likely to show learned helplessness. The idea, "poor me—I can't do it begins early in school." They respond to negative situations with resignation and tend to blame themselves when things go wrong.
- Women with ADHD think they cannot control the outcomes of their lives and that they are unable to accomplish anything.
- Women will be more likely to report depression and anxiety and have been in psychological treatment more often than women without ADHD.

Cultural expectations of women may also bring out obvious symptoms of ADHD. It may become critical for women in their late 40s and 50s. Women need managerial skills to manage families, joggle demands of a job, and juggle multiple activities. The symptoms of ADHD increase with obvious demand; women may turn to drugs, alcohol, or other self-destructive pursuits to cope.

Nicole Crawford (2003) calls ADHD a women's issue with gender bias in research on ADHD. She describes the studies of several psychologists and researchers, including an article by psychologist Stephen B. Hinshaw, who published one of the first studies of girls with ADHD in the *Journal of Consulting and Clinical Psychology*. Prior studies had focused on comparing girls to boys, using boys ADHD symptoms as the marker for measurement. Hinshaw concluded that girls experience significant symptoms that are often overlooked because they bear little resemblance to those of boys. This observation also highlights the fact that current diagnostic criteria as found in DSM-IV focus on male rather than females and parent and teacher referral patterns. The new DSM hopefully will address ADHD in girls and women.

Crawford also refers to the work of educational researcher Jane Adelizzi who theorizes that researchers have neglected women with ADHD because hyperactivity is usually missing in girls and they just have the inattention. She likened the unpleasant and stressful experiences of girls with ADHD in education to post traumatic stress disorder (PTSD). However, when they are undiagnosed, they will carry their problems into adulthood, and left untreated, their lives fall apart. They are then at risk for low self-esteem, underachievement, anxiety, depression, teen pregnancy, and underage smoking and drinking.

Treating women for ADHD is often more complicated than treating for men with ADHD. Prescribing any medication must take into consideration

Suffering in Silence: Women and ADHD

The feeling about women with adult ADHD is summed up in a book titled *Suffering in Silence: Women with Adult ADHD* by Lori-Lynn Dale. Lynn details how she appeared to handle herself so well but internally was overwhelmed by three jobs, school, and caring for a young son. She stayed awake days to finish projects. To ease frustration and deal with low self-esteem, she turned to alcohol and drugs.

She found relief in her 30s when she was diagnosed with adult ADHD when her two sons were diagnosed in school. She is convinced women with the disorder tend to suffer in silence compared to male counterparts. She tells how ADHD can silently follow adults for years, but there is help if you know the signs.

Source: Dale, Lori-Lynn. *Suffering in Silence: Women with Adult ADHD.*

all aspects of the women's life including treatment for coexisting conditions, including possible substance abuse and alcoholism. Considering hormonal fluctuations across the menstrual cycle and across the lifespan is imperative. According to a study by Quinn et al. (2002) reduced levels of the hormone estrogen may increase symptoms of ADHD. In some cases, hormone replacement therapy must be added to control hormonal fluctuations. Women with ADHD are usually treated with a combination of stimulant medications. ADD-focused psychotherapy, which is structured and goal-oriented, must accompany the medication.

Other treatment approaches may benefit the woman with ADHD:

- Parent training. Women are generally expected to be family managers and that requires organization and parenting skills. However, if the person has high levels of ADHD symptoms, the training may less effective.
- Group therapy. Social problems for women with ADHD develop early and appear to increase with age. Because many women with ADHD feel shame and rejection, group therapy sessions can provide a place where they are safe and understood.
- ADHD coaching. Coaching is a new profession that has developed in response to the need among some adults with ADHD for structure, support, and focus. Coaching may take place by telephone or e-mail.
- Professional organizing. The organizer profession has been made popular with television programs that help people organize their space and lives. A professional organizer may provide hand-on assistance at home and office for a system that is easy to manage and maintain.
- Career guidance. Women may need specific guidance about their careers. Some of the tasks involved in office management are challenging for a person with ADHD who must pay attention to detail, scheduling, paper work, and an organized workspace.

Further Readings: Biederman, J. et al. 2004. Gender effects of attention-deficit/hyperactivity disorder in adults, revisited. *Biological Psychiatry* 55.692–700; Brown, T. E. et al. 2006. ADHD gender differences in a clinic-referred sample. In *Attention-deficit* *hyperactive disorder: A handbook for diagnosis and treatment.* 3rd ed., edited by Russell Barkley. New York: Guilford Publications. Also presented at the annual meeting of the American Academy of Child and Adolescent Psychiatry, New York, October 1989; Crawford, Nicole. 2003. "ADHD: A women's issue: Psychologists are fighting gender bias in research on attention-deficit hyperactivity disorder." http://www.apa.org/monitor/feb03/adhd.html. Accessed 5/29/2008; National Resource Center on AD/HD. "Women and AD/HD: WWK19." http://www.help4adhd.org/en/living/womengirls/WWK19. Accessed 5/29/2008; Quinn, P. 2002. Hormonal fluctuations and the influence of estrogen in the treatment of women with ADHD. In *Gender issues and ADHD Research, diagnosis, and treatment,* edited by P. Quinn and K. Nadeau, 183–99. Silver Spring, MD: Advantage Books; Rucklidge, J. J., and R. Tannock. 2001. Psychiatric, psychosocial, and cognitive functioning of female adolescents with ADHD. *Journal of the American Academy of Adolescent Psychiatry* 40(5):530–40.

Working Memory. *See* Memory, Working.

X

XXY Syndrome. *See* Klinefelter Syndrome.

XYY Syndrome

47XYY syndrome may mimic ADHD, but they are two completely different conditions. In human beings females have one X chromosome inherited from their mothers and an X chromosome from the father. Males have an X chromosome from the mother and a Y chromosome from the father. There is a rare disorder in which the male may have an extra Y chromosome. Called the XYY trisomy syndrome, the individual may appear to be a normal male. The number 47 is placed in the name to indicate that there are 47 chromosome, rather than the normal 46 chromosomes. In the past it was thought that an excess of testosterone may be responsible for aggressive behaviors, but current studies have shown that this may not be the case. However, the extra Y chromosome has been associated with antisocial behavior and an increased risk for learning difficulties and delayed speech and language skills. The children may be taller than their age group and may also display behaviors of hyperactivity, aggressiveness, and attention deficit. This condition is not inherited but is a chromosomal aberration.

Rais (2008) found a study from the United Kingdom that estimates that 97 percent of XYY males may not appear any different from regular males. She has studied 47XYY males extensively and works with children who display tendencies for disobedience very early in life. For example, one boy had the diagnosis of XYY syndrome at the age of 6 because of his defiant behaviors, frequent temper tantrums, larger body size, self-mutilation, and delayed speech development. Stimulant medication and a host of psychotherapeutic drugs such as lithium did not improve his attention span and concentration ability. When they removed the two drugs, he improved. Although symptoms of ADHD may be present in 47XYY syndrome, the two really are not related.

ADHD is a genetic neurological condition relating to neurotransmitters; 47XYY is an anomaly of the entire chromosome.

Further Readings: Rais, Alina R. 2008. "Treatment of Pervasive Aggression in a Patient with 47XYY Karyotype." http://priory.com/psychiatry/XYY_aggression.htm. Accessed 8/4/2008; Genetics Home Reference. 2009. "47XYY Syndrome." http://www.ghr.nlm.nih.gov/condition=47xyysyndrome. Accessed 5/27/2009.

Y

Yeast Infections

The yeast *Candida albicans* can cause hyperactivity in children. The condition, called candidiasis, almost had some underlying cause that can produce behaviors seen in ADHD. The cause may be an immune disorder, a disorder affecting carbohydrate metabolism, or some other situation that alters blood sugar levels.

When children and adults exhibit listlessness and inattentiveness, they may have this yeast overgrowth, primarily in the intestinal tract. The presence of the yeast can create or aggravate a host of health problems including fibromyalgia, autism, hypoglycemia, ADD, ADHD, and adult ADD and ADHD. At one time only alternative practitioners talked about yeast infections, but with several recent research studies, medical doctors have considered the Candida connection.

In the intestines, numerous strains of bacteria, yeast, and other single-cell organisms reside. The organisms are called "flora," and they may be both friendly and unfriendly. When they are all living together in a normal, healthy environment, everything is normal, but if something happens to destroy the good flora, the bad ones may take over. Overuse of antibiotics may sometimes kill friendly bacteria, leaving the harmful organisms such as yeast to thrive and grow because the antibiotics do not affect them. Other medications such as oral contraceptives and prednisone may also upset this balance.

Yeasts get nourishment from sugar, and they give off waste products called metabolites that can damage the intestinal wall. The walls may develop small holes that allow food and toxic chemicals to get into the bloodstream. This "leaky gut" causes poor health conditions such as food allergies, attention disorders, and other conditions.

A simple blood test that measures the antibodies that have been built up against yeast detects candidiasis. The treatment is threefold:

- Stop feeding the yeast with the intake of the organism's favorite food: sugar.
- Kill the yeast with either a prescription drug or product recommended by a practitioner.
- Replace the yeast with acidophilus and bifidobacteria cultures.

The symptoms of candidiasis are similar to those of hypoglycemia, and both can be present together. Fatigue and sugar craving are common to both conditions.

Further Reading: RXAlternative Medicine. "Yeast and Candidiasis." 2006. http://www.rxalternativemedicine.com/articles/yeast_candidiasis.html. Accessed 5/27/2009.

APPENDIX A: IS IT REALLY ADHD? CONDITIONS THAT MAY BE CONFUSED WITH ADHD

Because health professionals must form opinions about ADHD as they observe children's behavior, they encounter many conditions that have some of the same symptoms as ADHD. Not knowing, parents sometimes settle prematurely for ADHD as a diagnosis before looking at everything. Many medical, biological, and mental conditions or disorders mimic symptoms of ADD or ADHD. Parents and diagnosticians should settle for a diagnosis of ADHD only after checking out as many as possible other answers. Most of the disorders listed below and how they are similar to ADHD are more fully described in separate entries in the Encyclopedia.

- Allergies (especially reactions to food dye, chocolate, and grains)[*]
- Anemias that reduce oxygen to the brain causing disturbance in the brain's chemistry[†]
- Bipolar disorder, early-onset[‡]
- Brain cysts[§]
- Brain tumors, early stage[§]
- B-Vitamin deficiencies[†]
- Carbon monoxide poisoning[†]
- Central Auditory Processing Disorder (CAPD)[†]
- Diabetes, early-onset (Type 1)[‡]
- Dietary factors, such as too much caffeine or sugar[†]
- Drugs (both prescription and illegal)[†]
- Emotional disturbances[†]
- Fetal alcohol syndrome (FAS)[†]
- Genetic defects (including mild forms of Turner's syndrome, sickle cell anemia, Fragile X syndrome, and others)[†]
- Gifted children[†]
- Head injuries[†]
- Hearing and vision problems[*]
- Heart disease and cardiac conditions[‡]

- Hypoglycemia (low blood sugar)[*]
- Infections, viral or bacterial[†]
- Intestinal parasites[§]
- Klinefelter syndrome[§]
- Lack of understanding and communication skills[†]
- Lead, high levels (even in the absence of clinical lead poisoning)[*]
- Learning disabilities[*]
- Malnutrition or improper diet[†]
- Manganese, high levels[†]
- Mercury, high levels[†]
- Metabolic disorders[†]
- Porphyria[§]
- Posttraumatic subclinical seizure disorder[‡]
- Seizure disorders[†]
- Sensory integration dysfunction (children are over- or undersensitive to touch, taste, smell, sound, or sight)[†]
- Sleeping disorders[†]
- Sniffing materials such as glue or other household products[†]
- Spinal problems[†]
- Spirited children[†]
- Spoiled and undisciplined children[†]
- Beta-Hemolytic streptococcus (Strep)[†]
- Temporal lobe seizures[§]
- Thyroid disease (hyper- or hypothyroidism)[*]
- Tourette's syndrome[†]
- Toxin exposures[†]
- Vitamins, excessive amounts[†]
- Worms[†]
- XYY disorder[§]
- Yeast infection (*Candida albicans*)[§]

---

[*]Conditions most often overlooked.

[†]Other conditions sometimes confused with ADHD.

[‡]Diagnoses worth considering, especially if a family history exists.

[§]Rare.

APPENDIX B: DIRECTORY OF ORGANIZATIONS

Adult ADHD Clinic
Department of Psychiatry
University of Massachusetts Medical Center
55 Lake Avenue North
Worchester, MA 01655
508-587-3700

American Academy of Medical Acupuncture (AAMA)
http://www.medicalacupuncture.org
800-521-2262

American Chiropractic Association
http://www.chiro.org

Attention Deficit Disorder Association (ADDA)
1500 Commerce Parkway, Suite C
Mount Laurel, NJ 08054
e-mail: mail@add.org
http://www.add.org
856-438-9099
(fax) 858-438-0525

ADDA is a nonprofit organization working to provide information, resources, and networking to help adults with ADHD lead better lives. Its mission is to generate hope, awareness, empowerment, and connections worldwide in the field of ADHD by bringing together science and the human experience for adults living with ADHD.

Attention Deficit Disorder Resources
223 Tacoma Avenue, Suite 100
Tacoma, Washington 98402
http://www.addresources.org

Attention Deficit Information Network (AD-IN)
475 Hillside Avenue
Needham, MA 02194
617-455-9895

This site provides support and education for those with ADD.

Born to Explore
http://www.borntoexplore.org

This Web site emphasizes the good and positive side of attention deficit disorder, supporting creativity, multiple intelligences, and turning the negative aspects into productive living.

The Reach Institute
Resources for Advancing Children's Health
708 Third Ave., 5th Floor
New York, NY 10017
212-947-REACH (7322)
http://www.thereachinstitute.net/index.html

Center for Science in the Public Interest (CSPI)
1875 Connecticut Avenue NW, Suite 330
Washington, DC 20009-5728
http://www.cspinet.org

C.H.A.D.D.
Children and Adults with Attention Deficit Disorder
8181 Professional Place, Suite 150
Landover, MD 20785
301-306-7070; 800-233-4050
http://www.chadd.org

CHADD is a support and research organization founded in 1987 by a small group of parents and two psychologists in Plantation, Florida. CHADD's mission is to provide a support network for parents and caregivers, to provide a forum for continuing education, to be a community resource for accurate information, and to give evidence-based information about ADHD to parents, educators, adults, professionals, and the media of behalf of the ADHD community. CHADD has local chapters throughout the United States; locations and contact names and phone numbers are available through National Headquarters.

Council for Exceptional Children
1920 Association Drive
Reston, VA 22091-1589
800-328-0272

Feingold Foundation
554 E Main Street, Suite 301
Riverhead, NY 11901
631 369-9340
http://www.feingold.org

Health Resource Center (National Clearing house for Postsecondary
Education for People with Disabilities)
1 DuPont Circle NW
Washington, DC 20038

Learning Disabilities Association of America
4156 Library Road
Pittsburgh, PA 15324-1349
412-341-1515
e-mail: info@ldaamerica.org
http://www.ldaamerica.org

National Alliance on Mental Illness
e-mail: info@nami.org
http://www.nami.org
1-800-950-NAMI (6264)

This is one of American's largest grassroots organizations dedicated to
improving the lives of persons living with serious mental illness. Information about ADHD is available.

National Center for Complementary and Alternative Medicine
National Library of Medicine
8600 Rockville Pike
Bethesda, MD 20894
http://www.nlm.nih.gov/medlineplus/complementaryandalternativemedicine.
html

National Center for Gender Issues and ADHD
3268 Arcadia Place NW
Washington, DC 20015
http://www.ncgiadd.org

This organization promotes awareness of research into and advocacy for
girls and women with ADHD.

National Center for Girls and Women with AD/HD
326 Arcadia Place NW
Washington, DC 20015
http://www.ncgiadd.org

The principal aims of the National Center for Girls and Women with AD/HD
are to raise awareness of the impact of ADHD on of girls and women and
to disseminate information about ADHD in females in to a broad spectrum

including families, medical and mental health professionals, educators, the media, and women of all ages.

National Center for Learning Disabilities
381 Park Avenue South, Suite 1401
New York, NY 10016
212-545-7510 or 888-575-7373
http://www.ld.org

National Institute of Mental Health (NIMH)
National Institutes of Health, DHHS
6001 Executive Blvd., Rm. 8184, MCS 9663
Bethesda, MD 20892-9663
301-443-4513 or 866-615-NIMH (6464)
e-mail: nimhinfo@nih.gov
http://www.nimh.nih.gov

National Information Center for Children and Youth with Disabilities (NICCHY)
P.O. Box 1492
Washington, DC 20013
800-695-0285

National Network of Learning Disabled Adults (NNLDA)
808 North 82nd Street, Suite F2
Scottsdale, AZ 85257
602-941-5112

National Resource Center on ADHD
818 Professional Place, Suite 150
Landover, MD 20785
800-233-4050
http://www.help4adhd.org

Orton Dyslexia Society (ODS)
8600 LaSalle Road
Chester Building, Suite 382
Towson, MD 21204
800-222-3123

Professional Group for ADD and Related Disorders (PGARD)
28 Fairview Road
Scarsdale, NY 10583
914-723-0118

Project Literacy US (PLUS)
4802 Fifth Avenue
Pittsburgh, PA 15213
412-622-1491

U.S. Department of Education Office of Vocational and Adult Education
Clearinghouse on Adult Education

MES Building, Room 4416
400 Maryland Avenue
Washington, DC 20202-5515
202-732-2410

U.S. Equal Employment Opportunity Commission (EEOC)
1-800-669-4000
This agency protects people who feel they have been targeted because of
their disability.

BIBLIOGRAPHY

Ackerman, Cheryl. "Identifying Gifted Adolescents Using Personality Characteristics: Dabrowski's Overexcitabilties." *Roeper Review—A Journal on Gifted Education* 19, no. 3 (1997): 229–36.

Adderall XR. "Adderall." http://www.adderallxr.com (accessed June 18, 2009).

"ADHD and Dyslexia." http://www.healthyplace.com/communities/add/judy/dyslexia_1.htm (accessed July 13, 2008).

ADHD Information Library. "ADHD vs. Drug Exposed Babies or Fetal Alcohol Syndrome." http://newideas.net/adhd/about-attention-deficit/fas-drug-exposed-adhd (accessed June 18, 2009).

ADHD Information Library. "Mercury Poisoning, Heavy Metal or Chemical Toxicity, and Brain Development." http://newideas.net/adhd/differential-diagnosis/mercury-chemical-toxicity (accessed June 18, 2009).

Amen, Daniel. *Healing ADD: The Breakthrough Program That Allows You to See and Heal the 6 Types of ADD.* New York: Berkley Books, 2001.

American Academy of Child and Adolescent Psychiatry. "Facts for Families: Lead Exposure in Children Affects Brain and Behavior" (updated 2004). http://www.aacap.org/cs/root/facts_for_families/lead_exposure_in_children_affects_brain_and_behavior (accessed June 18, 2009).

American Academy of Pediatrics. "AAP Policy: Clinical Practice Guidelines." http://aappolicy.aappublications.org/practice_guidelines/index.dtl (accessed May 20, 2009).

American Chiropractic Association. "Research." http://www.chiro.org/pediatrics/ADD.shtml (accessed July 23, 2008).

American Psychiatric Association. 2004. *Diagnostic and Statistical Manual of the American Psychiatric Association.* 4th ed. Arlington, VA: American Psychiatric Association.

Amethyst Natural Healing. "The Bowen Technique." http://www.amethystnatural-healing.co.uk/bowen.html (accessed June 18, 2009).

Anxiety-Panic.Com. http://www.anxiety-panic.com (accessed June 18, 2009).

Arnold, L. E. "Alternative Treatments for Adults with Attention-Deficit Hyperactivity Disorder (ADHD)." *Annals of New York Academy of Science* 931 (2001): 310–341.

Aston-Jones, G., J. Rajkowski, and J. Cohen. "Role of Locus Coeruleus in Attention and Behavioral Flexibility." *Biological Psychiatry* 46 (1999): 1309–20.

Attention Deficit Disorder Help Center. "Attention Deficit Disorder or Hypoglycemia?" http://www.add-adhd-help-center.com/newsletters/newsletter_15nov03.htm. Accessed 8/6/2008.

"Attention Deficit Hyperactive Disorder." In *Conn's Current Therapy*, edited by R. E. Rakel and E. T. Bope, 947–58. Philadelphia: Saunders, 2004.

Autism Speaks. "Treatments for Autism." http://www.autismspeaks.org/whattodo/index.php (accessed June 18, 2009).

Baldwin, Neill. *Edison: Inventing the Century.* New York: Hyperion, 1995.

Barkley, R. A. *ADHD Adolescents: Family Conflicts and their Management.* Grant from National Institute of Mental Health (MH41583), 1990.

Barkley, R. A. "ADHD and Accident Proneness." *The ADHD Report* May (2002): 2–5.

Barkley, R. A. *ADHD and the Nature of Self-Ccontrol.* New York: Guilford Press, 1997.

Barkley, R. A. *Attention-Deficit Hyperactivity Disorder: A Handbook for Diagnosis and Treatment.* 3rd ed. New York: Guilford Press, 2006.

Barkley, R. A. "Biography." WebMD. http://www.webmd.com/russell-a-barkley (accessed June 18, 2009).

Barkley, R. A. "International Consensus Statement on ADHD." *Clinical Child and Family Psychology Review* 5, no. 2 (2002): 218–43.

Barkley, R. A. *Taking Charge of ADHD.* New York: Guilford Press, 2000.

Barkley, R. A., G. J. DuPaul, and M. B. McMurray. "Comprehensive Evaluation of ADD with and without Hyperactivity as Defined by Research Criteria." *Journal of Consulting and Clinical Psychology* 58 (1990): 775–89.

Barkley, R. A. et al. "Does the Treatment of ADHD with Stimulant Medication Contribute to Illicit Drug and Abuse in Adulthood: Results from a 15-year Prospective Study." *Pediatrics* 111 (1990): 109–21.

Barkley, R. A., M. Fischer, C. S. Edelbrock, and L. Smallish. "The Adolescent Outcome of Hyperactive Children Diagnosed by Research Criteria: I. An 8-year Prospective Follow-up Study." *Journal of the American Academy of Child and Adolescent Psychiatry* 29 (1990): 546–57.

Barkley, R. A., M. Fischer, L. Smallish, and K. Fletcher. "Does the Treatment of Attention-Deficit/Hyperactivity Disorder with Stimulants Contribute to Drug Use/Abuse? A 13-year Prospective Study." *Pediatrics* 111 (2003): 97–109.

Barkley, R. A., D. C. Guevremont, A. D. Anastopoulos, G. J. DuPaul, and T. L. Shelton. "Driving-related Risks and Outcomes of Attention Deficit Hyperactivity Disorder in Adolescents and Young Adults: A 3–5 Year Follow-up Survey." *Pediatrics* 92, (2003): 212–18.

Barkley, R. A., K. R. Murphy, and M. Fischer. *ADHD in Adults: What the Science Says.* New York: Guilford Press, 2007.

Bazar, K. A., A. J. Yun, P. Y. Lee, S. M, Daniel, and J. D. Doux. "Obesity and ADHD May Represent Different Manifestations of a Common Environmental Oversampling Syndrome: A Model for Revealing Mechanistic Overlap among Cognitive, Metabolic, and Inflammatory Disorders." *Medical Hypotheses* 66, no. 2 (2006): 263–69.

Berman, T., Douglas V. I., and Barr, R. G. "Effects of Methylphenidate on Complex Cognitive Process in Attention-Deficit Hyperactive Disorder." *Journal of Abnormal Psychology* 108 (1998): 90–105.

Berridge, C. W., and B. D. Waterhouse. "The Locus Coeruleus-Noradrenergic System: Modulation of Behavioral State and State-dependent Cognitive Process." *Brain Research Review* 42 (2003): 33–84.

Bhatara V., R. Loudenberg, and R. Ellis. "Association of Attention Deficit Hyperactivity Disorder and Gestational Alcohol Exposure: An Exploratory Study." *Journal of Attention Disorders* 9 (2006): 515–22.

Biederman, J. "Breaking News: The Social and Economic Impact of ADHD." Discussion presented at the Attention Deficit Hyperactive Disorder (ADHD) AMA Briefing: September 9; New York, NY, 2004.

Biederman J., M. C. Monuteaux, E. Mick, et al. "Is Cigarette Smoking a Gateway to Alcohol and Illicit Drug Use Disorders? A Study of Youths with and without Attention Deficit Hyperactivity Disorder." *Biological Psychiatry* 59 (2006): 258–64.

Biederman, J., S. V. Faraone, M. C. Monuteaux, M. Bober, and E. Cadogen. "Gender Effects of Attention-Deficit/Hyperactivity Disorder in Adults, Revisited." *Biological Psychiatry* 55 (2004): 692–700.

Bird, H. R., G. Canino, M. Rubio-Stipec, et al. "Estimates of the Prevalence of Childhood Maladjustment in a Community Survey in Puerto Rico. The Use of Combined Measures." *Archives of General Psychiatry* 32 (1988): 361–68.

Birnbaum, H. G., R. C. Kessler, S. W. Lowe, et al. "Costs of Attention Deficit-Hyperactivity Disorder (ADHD) in the US: Excess Costs of Persons with ADHD and Their Family Members in 2000." *Current Medical Opinion* 21, no. 2, (2005): 195–205.

Born to Explore. "Can Allergies Cause Behavior Problems?" http://borntoexplore. org/allergies.
htm (accessed June 18, 2009).

Bouchez, Colette. "Seasonal Allergies Affect ADHD." http://www.redorbit.com/ news/science/4675/seasonal_allergies_affect_adhd/index.html (accessed June 18, 2009).

Boutros, N., L. Fraenkel, and A. Feingold. "A Four-step Approach for Developing Diagnostic Tests in Psychiatry: EEG in ADHD as a Test Case." *Journal of Neuropsychiatry Clinical Neuroscience* 17, no. 4 (2005): 455–64.

Bratman, Steven. *The Alternative Medicine Sourcebook*. Los Angeles: Lowell House, 1997.

Braun J. M., R. S. Kahn, T. Froehlich, P. Auinger, and B. P. Lanphear.
"Exposures to Environmental Toxicants and Attention Deficit Hyperactivity Disorder in U.S. Children." *Environmental Health Perspectives* 114, no. 12, (2006): 1904–09.

Bright, G. M. "Medication/Substance Abuse Issues in ADHD." Discussion presented at the Attention Deficit Hyperactive Disorder (ADHD) AMA Media Briefing; September 9. New York, NY, 2004.

Brown, Thomas E. *Attention Deficit Disorder: The Unfocused Mind in Children and Adults*. New Haven: Yale University Press, 2005.

Brown, Thomas E., ed. *Attention-deficit Disorders and Comorbidities in Children, Adolescents, and Adults*. Washington, DC: American Psychiatric Press, 2000.

Brown, Thomas E. "Attention-Deficit/Hyperactivity Disorders with Obsessive-Compulsive Disorder." In *Attention-Deficit Disorders and Comorbidities in Children Adolescents and Adults,* edited by T. E. Brown, 209–30. Washington, DC: American Psychiatric Press, 2000.

Brown, Thomas E. "A New Approach to Attention Deficit Disorder." *Educational Leadership* 64, no. 5 (2007): 22–27. http://www.ascd.org/publications/educational_ leadership/feb07/vol64/num05/abstract.aspx#A_New_Approach_to_Attention_ Deficit_Disorder (accessed May 18, 2009).

Brown, Thomas E. Official Web site. http://www.drthomasbrown.com (accessed May 18, 2009).

Brown, Thomas E. et al. "ADHD Gender Differences in a Clinic-referred Sample." In *Attention-Deficit Hyperactivity Disorder: A Handbook for Diagnosis and Treatment.* 3rd ed., edited by Russell Barkley. 108. New York: Guilford Press,

2006. Also presented at the annual meeting of the American Academy of Child and Adolescent Psychiatry, New York, October 1989.

Brown, Thomas E. et al. "Attention-Activation Disorder in Hi-IQ Underachievers." Abstract. *Proceedings of American Psychiatric Association* 145th Annual Meeting. Washington, DC, May 1992.

Burden, Paul. *Classroom Management: Creating a Successful K-12 Learning Community.* New York: John Wiley & Sons, 2006.

Burke, J. D. et al. "Developmental Transitions among Affective and Behavioral Disorders in Adolescent Boys." *Journal of Child Psychology and Psychiatry* 45 (2005): 577–88.

Burney, Fanny. "Diary of Fanny Burney." http://www.edprint.demon.co.uk/johnson/sam-fanny.html

Busco, Marlene. "Adult ADHD Is Common Among Patients in Anxiety-Disorders Clinic." (2008). http://www.medscape.com/viewarticles/571537 (accessed May 19, 2008).

Cadena, Christine. "Food Intolerance & Allergies in the ADHD Child." Associated Content. (March 2007). http://www.associatedcontent.com/article/155824/food_intolerance_allergies_in_the_adhd.html?cat=25 (accessed June 18, 2009).

Cauldwell, K. (2006). "Acupuncture for Attention Deficit Disorder and ADHD." http://www.associatedcontent.com/article/31125/acupuncture_for_attention_deficit_disorder.html?cat=5 (accessed June 18, 2009).

Center for Science in the Public Interest (CSPI). http://www.cspinet.org (accessed July 13, 2008).

Centers for Disease Control and Prevention. "ADHD and Risk of Injuries." http://www.cdc.gov/ncbddd/adhd/facts.html (accessed June 18, 2009).

Child Development Institute. "Facts About Fragile X Syndrome." http://www.childdevelopmentinfo.com/disorders/facts_about_fragile_x_syndrome.htm (accessed June 18, 2009).

Children and Adults with Attention Deficit/Hyperactivity Disorder. http://chadd.org (accessed June 18, 2009).

Chiro.Org. "Attention Deficit Disorder (ADD)." http://www.chiro.org/pediatrics/ADD.shtml (accessed June 18, 2009).

"Clinical Trials": Attention Deficit Hyperactive Disorder." http://www.nimh.nih.gov/studies/studies_ct.cfm?id=2&Output=Print Accessed 6/16/2008.

Cohen, Don, and Fred Volmar. *The Handbook of Autism and Pervasive Development Disorders.* 3rd ed. New York: Wiley Press, 2005.

Comings, D. E. "Attention-Deficit/Hyperactivity Disorder with Tourette Syndrome." In *Attention-Deficit Disorders and Comorbidities in Children, Adolescents, and Adults,* edited by Thomas Brown, 363–92. Washington, DC: American Psychiatric Press, 2000.

"Computed Tomography." http://www.en.wikipedia.org/wiki/Computed_tomography. Accessed 6/26/2008

Conners, C. Keith. (2008). "CRS-R (Conner's Rating Scales-Revised)." http://www.pearsonassessments.com/crsr.aspx (accessed June 19, 2009).

Cooper, Paul, and Katherine Bilton. *ADHD: Research, Practice and Opinion.* London: Whurr Publishers, 1999.

Coren, Stanley. *The Left-handed Syndrome: The Causes and Consequences of Left-Handedness.* New York: Macmillan, 1992.

Corman, C. A., and E. Hallowell. *Positively ADD: Real Stories to Inspire Your Dreams.* New York: Walker and Company, 2006.

Cramond, Bonnie. (1995). "The Coincidence of Attention Deficit Hyperactivity Disorder and Creativity." Born to Explore. http://www.borntoexplore.org/adhd.htm (accessed June 18, 2009).

Crawford, Nicole. (2003). "ADHD: A women's issue. Psychologists are fighting gender bias in research on attention-deficit hyperactivity disorder." APA Online. http://www.apa.org/monitor/feb03/adhd.html (accessed June 18, 2009).

Dalby, J. T. "Will Population Decreases in Caffeine Consumption Unveil Attention Deficit Disorder in Adults?" *Medical Hypotheses* 18, no. 2, (2002): 163–67.

Davis, P., and Waldron Saffron. *Aromatherapy from A-Z*. Essex, England: Daniel Publishers, 1988.

deGraaf, R., R. C. Kessler, J. Fayyad, et al. "The Prevalence and Effects of Adult Attention-Deficit/Hyperactivity Disorder (ADHD) on the Performance of Workers: Results from the WHO Mental Health Survey Initiative." *Occupational and Environmental Medicine* 65 (2008): 835–42.

Delisle, J. R., J. R. Whitmore, and R. P. Ambrose. "Preventing Behavior Problems with Gifted Students." *Teaching Exceptional Children* 19 (1987).

Diller, Lawrence H. *The Last Normal Child: Essays on the Intersection of Kids, Culture, and Psychiatric Drugs*. Westport, CT: Praeger, 2006.

Donnay, Albert. (2006). "Background on Sources, Symptoms, Biomarkers, and Treatment of Chronic Carbon Monoxide Poisoning." Multiple Chemical Sensitivity. http://www.mcsrr.org/resources/articles/P11.html (accessed. June 18, 2009).

Donovan, Jennifer. (1997). "Hyperactivity Linked to Thyroid Hormones." Science Daily. http://www.sciencedaily.com/releases/1997/03/970312165726.htm (accessed June 18, 2009).

Douglas, V. I. "Cognitive Control Processes in Attention-Deficit Hyperactive Disorder." In *Handbook of Disruptive Behavior Disorders*, edited by H. C. Quay and A. E. Hogan, 105–38. New York: Plenum Publishing, 1998.

Dr. X's Free Associations. "Sugar and ADHD." (2008) http://drx.typepad.com/psychotherapyblog/2008/06/sugar-and-adhd.html (accessed June 18, 2009).

Drug Enforcement Administration, U.S. Department of Justice. "Controlled Substance Schedules." http://www.deadiversion.usdoj.gov/schedules/schedules.htm (accessed June 18, 2009).

Drugs.com. "Cylert." http://www.drugs.com/pro/cylert.html (accessed June 18, 2009).

Duke, M. *Acupuncture, The Chinese Art of Healing*. London: Constable, 1973.

Dye, John M. "Herbal Medicine and Treatments for ADHD." (2000). Healing Center On-Line. http://www.healing-arts.org/children/ADHD/herbal.htm (accessed June 18, 2009).

eHow. "How to Treat ADHD with Homeopathy." (2006) http://www.ehow.com/how_2052053_treat-adhd-homeopathy.html (accessed August 3, 2008).

Enstrom, E. A., and Doris C. Enstrom. "Reading Help for Lefties." *Reading Teacher* 25 (1971): 41–44.

Epstein, M. A., S. E. Shaywitz, B. A. Shaywitz, and J. L. Woolston. "The Boundaries of Attention Deficit Disorder." *Journal of Learning Disabilities* 24 (1991): 110–20.

Faraone, Stephen. (2007). "ADHD in Children with Comorbid Conditions: Diagnosis, Misdiagnosis, and Keeping Tabs on Both." *Medscape Psychiatry and Mental Health* http://www.medscape.com/viewarticle/555748 (accessed May 19, 2008).

Faraone, S. V., T. J. Spencer, C. B. Montano, J. Biederman. "Attention-Deficit/Hyperactivity Disorder in Adults: A Survey of Current Practice in Psychiatry and Primary Care." *Archives of Internal Medicine* 164, no. 11 (2004): 1221–26.

Faraone, S. V. "Advances in the Genetics and Neurobiology of Attention Deficit Hyperactivity Disorder." *Biological Psychiatry* 60, no. 10 (2006): 1025–27.

FDA News Release. "FDA Approves Methylphenidate Patch to Treat Attention Deficit Hyperactivity Disorder in Children" (April 10, 2006.) http://www.fda.gov/NewsEvents/Newsroom/PressAnnouncements/2006/ucm108633.htm (accessed June 18, 2009).

Feingold, B. F. *The Feingold Cookbook for Hyperactive Children.* New York: Random House, 1979.

Feingold, B. F. *Introduction to Clinical Allergy.* New York: Charles C. Thomas, 1973.

Feingold, B. F. *Why Your Child Is Hyperactive.* New York: Random House, 1974.

Findling, Robert. "AHA Recommendations on Cardiovascular Monitoring in Patients with ADHD and Heart Disease." (2008). Medscape Psychiatry and Health. http://www.mcdscape.com/viewarticle/574540_print (accessed August 11, 2008).

Frazier, T. W., H. A. Demaree, and E. A. Youngstrom. "Meta-analysis of Intellectual and Neuropsychological Test Performance in Attention-Deficit/Hyperactivity Disorder." *Neuropsychology* 18 (2004): 543–55.

Frick, P. J., R. W. Kamphaus, B. B. Lahey, et al. "Academic Underachievement and the Disruptive Behavior Disorders." *Journal of Consulting and Clinical Psychology* 59 (1991): 289–94.

Friedman, H. S., J. S. Tucker, J. E. Schwartz, et al. "Psychosocial and Behavioral Predictors of Longevity: The Aging and Death of the 'Termites.'" *American Psychologist* 50 (1995): 69–313.

Gantos, Jack. *Joey Pigza Swallowed the Key.* New York: Farrar, Strauss, and Giroux, 1998.

Garber, Kent. "Who's Behind the Bible of Mental Illness?" *U.S. News &World Report,* December 31, 2007.

Gardner, Howard. *Creating Minds: An Anatomy of Creativity Seen through the Lives of Freud, Einstein, Picasso, Stravinsky, Eliot, Graham, and Gandhi.* New York: Basic Books.

Gardner, Howard. *Frames of Mind: The Theory of Multiple Intelligences.* 10th ed. New York: Basic Books, 1993.

Garfinkel, B. D., C. D. Webster, and L. Sloman. Responses to methylphenidate and varied doses of caffeine in children with attention deficit disorder. *Canadian Journal of Psychiatry* 26, no. 6 (1981): 395–401.

Gaub, M., and C. L. Carlson. "Gender Differences in ADHD: A Meta-analysis and Critical Review." *Journal of the American Academy of Child and Adolescent Psychiatry* 36 (1997): 1036–45.

Gavin, Kara. (2006). "Kids Behave and Sleep Better after Tonsillectomy, University of Michigan Study Finds." University of Michigan Health System. http://www.med.umich.edu/opm/newspage/2006/sleep.htm (accessed June 18, 2009).

Genetics Home Reference. "47,XYY Syndrome." http://ghr.nlm.nih.gov/condition=47xyysyndrome (accessed May 18, 2009).

Geschwind, N., and P. Behan. "Lefthandedness: Association with Immune Disease, Migraine, and Developmental Learning Disorder." *Proceedings of the National Academy of Sciences USA* 79 (1982): 5097–100.

Gilman, Lois. "Career Advice from Powerful ADHD Executives." *ADDitude,* December/January 2005. http://www.additudemag.com/adhd/article/754.html (accessed June 18, 2009.

GlaxoSmithKline. "Dexedrine Prescribing Information." (2008) http://us.gsk.com/products/assets/us_dexedrine.pdf (accessed June 18, 2009).

"Global ADHD Working Group. Global Consensus on ADHD/HKD." *European Child Adolescent Psychiatry* 14 (2005): 127–37.

Gold Bamboo. "Bowen Technique". http://goldbamboo.com/topic-t6723-a64022.html (accessed June 18, 2009).

Goldstein, S. *Managing Attention and Learning Disorders in Late Adolescence and Adulthood.* New York: Wiley, 1997.

Goldstein, S., and A. J. Schwebach A. J. "The Comorbidity of Pervasive Developmental Disorder and Attention Deficit Hyperactive Disorder: Results of a Retrospective Chart Review." *Journal of Autism and Developmental Disorders* 34 (2004): 328–39.

Gonzalez-Lima, F. "Cortical and Limbic Systems Mediating the Predisposition to Attention Deficit and Hyperactivity." In *Attention Deficit Hyperactivity Disorder Research,* edited by Michelle P. Larimer, 1–18. New York: Nova Science Publishers, 2005.

"Good News for South Paws: Mortality of Left-Handed People." *University of California-Berkeley Wellness Letter* 8 (February 1992): 2.

Goodman, Alice. "Study Offers Suggestions for Differentiating between Pediatric Seizures and ADHD." *Neurology Today* 2, no. 2 (2002): 36.

Gozal, David, and Dennis L. Molfese, eds. *Attention Deficit Hyperactive Disorder: From Genes to Patients.* Totowa, NJ: Humana Press, 2005.

Gross, Monroe. (2007). "A History of Bedwetting Is a Very Strong Clue to the Diagnosis of ADD/ADHD." http://www.addmtc.com/bedwet (accessed July 13, 2008).

Hallowell, E. M., and R. J. Ratey. *Driven to Distraction: Recognizing and Coping with Attention Deficit Disorder from Childhood through Adulthood.* New York: Touchstone, 1994.

Hartmann, Thom. *Attention Deficit Disorder: A Different Perception.* Grass Valley, CA: Mythical Intelligences Press, 1997.

Hartmann, Thom. *Beyond ADD: Hunting for Reasons in the Past and the Present.* Grass Valley, CA: Mythical Intelligences Press, 1996.

Hartsough, C. S., and N. M. Lambert. "Medical Factors in Hyperactive and Normal Children: Prenatal, Developmental, and Health History Findings." *American Journal of Orthopsychiatry* 55 (1985): 190–210.

Healing Center On-Line. "Bach Flower Essences for the Treatment of ADHD." http://www.healing-arts.org/index2.htm (accessed June 18, 2009).

Health Consumer. "Gifted Children with ADHD." http://www.athealth.com/consumer/disorders/adhdgifted.html (accessed June 29, 2008).

Health Guidance. "ADHD and Diet: Is there a Link Between Sugar and Hyperactivity?" http://www.healthguidance.org/entry/1563/1/ADHD-and-Diet-Is-There-a-Link-Between-S (accessed July 30, 2008).

Heijtz, R. D. et al. "Motor Inhibitory Role of Dopamine D1 Receptors: Implications for ADHD." *Physiological Behavior* 92, no. 1-2 (2007): 155–60.

Hitti, Miranda. "New Heart Alert for Some ADHD Drugs." (2006) http://www.webmd.com/add-adhd/news/2006822/geart-alert-adhd-drugs (accessed August 11, 2008).

Hoffman, Martin. "Treatment of ADHD in Children with Seizure Disorders." (2006) http://www.medscape.com/viewarticle/536122 (accessed August 8, 2008).

Holos, Health for the Whole Person."The Homeopathic Treatment of Children with ADHD and Similar Behavioural Learning Disorders." http://www.holos-homeopathy.com/ADHD_information_1.htm (accessed May 18, 2009).

Hughes, Sue. "Children with ADHD Should Have ECG before Taking Stimulant Drugs." (2008) http://www.theheart.org/article/858823.do (accessed August 11, 2008).

Hunt, Robert D. "Functional Roles of Norepinephrine and Dopamine in ADHD." *Medscape Medical Psychiatry and Mental Health*, 11, no. 1 (2006). http://www.medscape.com/viewarticle/523887_print.

Iannelli, Vincent. "Sensory Integration Disorder." http://www.pediatrics.about.com/od/weeklyquestion/a/94_sensory_intg.htm (accessed August 9, 2008).

Incredible Horizons. "Signs, Symptoms, and Background Information on Sensory Integration." http://www.incrediblehorizons.com/sensory-integration.htm (accessed May 27, 2009).

"International Consensus Statement of ADHD." *Clinical Child and Family Psychological Review* 5, no. 2 (2002): 89–111.

"The Intuitive Brain." http://borntoexplore.org/addint.htm (accessed February 3, 2008).

Jensen, P. S. et al. "Findings from the NIMH Multimodal Treatment Study of ADHD (MTA): Implications and Applications for Primary Care Providers." *Journal of Behavior Pediatrics* 22 (2001): 60–72.

Johnson, C. "Smart Kids Have Problems, Too." *Today's Education* 70 (1981): 22–27, 29.

Johnston, L. D. et al. "Monitoring the Future: National Results on Adolescent Drug Use." Bethesda, MD: National Institute on Drug Abuse, 2006. http://www.monitoringthefuture.org/new.html (accessed May 18, 2009).

Jones, K. L., and D. W. Smith. "Recognition of the Fetal Alcohol Syndrome in Early Infancy." *Lancet* 2 (1973): 1267–71.

Kane, Anthony. "The Role of Sugar in ADHD." EmaxHealth. http://67.192.78.234/37/894.html (accessed June 18, 2009).

Karl Harrison. "Dextroamphetamine Molecule: Dexedrine, Dextrostat, D-Amphetamine, and Dexamphetamine." http://www.3dchem.com/molecules.asp?ID=401 (accessed June 18, 2009).

Katusic, S. K. et al. "Case Definition in Epidemiologic Studies of ADHD." *Annals of Epidemiology* 15 (2005): 430–37.

Kaufman, F. et al. *Attention Deficit Disorder and Gifted Students: What Do We Know?* Storrs, CT: National Research Center on Gifted and Talented, University of Connecticut, 2000.

Kelly, Evelyn B. *Left-Handed Students: A Forgotten Minority*. Bloomington, IN: Phi Delta Kappa Foundation, 1996.

Kelly, Evelyn B. *Legal Basics: A Handbook for Educators*. 2nd ed. Bloomington, IN: Phi Delta Kappa International, 2006.

Kennedy, Diane. *The ADHD Autism Connection*. Colorado Springs, CO: Waterbrook Press, 2002.

Kessler, R. C. et al. "Lifetime Prevalence and Age-of-Onset Distributions of DSM-IV Disorders in the National Comorbidity Survey Replication." *Archive General Psychiatry* 62 (2005): 593–602.

Kidd, P. M. "Attention Deficit/Hyperactivity Disorder (ADHD) in Children: Rationale for Its Integrative Management." *Alternative Medicine Review* 5, no. 5 (2000): 402–28.

Kirley, Aiveen. "Scanning the Genome for Attention Deficit Hyperactivity Disorder." In *Attention Deficit Hyperactivity Disorder: From Genes to Patients*, edited by David Gozal and Dennis Molfese. Totawa, NJ: Humana Press, 2005.

Knight, J. R. et al. "Barriers to Screening Teens for Substance Abuse in Primary Care." Poster presentation, American Society of Pediatrics Annual Meeting, May 14, Washington, DC, 2005.

Knight, J. R. et al. "Validity of the CRAFFT Substance Abuse Screening Test among Adolescent Clinic Patients." *Archives of Pediatric Adolescent Medicine* 156 (2002): 607–14.

"Know Your Children's Educational Rights." *ADDitude* (August/September 2006). http://www.addiitudemag.com/adhd/article/1623.html (accessed May 19, 2009).

Kollins, S. H., F. J. McClernon, and B. F. Fuemmeler. "Association between smoking and attention-deficit/hyperactivity disorder symptoms in a population-based sample of young adults." *Archives of General Psychiatry* 62 (2005): 1142–47.

Konofal, E. et al. "Iron Deficiency in Children." *Archives of Pediatric Adolescent Medicine* 158, no. 12 (2004): 1113–15.

Kunwar, A. et al. "Treating Common Psychiatric Disorders Associated with Attention-Deficit/Hyperactive Disorder." *Expert Opinion Pharmacotherapy* 8 (2007): 555–62.

Kutscher, Martin L. (2002). *The ADHD e-Book.* http://www.booklocker.com/p/books/952.html?s=pdf (accessed May 19, 2009).

Kutscher, Martin. *Kids in the Syndrome Mix of ADHD, LD, Asperger's, Tourette's, Bipolar and More: The One Stop Guide for Parents, Teachers, and Other Professionals.* Philadelphia: Jessica Kingsley, 2006.

Lang, Susan. "Study Suggests Link between Maternal Cocaine Use, Attention Dysfunction in Kids." (2000). http://www.news.cornell.edu/Chronicle/00/6.15.00/cocaine.html (accessed February 3 2008).

LD Research Foundation. "Famous People with ADHD and Dyslexia." http://www.ldrfa.org/pID=34 (accessed June 19, 2009).

Little, Nan. "What is Color Therapy?" http://www.anxiety-and-depression-solutions.com/articles/complementary_alternative_medicine/color_therapy/color_therapy.php (accessed May 20, 2009).

Low, Keith. "Understanding and Nurturing Your Child's Creativity." http://www.add.about.com/od/childrenandteens/a/creativity2.htm (accessed June 29, 2008).

Lyon, Michael. *Healing the Hyperactive Brain: Through the New Science of Functional Medicine.* Calgary, AB, Canada: Focused Publishing, 2000.

Martino, Davide. "Antibasal Ganglia Antibodies and Their Relevance to Movement Disorders." *Current Opinion in Neurology* 17, no. 4 (2004): 425–32.

McCauley, E. et al. "Self-esteem and Behavior in Girls with Turner Syndrome." *Journal of Developmental and Behavioral Pediatrics* 16, no. 2, (2002): 82–88.

"Medical Acupuncture Treats ADHD without Drugs." (2000). http://www.medicalacupuncture.org/acu_info/pressrelease/adhd.html (accessed April 26, 2008).

Medical News Today. "Attention Seeking Confused with ADHD." http://www.medicalnewstoday.com/articles/93732.php (accessed June 18, 2009).

Medical News Today. "Children with Both Autism and ADHD Often Bully, Parents Say." http://www.medicalnewstoday.com/articles/71296.php (accessed June 18, 2009).

Medical News Today. "Dore: Ground Breaking Drug-Free Treatment for ADHD, USA." (2007) http://www.medicalnewstoday.com/articles/90429.php (accessed June 18, 2009).

Medical News Today. "For Boys with Fragile X Syndrome and ADHD, New Hope Found in Non-Stimulant Medication." (2008) http://www.medicalnewstoday.com/articles/98191.php (accessed June 18, 2009).

Medical News Today. "FDA Approves VYVANSE(TM) (lisdexamfetamine Dimesylate), the First and Only Once-Daily Prodrug Stimulant to Treat ADHD in Adults." (2008) http://www.medicalnewstoday.com/printerfriendlynews.php?newsid=105131 (accessed June 18, 2009).

Medical News Today. "How Best to Treat Preschoolers with ADHD? The Harvard Mental Health Letter Discusses the Options." (2007) http://www.medicalnewstoday.com/articles/81498.php (accessed June 18, 2009).

Medical News Today. "New Analysis in Boys and Girls Shows the ADHD Patch, DAY-TRANA(TM) (methylphenidate Transdermal System), Offered ADHD Symptom Control for 12 Months." (2008) http://www.medicalnewstoday.com/articles/106671.php (accessed June 18, 2009).

Medical News Today. "New Study Finds Working Memory Training Procedures Lasting Improvements in Kids with Attention Deficits." (2007) http://www.medicalnewstoday.com/articles/90426.php (accessed June 18, 2009).

Medical News Today. "Research Identifies New Feature of Brain Structure That May Lead to ADHD." http://www.medicalnewstoday.com/articles/89793.php (accessed May 19, 2009).

Medical News Today. "Sciele Pharma Announces That Addrenex Has Completed Enrollment of Pivotal Phase III Trial for Clonicel for ADHD." http://www.medicalnewstoday.com/articles/109952.php (accessed May 19, 2009).

Medical News Today. "Shire Investigational Nonstimulant INTUNIV Showed Significant Efficacy in Reducing ADHD Symptoms." http://www.medicalnewstoday.com/articles/106801.php (accessed May 28, 2008).

Medical.Webends.com. "Ventral Tegmental Area." http://medical.webends.com/kw/Ventral%20Tegmental%20Area (accessed June 18, 2009).

"Medication Guide: Concerta." Ortho-McNeill-Janssen Pharmaceuticals. http://www.concerta.net (accessed May 18, 2009).

"Medication Guide: Vyvanse." Shire US. http://www.Vyvanse.com (accessed May 18, 2009).

MedicineNet.com. "Definition of Dopamine." http://www.medterms.com/script/main/art.asp?articlekey=14345 (accessed June 18, 2009).

"Medline Abstracts: Complementary and Alternative Therapies for ADHD." http://www.medscape.com/viewarticle/438960_print.

Medline Plus. "Complementary and Alternative Medicine." http://www.nlm.nih.gov/medlineplus/complementaryandalternativemedicine.html (accessed June 18, 2009).

Michigan Department of Community Health. "What is Turner Syndrome?" http://www.michigan.gov/documents/Turner_factsheet_160406_7.pdf (accessed June 18, 2009).

Michigan State University. "MSU Researchers Link Low Lead Exposure to ADHD." (2007). http://news.msu.edu/story/963/&topic_id=11 (accessed June 18, 2009).

Molina, B. S. et al. "Childhood Predictors of Adolescent Substance Use in a Longitudinal Study of Children with ADHD." *Journal of Abnormal Psychology* 112 (2003): 497–507.

Moon, S. "Gifted Children with Attention Deficit/Hyperactivity Disorder." In *The Social and Emotional Development of Gifted Children: What Do We Know?* edited by M. Niehart et al., 193–204. Waco, TX: Prufrock Press, 2002.

Moving Mountains for Kids. "Turner Syndrome." http://movingmountainsforkids.com/turnersyndrome.asp (accessed June 18, 2009).

MTA Cooperative Group. "A 14-month Randomized Clinical Trial of Treatment Strategies for Attention-Deficit/Hyperactivity Disorder (ADHD)." *Archives of General Psychiatry* 56 (1999): 1073–86.

Myers, Martin, and Diego Pineda. *Do Vaccines Cause That?* Galveston, TX: Immunizations for Public Health (i4ph), 2008.

Myomancy. "Caffeine and ADHD." http://www.myomancy.com/2006/07/caffeine_and_ad (accessed June 18, 2009).

Myomancy. "The Corpus Callosum, Dyslexia, and ADHD." http://www.myomancy.com/2008/01/the-corpus-callosum-dyslexia-and-adhd (accessed June 18, 2009).

"Myth: Sugar and Food Additives Cause ADHD." (2007). http://www.healthcentral. com/adhd/c/1443/14464/myth-sugar-food-adhd/pf/ (accessed July 30, 2008).

Nadeau, K. *A Comprehensive Guide to Adults with Attention Deficit Hyperactivity Disorder.* New York: Brunner/Mazel, 1995.

National Alliance on Mental Illness. "Attention-Deficit/Hyperactivity Disorder." www. nami.org/helpline/adhd.htm (accessed June 18, 2009).

National Resource Center on AD/HD. http://www.help4ADHD.org (accessed June 18, 2009).

Needleman, H. L. "Childhood Lead Poisoning." *Current Opinion in Neurology* 7, no. 2 (1994): 187–90.

Newsmax.com. "Chiropractic Care May Help Adult ADHD" (2007). http://www.newsmax.com/health/adult_ADHD_chiropractic/2007/09/06/30292.html (accessed June 18, 2009).

Niehart, M. et al. *The Social and Emotional Development of Gifted Children: What Do We Know?* Waco, TX: Prufrock, 2002.

Novartis Pharmaceuticals Corp. "Focalin Prescribing Information." (April 2007). http://www.pharma.us.novartis.com/product/pi/pdf/focalin.pdf (accessed June 18, 2009).

Oades, Robert D. "The Role of the Serotonin System in ADHD: Treatment Implications." *Expert Reviews of Neurotherapy* 7, no. 10 (2007): 1357–74.

Oatis, M. D. "Treatment-pharmacology." Discussion presented at the Attention Deficit Hyperactivity Disorder (ADHD) AMA Media Briefing, September 9, New York, NY, 2004.

Optometrists Network. "What is Vision Therapy or Visual Training?" (2007) http://www.add-adhd.org/vision_therapy_FAQ.html (accessed June 18, 2009).

Norvilitis, Jill, and Howard M. Reid. "Laterality and perceptual bias in ADHD." In *Attention Deficit Hyperactivity Disorder (ADHD) Research*, edited by Michelle Larimer. New York: Nova Science Publishers, 2005.

"Parasites." http://www.symmetry4u.com/Info/parasites.htm (accessed August 7, 2008).

Partners Resource Network, Texas. http://www.PartnersTX.org (accessed June 18, 2009).

Perrin, J. M. et al. "Clinical Practice Guideline: Treatment of School Aged Children with Attention Deficit/Hyperactivity Disorder." *Pediatrics* 108, no. 4 (2001): 1033–44.

Peterson, B. S. et al. "Prospective, Longitudinal Study of Tic, Obsessive-Compulsive and Attention-Deficit/Hyperactivity Disorder in an Epidemiological Sample." *Journal of the American Academy of Child and Adolescent Psychiatry* 40 (2001): 685–95.

Piano, Marina. "Scientists Use MRIs to Study ADHD, Depression in Children." San Antonio Express-News (Texas), May 19, 2003, F1.

Plesman, Jurriaan. "The Serotonin Connection." http://www.hypoglycemia.asn.au/articles/serotonin_connection.html (accessed June 18, 2009).

Popham, W. James. *Assessing Students with Disabilities*. New York: Routledge, 2006.

Popham, W. James. *Modern Educational Measurement*. 3rd ed. Boston: Allyn & Bacon, 2000.

"Porphyria Disease." http://www.depression-guide.com/porphyria.htm (accessed August 11, 2008).

"Preschoolers with ADHD Improve with Low Doses of Medication." http://www.nimh.nih.gov/press/preschooladhd.cfm?Output=Print (accessed April 12, 2007).

Quinn, P. "Hormonal Fluctuations and the Influence of Estrogen in the Treatment of Women with ADHD." In *Gender Issues and ADHD Research, Diagnosis, and Treatment,* edited by P. Quinn and K. Nadeau, 183–99. Silver Spring, MD: Advantage Books, 2002.

Quist, J. F., and J. L. Kennedy. "Genetics of Childhood Disorders: XXIII. ADHD, Part 7: The Serotonin System." *Journal of the American Academy of Child and Adolescent Psychiatry* 40, no. 2 (2001): 253–56.

Rabiner, David. "The Role of Neurofeedback in the Treatment of ADHD." http://www.add.org/articles/TheRoleofNeurofeedbackintheTreatmentofADHD.html (accessed May 27, 2009).

Radiological Society of North America. "Functional MR Imaging (fMRI)- Brain." Radiology Info. (2008) http://www.radiologyinfo.org/en/info.cfm?pg=fmribrain&bhcp=1 (accessed July 13, 2008).

Rais, Alina R. "Treatment of Pervasive Aggression in a Patient with 47 XYY Karyotype." http://priory.com/psychiatry/XYY_aggression.htm (accessed June 18, 2009).

Ramirez, P. M. et al. "EEG Biofeedback Treatment of ADD. A Viable Alternative to Traditional Medical Intervention?" *Annals of the New York Academy of Science* 931 (2001): 342–58.

Ray, G. T. et al. "Attention Deficit/Hyperactivity Disorder in Children: Excess Costs Before and After Initial Diagnosis and Treatment Cost Differences by Ethnicity." *Archives of Pediatric Adolescent Medicine* 160 (2006): 1063–69.

Reid, Brian et al. "Square Pegs in Round Holes—These Kids Don't Fit: High Ability Students with Behavior Problems." The National Research Center on the Gifted and Talented, University of Connecticut, 1995.

Reinberg, Steven. "ADHD Might Raise Kids' Obesity Risk." http://abcnews.go.com/Health/Healthday/story?id=5322482&page=1 (accessed June 18, 2009).

"Reuptake." http://www.medicine.net.com (accessed July 8, 2008).

Rietveld, M. J. et al. "Heritability of Attention Problems in Children: Longitudinal Results from a Study of Twins, age 3 to 12." *Journal of Child Psychology and Psychiatry* 45 (2004): 577–88.

Roessner et al. " First-Onset Tics in Patients with Attention-Deficit-Hyperactivity Disorder: Impact of Stimulants." *Developmental Medicine in Child Neurology* 48 (2006): 616–21.

Rowe, R. et al. "Childhood Psychiatric Disorder and Unintentional Injury: Findings from a National Cohort Study." *Journal of Pediatric Psychology* 29 (2004): 119–30.

Rucklidge, J. J., and R. Tannock. "Psychiatric, Psychosocial, and Cognitive Functioning of Female Adolescents with ADHD." *Journal of the American Academy of Adolescent Psychiatry* 40, no. 5 (2001): 530–40.

Rutherford, Dan. "Carbon Monoxide Poisoning." (2005). http://www.netdoctor.co.uk/health_advice/facts/carbonmonoxide.htm (accessed August 8, 2009).

Rydberg, Michelle. "ADHD can inspire creativity." LaVoz, June 16, 2008. http://www.lavozdeanza.com/home/index.cfm?event=displayArticlePrinterFriendly&uStor (accessed June 29, 2008).

Safren, S. A. et al. "Cognitive-Behavioral Therapy for ADHD in Medication-treated Adults with Continued Symptoms." *Behavior Research Therapy* 43 (2005): 831–42.

Scheffler, R. M., S. P. Hinshaw, S. Modrek, and P. Levine. "The Global Market for ADHD Medications." *Health Affairs* 26, no. 2 (2007): 450–57.

Schram, Thomas D. "The Eyes Have It in Attention Disorders: Visual Focus May be Affecting Mental Issues" (2000). http://www.add-adhd.org/textonlty/convergence_insufficiency.html (accessed August 7, 2008).

Scott, Julian, and Teresa Barlow. *Acupuncture in the Treatment of Children.* Vista, CA: Eastland Press, 1999.

Sellar, Wanda. *The Directory of Essential Oils.* London: C. W. Daniel Co., 1992.

"Sensory Integration Disorder." http://www.healthatoz/Atoz/common/standard/transform.jsp?requestURL=h (accessed August 9, 2008).

Serfontein, G. *The Hidden Handicap: Dyslexia and Hyperactivity in Children.* Auckland, New Zealand: Bateman, 1989.

Shire US Inc. "Daytrana Prescribing Information." Revised 5/2009. http://www.daytrana.com/prescribing-information/ (accessed June 18, 2009).

Silva, R. R., D. M. Munoz, and M. Alpert. "Carbamazepine Use in Children and Adolescents with Features of Attention-Deficit Hyperactivity Disorder: A Meta-analysis." *Journal of the American Academy of Child and Adolescent Psychiatry* 35, no. 3 (1996): 352–58.

Smalley, S. L. et al. "Genetic Linkage of Attention-Deficit/Hyperactivity Disorder on Chromosome 16p13 in a Region Implicated in Autism." *American Journal of Human Genetics* 71 (2002): 959–63.

Spencer, T. et al. "ADHD and Thyroid Abnormalities: A Research Note." *Journal of Child Psychology and Psychiatry* 86, no. 5 (2006): 879–85.

Steele, Robert. "Can Lead Exposure Cause ADHD?" http://parenting.ivillage.com/baby/bsafety/0,,3q63-p,00.html (accessed August 8, 2008).

Stein D. et al. "Sleep Disturbances in Adolescents with Symptoms of Attention-Deficit/Hyperactivity Disorder." *Journal of Learning Disabilities* 35 (2002): 268–75.

Stewart, M. A. et al. "The Hyperactive Child Syndrome." *American Journal of Orthopsychiatry* 36 (1966): 861–67.

"Study: Tonsil, Adenoid Removal Could Aid in ADHD Treatment." http://www.10news.com/health/9948935/detail.html (accessed June 8, 2008).

"Sugar: Does it Cause ADHD?" http://www.riversideonline.com/health_reference/Childrens-Healthy/AN00583.cfm (accessed July 18, 2008).

Swanson, J. M., G. R. Elliott, L. L. Greenhill, et al. "Effects of Stimulant Medication on Growth Rates across 3 Years in the MTA Follow-Up." *Journal of the American Academy of Child and Adolescent Psychiatry* 46 (2007): 1015–27.

Swensen, A. R. et al. "Incidents and Costs of Accidents among Attention-Deficit/Hyperactivity Disorder Patients." *Journal of the American Academy of Child and Adolescent Psychiatry* 42(2004): 21415–423.

"Tegretol (Carbamazepine) for ADHD." http://www.revolutionhealth.com/blogs/earthling/tegretol-etc-carbam-4851 (accessed May 20, 2008).

Thompson, Sandra J. et al. *Accommodations Manual: How to Select, Administer, and Evaluate Use of Accommodations for Instruction and Assessment of Students with Disabilities.* 2nd ed. Washington, DC: The Council of Chief State School Officers, August, 2005.

Thurnell-Read, Jane. "9 Allergy Signs in Children." http://ezinearticles.com/?9-Allergy-Signs-In-Children&id=97360 (accessed May 18, 2009).

"Tonsil Removal and ADHD: Connected?" http://globalrph.healthology.com/main/article_print.aspx?content_id=3485 (accessed June 9, 2008).

"Treating ADHD &ADD with Acupuncture." (2007) http://www.healthy.net/scr/news/asp?id=9235&action=print (accessed April 26, 2008).

"Treatment for Fetal Alcohol Syndrome May Be Inappropriate" (1997) http://emory.edu/EMORY_REPORT/erarchive/1997/April/erapril.14/4_14_97Fetal (accessed July 13, 2008).

Ulrich, Margie. "ADHD/ADD or Hearing Loss?" http://www.healtharticles.org/adhd_add_hearing_loss_071304.html (accessed August 9, 2008).

University of Michigan Health System. "Fragile X Syndrome." http://www.med. umich.edu/yourchild/topics/fragilex.htm (accessed Jun 18, 2009).

Upadhyaya, H. P. et al. "Attention Deficit/Hyperactivity Disorder, Medication Treatment, and Substance Use among Adolescents and Young Adults." *Journal of Child and Adolescent Psychopharmacology* 15 (2005): 799–809.

Upledger, John. "Craniosacral Therapy and the Central Nervous System." http://www.latitudes.org/articles/cranio_upledger_ld.html (accessed May 19, 2009).

U.S. Food and Drug Administration. "Adderall and Adderall XR (amphetamines) Information." http://www.fda.gov/Drugs/DrugSafety/PostmarketDrugSafetyInformationforPatientsandProviders/ucm111441.htm (accessed June 18, 2009).

U.S. Food and Drug Administration. "Aromatherapy." http://www.fda.gov/Cosmetics/ProductandIngredientSafety/ProductInformation/ucm127054.htm (accessed June 18, 2009).

U.S. Food and Drug Administration. "Patient Information Sheet: Adderall and Adderall XR Extended-Release Capsules." http://www.fda.gov/cder/drug/infopage/adderall/default.htm (accessed February 2, 2008).

"Vitamin B Deficiency." http://www.depression-guide.com/vitamin-b-deficiency.htm (accessed August 9, 2008).

Watkins, Carol."ADHD and Enuresis (Bedwetting)." (2000) http://www.baltimorepsych.com/adhd_and_bedwetting.htm (accessed June 18, 2009).

Watkins, Carol. "The Gifted Student with ADD: Between Two Worlds." (2006). http://www.ncpamd.com/Gifted_ADD.htm (accessed May 20, 2009).

WebMD. "What is Klinefelter Syndrome?" Men's Health. http://www.men.webmd.com/tc/klinefelter-syndrome-topic-overview (accessed August 11, 2008).

Wehrspann, Bill. "ADHD Related to Fetal Alcohol Syndrome." *Medscape Psychiatry & Mental Health* 11, no. 2 (2006). http://cme.medscape.com/viewarticle/546475.

Wender, Paul. *Attention-Deficit Hyperactivity Disorder in Adults.* New York: Oxford University Press, 1995.

Wender, Paul H. *The Hyperactive Child, Adolescent, and Adult: Attention Deficit Disorder through the Lifespan.* New York: Oxford University Press, 1987.

West, Thomas. *In the Mind's Eye: Visual Thinkers, Gifted People with Dyslexia and Other Learning Difficulties, Computer Images and the Ironies of Creativity.* New York: Prometheus Books, 1997.

"What You Need To Know about the Americans with Disabilities Act." *ADDitude* http://www.additudemag.com/adhd-web/article/pront/674.html (accessed May 20, 2009).

"White House Commission on Complementary and Alternative Medicine Policy." Final report: March 2002. Washington, DC http://www.whccamp.hhs.gov/ (accessed May 18, 2009).

Wigal, S., J. M. Swanson, D. Feifel, et al. "A Double-blind, Placebo-controlled Trial of Dexmethylphenidate Hydrochloride and d,l-threo-methylphenidate Hydrychoroide in Children with Attention-Deficit/Hyperactivity Disorder." *Journal of the American Academy of Child and Adolescent Psychiatry* 43, no. 11 (2004): 1406–14.

Wilens, T. "Attention-Deficit/Hyperactivity Disorder and the Substance Abuse Disorders: The Nature of the Relationship, Subtypes at Risk, and Treatment Issues." *Psychiatric Clinic North America* 27 (2004): 283–301.

Wilens, T. E. et al. "Does Stimulant Therapy of Attention Deficit/Hyperactivity Disorder Beget Later Substance Abuse? A Meta-analytic View of the Literature." *Pediatrics* 111 (2003): 179–85.

Wilens T. E., et al. "Psychiatric Comorbidity and Functioning in Clinically Referred Preschool Children and School-Age Youths with ADHD." *Journal of the American Academy of Child and Adolescent Psychiatry* 41 (2002): 262–68.

Wills, P. *Color Therapy: The Use of Color for Health and Healing.* Shaftsbury, Dorset: Element Books, 1993.

World Health Organization. "F84 Pervasive Development Disorders." *International Statistical Classification of Diseases and Related Health Problems.* 10th ed. (ICD-10), Geneva, Switzerland, WHO, 2006.

Wormwood, V. A. *The Fragrant Pharmacy: A Complete Guide to Aromatherapy and Essential Oils.* London: Bantam, 1991.

Wozniak, J. et al. "Antecedents and Complications of Trauma in Boys with ADHD: Findings from a Longitudinal Study." *Journal of the American Academy of Child and Adolescent Psychiatry* 38 (1999): 48–55.

"Yeast and Candidiasis." RXAlternative Medicine. (2006) http://www.rxalternative-medicine.com/articles/yeast_candidiasis.html (accessed August 6, 2006).

Zametkin, A. J. et al. "Cerebral Glucose Metabolism in Adults with Hyperactivity of Childhood Onset." *New England Journal of Medicine* 323 (1990): 1361–66.

Zaslow, Jeffrey. "What if Einstein Had Taken Ritalin? ADHD's Impact on Creativity." *The Wall Street Journal* http://online.wsj.com/article/SB110738397416844127.html (accessed June 18, 2009).

Zimney, Ed. "Dr. Z's Medical Report: Carbon Monoxide Poisoning." (2006) http://www.blog.healthtalk.com/zimney/carbon-monoxide-poisoning/ (accessed May 18, 2009).

Zirkle, Perry A. *Section 504: Student Issues, Legal Requirements, and Practical Recommendations.* Bloomington, IN: Phi Delta Kappa Educational Foundation, 2005.

INDEX

About the Author

EVELYN B. KELLY is an independent scholar who has written more than 16 books and over 400 journal articles. She is a member of the National Association of Science Writers; is past president of the American Medical Writer's Association, Florida chapter; and is a member of the American Society of Journalists and Authors. Kelly is an adjunct professor of education at St. Leo University.